BREAST
CANCER
JOURNEY

BREAST CANCER JOURNEY

THIRD EDITION

THE ESSENTIAL GUIDE TO TREATMENT AND RECOVERY

Ruth O'Regan, MD

Sheryl G. A. Gabram-Mendola, MD, FACS

Terri Ades, DNP, FNP-BC, AOCN

Rick Alteri, MD

Joan L. Kramer, MD

Kimberly A. Stump-Sutliff, MSN, RN, AOCNS

Published by the American Cancer Society
Health Promotions
250 Williams Street NW
Atlanta, GA 30303-1002

Printed in the United States of America

Cover design and composition by LaShae Ortiz
Copy editing by Patricia A. French, Left Lane Communications
Illustrations by Samuel K. Collins, CMI, FAMI, and Amy P. Collins, FAMI
Indexing by Bob Land

1 2 3 4 5   13 14 15 16 17

Library of Congress Cataloging-in-Publication Data
    O'Regan, Ruth.
Breast cancer journey : the essential guide to treatment and recovery.—Third edition /
Ruth O'Regan, MD [and five others].
    pages cm
Includes bibliographical references and index.
ISBN 978-1-60443-030-1 (pbk. : alk. paper)—ISBN 1-60443-030-3 (pbk. : alk. paper)
1. Breast—Cancer—Popular works. I. American Cancer Society. II. Title.
RC280.B8B6876 2013
616.99'449—dc23
                       2013019504

Quantity discounts on bulk purchases of this book are available. Book excerpts can also be created to fit specific needs. For information, please contact the American Cancer Society, Health Promotions Publishing, 250 Williams Street NW, Atlanta, GA 30303-1002, or send an e-mail to trade.sales@cancer.org.

American Cancer Society

Managing Director, Content: Chuck Westbrook

Director, Book Publishing: Len Boswell

Managing Editor, Book Publishing: Rebecca Teaff, MA

Senior Editor, Book Publishing: Jill Russell

Book Publishing Coordinator: Vanika Jordan, MSPub

Editorial Assistant, Book Publishing: Amy Rovere

Table of Contents

PART II: Preparing for Treatment

Chapter 4: Understanding Your Diagnosis

Chapter 5: Coping with Your Diagnosis and Moving Forward

Chapter 6: Making the Medical System Work for You

PART III: Treatment

Chapter 7: Exploring Treatment Options

Chapter 8: Surgery

Chapter 9: Other Treatments for Breast Cancer

Chapter 10: Treatment Options Based on Your Situation

Chapter 11: Clinical Trials

Chapter 12: Complementary and Alternative Therapies

PART IV: Living with the Effects of Treatment

Chapter 13: Coping with Symptoms and Side Effects

Chapter 17: Insurance and Your Rights

Chapter 18: Finances and Cancer Treatment

Special Caregiver's Section: Supporting the Woman with Cancer

Supporting the Woman with Cancer

PART VI: Life After Cancer

Chapter 19: Taking Care of Yourself After Cancer: Health and Wellness

Chapter 20: Emotional Wellness After Treatment: Moving On

Chapter 21: Intimacy After Cancer Treatment

American Cancer Society

Chapter 22: The Possibility of Facing Cancer Again

NOTE TO THE READER

The treatment information in this book is not official policy of the American Cancer Society and is not intended as medical advice to replace the expertise and judgment of your cancer care team. It is intended to help you and your family make informed decisions, together with your doctor.

For more information about breast cancer, contact your American Cancer Society at 800-227-2345 or www.cancer.org.

INTRODUCTION

"You have breast cancer." Hearing those words changes everything and triggers a flood of emotions. You may suddenly feel shock, anger, fear, or sadness. You may question why this has happened to you. You may wonder how you are going to manage your life and cope with this new reality. These are all normal reactions to receiving a diagnosis of cancer. And there may be times, in the days and months ahead, that you will feel overwhelmed in trying to orient yourself to the changes in your life.

In the midst of all the pressure and upheaval a cancer diagnosis brings, remember that there is hope. Today, more is known about breast cancer and its treatment than ever before. Many women who receive a diagnosis of breast cancer will be cured by standard medical treatments. Many women recover completely, and others live for years with their cancer well under control. Each person's cancer is different; therefore, the way your body responds to cancer and its treatment will also be unique.

Beginning to inform yourself about your disease and your health is an important step in your journey forward. Making informed decisions will help you feel more in control of your life—at a time when everything around you feels out of control!

From the perspective of a pathology report or a medical textbook, breasts are simply parts of the body. But in reality, breasts are more than that. Throughout life, the breasts are integral to a woman's personal experiences—of puberty, sex, motherhood, health, and aging. They are symbolic of sexuality, beauty, power, desire, femininity, pleasure, and comfort. Coming to terms with a breast cancer diagnosis can bring with it the recognition that having this disease may affect the way you see yourself as a woman.

Breast Cancer Journey: The Essential Guide to Treatment and Recovery explores the experiences and challenges you're likely to face during your breast cancer experience. In this revised edition, you'll learn how cancer and its treatment can affect your body, your emotions, your family, and your life in general. The book covers these crucial topics:

- breast cancer treatment options and potential side effects, including the latest surgical techniques, drug therapies, and complementary and alternative therapies
- the physical and emotional side effects associated with breast cancer and its treatment and how to manage them

- intimacy, fertility, lymphedema, and other issues of importance for breast cancer patients and survivors
- the latest surgical techniques for breast reconstruction
- updated and expanded information on life after cancer treatment
- detailed questions to ask your medical team

How to Use This Book

This new edition of *Breast Cancer Journey* is designed to help you through each phase of diagnosis and treatment. This is your book. Use it. Bend the pages. Make notes in it. You might prefer to read it from cover to cover or read only the parts that apply to you.

Part I: Understanding Breast Cancer

Part I outlines the basics of breast cancer: what it is, what the risk factors are, and the most common diagnostic tests and procedures used when breast cancer is suspected. Not every person will want or need to read these first few chapters, depending on where she is in the process. However, for some, becoming more familiar with the basic anatomy and terminology will help you make more informed decisions about your care.

Part II: Preparing for Treatment

Part II will help you better understand your diagnosis and prepare for treatment. This section begins with an explanation of the staging system used for breast cancer and then moves to a discussion of how you can begin to get ready for treatment: educating yourself, talking with friends and family, building your support network, and—if you have young children—helping them cope with your illness. Part II also will help you navigate an often complex and confusing medical system, from getting a second opinion to becoming an active participant in your care.

Part III: Treatment

Part III provides an overview of various treatment options for breast cancer, including surgery, chemotherapy, radiation therapy, hormone therapy, targeted therapy, and drugs to protect the bones. Each treatment is examined, along with its benefits, risks, and side effects. Additional information on clinical trials and complementary and alternative therapies is provided to help you learn about all types of treatment options.

Part IV: Living with the Effects of Treatment

The chapters in part IV address what to expect during and immediately after treatment. They include information on managing side effects and symptoms and maintaining your emotional health. This section also details the latest options for breast reconstruction.

Part V: Practical Matters: Work, Insurance, and Finances

The chapters in part V explore many of the practical challenges that can come with cancer treatment, such as work issues and managing insurance and financial matters.

Part VI: Life After Cancer

Part VI focuses on physical, emotional, and spiritual wellness after cancer treatment. This section provides suggestions for maintaining your health and receiving follow-up care, eating well and staying physically active, and finding renewed meaning in life after cancer. Post-treatment issues such as adjusting to life after treatment, intimacy and sexuality, and the possibility of recurrence are also covered.

A Special Section for Caregivers

This special section, written specifically for caregivers, discusses the most common challenges that caregivers face, and it provides tools to help them support a woman with breast cancer. Topics include supporting the woman before, during, and after treatment; balancing caregiving and other responsibilities; and the importance of seeking support from others. Issues of intimacy and adjusting to life after cancer are also addressed.

Finally, an extensive resource guide provides contact information for organizations that may be helpful to you and your loved ones. You'll also find an updated glossary, the American Cancer Society Recommendations for Early Breast Cancer Detection, information on the Women's Health and Cancer Rights Act, a section on benign breast conditions and their relationship to cancer risk, and the American Cancer Society Guidelines on Nutrition and Physical Activity for Cancer Prevention.

Your Unique Journey

No one deserves to have breast cancer. *Breast Cancer Journey* was created to help you get through it with all the latest knowledge and tools available. Each person is different, and your cancer experience will be unique. However, by becoming informed, you can be an active participant in your care and recovery and feel confident of meeting the challenges ahead. Let this book serve as your guide.

PART ONE

Understanding Breast Cancer

Breast cancer is a complex disease, with different types, different characteristics, and different treatments. It occurs in women of all ages and ethnicities, and for each woman, the experience will be different.

These first three chapters of *Breast Cancer Journey* outline the basics of breast cancer, the different types of breast cancer, and what factors affect breast cancer risk. We describe the main tests and procedures that you might experience during diagnosis and treatment and what the test results mean.

You may have already done some research and familiarized yourself with the information covered here. As we discussed in the introduction, this is your book—use it in the way that is most helpful to you. Depending on where you are in your experience, you may wish to skip forward to the next section, where we discuss understanding your diagnosis and gearing up for treatment.

Many women with breast cancer report that spending time educating themselves about their disease and taking an active role in decisions about their health has helped them in their breast cancer journey. Knowledge can be empowering. Beginning to understand what is happening in your body can help you orient yourself in this new and unfamiliar landscape.

CHAPTER 1

What Is Cancer?

Cancer is not just one disease; it is more than one hundred different diseases with one thing in common: out-of-control growth and spread of abnormal cells that occur because of gene mutations, or changes.

Normal cells grow, divide, and die in an orderly fashion. During the early years of a person's life, normal cells divide more rapidly to allow the person to grow. After that, in most tissues, normal cells divide only to replace worn-out or dying cells and to repair injuries.

Cancer cell growth is different from normal cell growth. Instead of dying, cancer cells continue to grow and form new, abnormal cells. Cancer cells can also invade other tissues, something that normal cells cannot do. Growing out of control and invading other tissues are what makes a cell a cancer cell.

In most cases, cancer cells form a tumor. But not all tumors are cancerous. A cancerous tumor is called malignant. Tumors that are not cancerous are called benign. Benign tumors can cause problems—they can grow very large and press on healthy organs and tissues—but they cannot invade, or grow into, other tissues. Because they cannot invade, they also cannot metastasize, or spread, to other parts of the body. These tumors are almost never life-threatening.

Cells become cancer cells because of damage to DNA. DNA is the genetic "blueprint" found in the nucleus of every cell and directs all its actions. In a normal cell, when DNA gets damaged, either the cell repairs the damage or the cell dies. In cancer cells, the damaged DNA is not repaired, but the cell does not die as it should. Instead, the damaged cell goes on making new cells that the body does not need. These new cells will all have the same damaged DNA as the first cell.

People can inherit damaged DNA, but most DNA damage is caused by mistakes that happen while the normal cell is reproducing. Sometimes the cause of the DNA damage is something that can be identified, such as cigarette smoking. But often no clear cause is found.

If cancer cells travel through the bloodstream or lymph vessels, they can spread to other parts of the body, where they can continue to grow and form new tumors. This process is called metastasis.

When cancer spreads, however, it is still named after the part of the body where it started. If breast cancer spreads to the lungs, it is still called breast cancer, not lung cancer. Different types of cancer behave very differently. For example, lung cancer and breast cancer are very different diseases. They grow at different rates and respond to different treatments. That is why people with cancer need treatment that is aimed at their particular type of cancer.

What Is Breast Cancer?

Breast cancer is a malignant tumor that has developed from cells of the breast. The disease occurs almost entirely in women, but men can have breast cancer, too. Although breast cancer can develop from any of the cells in the breast, doctors use the term "breast cancer" most often to mean cancers that start in the cells lining the ducts or lobules of the breast. These cancers are a type of cancer called carcinoma. Other types of cancer, such as sarcomas and lymphomas, can start in the breast. However, because these types of cancer occur much less frequently and have different causes and treatments, they are considered different diseases and are not grouped with breast carcinomas. In these cases, a doctor would say that a woman has lymphoma of the breast or sarcoma of the breast.

To understand breast cancer, it helps to have some basic knowledge about the normal structure and function of the breasts.

Normal Breast Tissue

There are three main components of the female breast:
- **lobules**, the glands that produce milk;
- **ducts**, the passages that carry the milk from the lobules to the nipple; and
- **stroma**, the fatty and connective tissues surrounding the ducts and lobules, blood vessels, and lymph vessels.

Most types of breast cancer begin in the cells that line the ducts (called ductal cancer). Some types begin in the cells that line the lobules (called lobular cancer), but a small number of breast cancers start in the cells of the stroma of the breast.

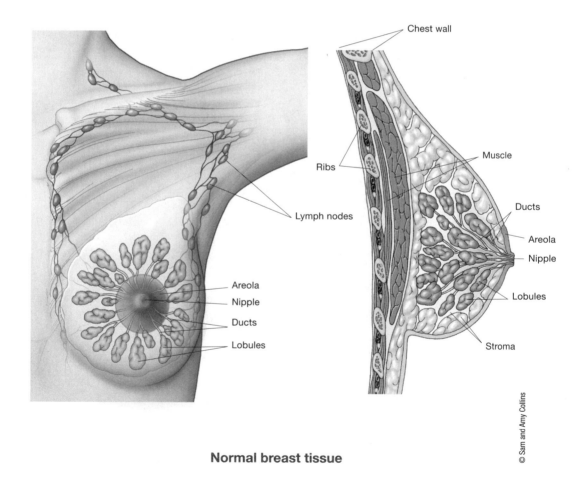

Normal breast tissue

© Sam and Amy Collins

The Lymphatic System

The lymphatic system is important to understand because it is one of the pathways by which breast cancer can spread. The lymphatic system has two main parts: lymph nodes and lymph vessels. Lymph nodes are small, bean-shaped collections of immune system cells, which are important in fighting infections. Lymph nodes are connected by lymph vessels. Lymph vessels are similar to veins, except they carry lymph instead of blood. Lymph is a clear fluid that contains tissue fluids, waste products, and immune system cells. Cancer cells can invade lymph vessels and spread to lymph nodes, where they can settle and grow.

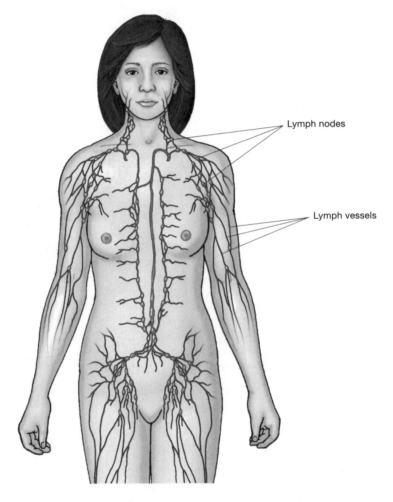

Lymph nodes

Lymph vessels

© Sam and Amy Collins

The lymphatic system

Lymph nodes in relation to the breast

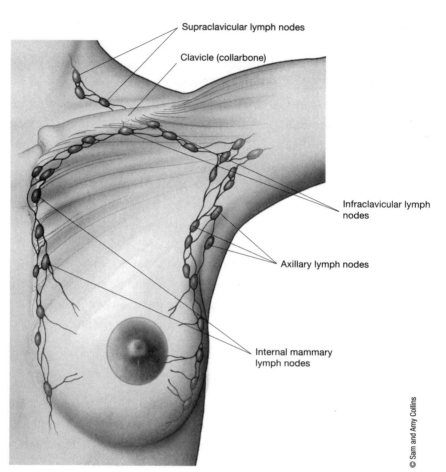

Most lymph vessels of the breast drain to the lymph nodes under the arms, called the axillary lymph nodes. Lymph nodes in this area are often removed to check for cancer cells. Lymph vessels of the breast can also drain to lymph nodes within the chest, called internal mammary lymph nodes, or to the lymph nodes near the collarbone, called the supraclavicular and infraclavicular lymph nodes. These other sets of lymph nodes are checked less often for signs of metastasis.

In the early stages of the disease, any spread of cancer cells to lymph nodes can be detected only by removing the lymph nodes and examining them with a microscope. With time, though, the cancer cells can grow and multiply, causing the lymph nodes to enlarge. They might grow large enough to be detected by a doctor feeling for lumps under the skin or seen on an imaging test. It is important to determine whether breast cancer has spread to any axillary lymph nodes, because metastasis to these lymph nodes means that the cancer is also more likely to have spread to other organs of the body.

Benign Breast Conditions

Most breast lumps are benign (not cancerous). However, tissue samples may need to be taken from the lumps and viewed under a microscope to prove they are not cancerous. Most lumps in the breast are caused by fibrosis and/or cysts (in the past, often referred to as fibrocystic changes). Fibrosis refers to connective tissue or scar tissue formation, and cysts are fluid-filled sacs. Fibrosis and cysts can cause breast swelling and pain, which are often worse just before a woman's menstrual period is about to begin. They may cause the breasts to feel lumpy, and the woman may also notice a clear or slightly cloudy nipple discharge.

Benign breast tumors, such as fibroadenomas and intraductal papillomas, are abnormal growths, but they are not cancerous and do not spread outside of the breast. They are not life-threatening. Still, some benign breast conditions are important because women with these conditions have a higher risk of developing breast cancer. For more information on these breast conditions, see pages 435–440.

Types of Breast Cancer

There are several types of breast cancer, some of which are quite rare. In some cases, a single breast tumor can have a combination of different types of cancerous cells or have a mixture of invasive and in situ cancer. It is important to understand some of the key terms that will be used to describe the type of breast cancer you have, as your type will determine your prognosis and treatment options.

Nearly all breast cancers are carcinomas—either ductal carcinoma or lobular carcinoma. This type of cancer begins in the lining layer—the epithelial cells—of such organs as the breast. Other types of cancer, such as sarcomas and lymphomas, can also start in the breast.

Not only are most breast cancers carcinomas, most are a certain type of carcinoma called adenocarcinoma. An adenocarcinoma is a type of carcinoma that starts in glandular tissue; adeno is the medical term for gland, the tissue that makes and releases a substance. The ducts and lobules of the breast are glandular tissue—they make breast milk. And nearly all breast cancers start in the cells of either the ducts or the lobules. The two main types of breast adenocarcinoma are ductal carcinoma and lobular carcinoma. There are also several subtypes of ductal carcinoma, some of which have important implications for prognosis and treatment.

In Situ Cancer

"In situ" is a term used for an early stage of cancer in which cancer cells are confined to the immediate part of the breast (such as the duct or lobule) where they began. In breast cancer, it means that the cancer cells are only in the ducts (ductal carcinoma in situ) or lobules (lobular carcinoma in situ) where they started. The cells have not invaded the nearby stroma, nor have they spread to other organs in the body. Because the cancer cells have not yet invaded other tissues of the breast, in situ cancer is often described as noninvasive cancer.

Ductal Carcinoma in Situ (DCIS)

Also known as intraductal carcinoma, ductal carcinoma in situ (DCIS) is the most common type of noninvasive breast cancer. In DCIS, cancer cells are found inside the ducts, but they have not spread through the walls of the ducts into the stroma (see illustration, next page). Because DCIS is noninvasive, it has not spread to lymph nodes or distant sites, and it does not cause cancer death. Still, sometimes an area of DCIS will contain an area of invasive cancer. This area can range in size from a small tumor to a tiny spot where cancer cells have grown through the duct wall, called a microinvasion. The chance that DCIS will contain an invasive cancer is higher if the area of DCIS is large or the DCIS cells are considered high grade, meaning they look very abnormal under the microscope. DCIS is sometimes subclassified based on its grade and type to help determine the most appropriate treatment and to help predict the risk for cancer recurrence. There are several types of DCIS, but one important distinction among them is whether there are areas of dead or degenerating cancer cells, known as tumor cell necrosis. The term comedocarcinoma is often used to describe DCIS with necrosis. Because DCIS can continue to grow and become an invasive cancer, it is important that it be treated. Nearly all women with a DCIS diagnosis can be cured. DCIS is often found on a mammogram, an x-ray of the breast. With more women getting mammograms each year, the number of DCIS diagnoses is also increasing.

Ductal carcinoma in situ

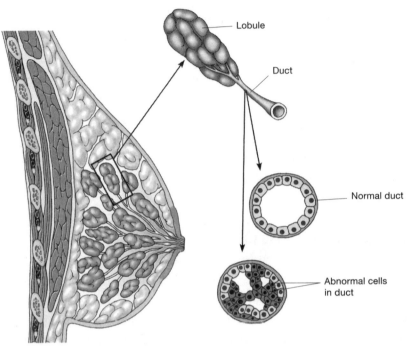

In ductal carcinoma in situ, cancer cells are found inside the ducts but have not spread through the walls of the ducts.

Lobular Carcinoma in Situ (LCIS)

Lobular carcinoma in situ (LCIS) is not a true cancer or precancer. Also called lobular neoplasia, LCIS is sometimes grouped with ductal carcinoma in situ as a noninvasive breast cancer, but it differs from DCIS in that it does not seem to become an invasive cancer if it is not treated. That is why it is not considered a true cancer. However, women with LCIS have a higher risk of invasive breast cancer developing in either breast.

Infiltrating (or Invasive) Carcinoma

Infiltrating (or invasive) carcinoma starts in the cells lining a duct (milk passage) or lobule (milk-producing gland) of the breast, and then breaks through this layer of cells to grow into the stroma of the breast. At this point, the cancer can spread to other parts of the body through the lymphatic system and bloodstream. There are two main types of invasive breast carcinoma: infiltrating ductal carcinoma and infiltrating lobular carcinoma.

American Cancer Society

Lobular carcinoma in situ

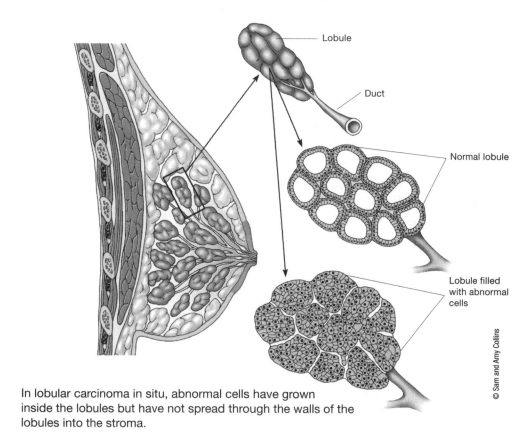

Lobule

Duct

Normal lobule

Lobule filled
with abnormal
cells

© Sam and Amy Collins

In lobular carcinoma in situ, abnormal cells have grown
inside the lobules but have not spread through the walls of the
lobules into the stroma.

Infiltrating Ductal Carcinoma

Infiltrating ductal carcinoma (IDC) is the most common type of breast cancer. It represents about 80 percent of invasive breast carcinomas. This type of cancer starts in the
cells lining a duct and grows into the stroma.

Some invasive carcinomas have features that make them different from the typical
infiltrating ductal carcinoma. These subtypes of invasive carcinoma are often named
after features seen when they are viewed under the microscope, such as the way the cells
are arranged. They are rare. In general, these subtypes are still treated like standard infiltrating ductal carcinoma.

The following subtypes tend to have a better prognosis than standard infiltrating
ductal carcinoma:

- adenoid cystic (or adenocystic) carcinoma

- low-grade adenosquamous carcinoma (a type of metaplastic carcinoma)
- medullary carcinoma
- mucinous (or colloid) carcinoma
- papillary carcinoma
- tubular carcinoma

Some subtypes have the same or possibly a worse prognosis than standard infiltrating ductal carcinoma:
- metaplastic carcinoma (most types, including spindle cell and squamous)
- micropapillary carcinoma
- mixed carcinoma (has features of both invasive ductal and lobular)

More information about these kinds of breast cancer can be found in the glossary, starting on page 499.

Triple-negative breast cancer: The term triple-negative breast cancer is used to describe breast cancers (usually invasive ductal carcinomas) whose cells lack estrogen receptors and progesterone receptors and do not have an excess of the HER2 protein on their surfaces. Because the tumor cells lack the necessary receptors, common treatments such as hormone therapy and drugs that target estrogen, progesterone, and HER2 are ineffective in treating triple-negative breast cancer. Chemotherapy is the most effective treatment for this type of cancer. For more information on triple-negative breast cancer, see page 50.

Infiltrating Lobular Carcinoma

Infiltrating lobular carcinoma (ILC) starts in a milk-producing gland of the breast. Like infiltrating ductal carcinoma, ILC has the potential to spread elsewhere in the body. About 10 to 15 percent of invasive breast cancers are invasive lobular carcinomas. Most patients with ILC present with physical symptoms, and it can be harder to detect on screening mammograms than infiltrating ductal carcinoma.

Inflammatory Carcinoma

Inflammatory carcinoma, or inflammatory breast cancer, is a rare and very aggressive form of breast cancer. It accounts for about 1 to 3 percent of all breast cancers. Inflammatory breast cancer does not present as a breast lump. Instead, it makes the skin of the breast look red and feel warm, as if it were infected and inflamed. The entire breast can swell, and the skin has a thick, pitted appearance that doctors often describe as resembling an orange peel, called p'eau d'orange. Sometimes the skin develops ridges and small bumps that look like hives. Although this type of breast cancer is called "inflammatory," the changes associated with it are not due to inflammation or infection. The breast becomes red and swollen, or "inflamed," because cancer cells are blocking the lymph vessels in the breast. Inflammatory carcinoma tends to grow and spread very quickly, and it has a worse prognosis than more common breast cancers. This type of breast cancer requires aggressive treatment, often with a combination of chemotherapy, radiation therapy, and surgery.

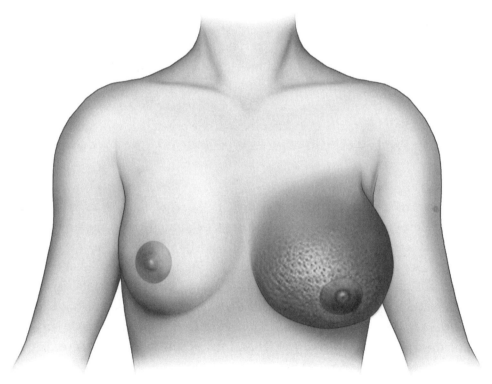

© Sam and Amy Collins

The signs of inflammatory breast cancer can include redness, warmth, and swelling. The skin of the breast may appear thick and pitted like the peel of an orange (called p'eau d'orange), or it can develop ridges or bumps.

Paget Disease of the Nipple

Paget disease of the nipple (also known as Paget disease of the breast) is a type of breast cancer that starts in the ducts of the breast and spreads to the skin of the nipple and the areola (the dark circle around the nipple). It is rare, accounting for only 1 percent of all breast cancer cases. The skin of the nipple and areola often appears crusty, scaly, and red, with areas of bleeding or oozing. The woman might notice burning or itching. Paget disease of the nipple can be associated with in situ carcinoma or with infiltrating breast carcinoma. If no lump can be felt in the breast tissue and the biopsy shows DCIS but no invasive cancer, the woman's prognosis is excellent. If invasive cancer is present, the prognosis is not as good, and the cancer will need to be staged and treated like any other invasive cancer.

Lymphoma

Lymphoma is a cancer of the lymphocytes; these cells are an important part of the immune system. Most lymphomas affect the bone marrow or lymph nodes, but, in rare cases, a lymphoma can develop in the breast. It most often presents as a single tumor and is found on biopsy to be a lymphoma. Lymphoma of the breast has a different prognosis and is treated differently than carcinoma of the breast. For more information on lymphoma, contact the American Cancer Society at 800-227-2345 or www.cancer.org.

Sarcoma

Sarcomas are cancers that start in connective tissues, such as muscle, fat, and blood vessels. Sarcomas of the breast are rare, the most common being angiosarcoma. An angiosarcoma starts from cells that line blood vessels or lymph vessels. It is rare, but when it does occur, it usually develops as a complication of previous radiation therapy to the breast. This is an extremely rare complication of breast radiation therapy and can develop about five to ten years after radiation treatment. Angiosarcoma can also occur in the arm of a woman who has had lymphedema caused by lymph node surgery or radiation therapy to treat breast cancer. These cancers tend to grow and spread quickly. Treatment is generally the same as for other sarcomas.

Malignant Phyllodes Tumor

A type of sarcoma, malignant phyllodes tumors are rare. This type of breast tumor forms in the stroma of the breast, in contrast to carcinomas, which develop in the ducts or lobules. Phyllodes (also spelled phylloides) tumors are usually benign but on rare occasions can be malignant. Benign phyllodes tumors are treated by removing the mass and a margin of normal breast tissue. Malignant phyllodes tumors are treated by removing the tumor and a wider margin of normal tissue or by mastectomy. They do not respond to the chemotherapy or hormone therapy used to treat most types of breast cancer, and they often do not respond well to radiation therapy. In the past, both benign and malignant phyllodes tumors were referred to as cystosarcoma phyllodes.

CHAPTER 2

Who Gets Breast Cancer?

Breast cancer is the most common cancer among American women (except for skin cancers). It accounts for more than one of every four cancers diagnosed in women in the United States. Currently, women living in the United States have about a 12 percent average lifetime risk of developing breast cancer, or a little less than one in eight. The American Cancer Society estimates that in 2013 about 232,340 new cases of invasive breast cancer and 64,640 cases of noninvasive (in situ) breast cancer will be diagnosed among women in the United States. An estimated 2,240 cases will be diagnosed among men.

Why Me?

One of the first questions you may have asked after your breast cancer diagnosis is, "Why me?" The short answer is, "We don't know." This answer is not very satisfying—most women want a better explanation. Most want to be able to point to a specific cause. Many women have their own ideas about why they have the disease. Some women believe they are being punished for something they did or did not do in the past. Some wonder whether they did something to cause the cancer. Others think they could have prevented the disease if they had done something differently. While these reactions to a cancer diagnosis are understandable, it will be harder to cope with your cancer if you blame yourself. Some of the risk factors that affect a woman's chance of getting breast cancer are known. The cause of most breast cancers, however, is unknown. More information is becoming available as scientists study potential causes and effects.

Not everyone will want to read about the risk factors for breast cancer; however, for others, this information can be a useful way to understand more about this disease.

What Are the Risk Factors for Breast Cancer?

A risk factor is anything that affects your chance of getting a disease, such as cancer. Different cancers have different risk factors. For example, frequent, unprotected exposure to sunlight is a risk factor for skin cancer, and smoking is a risk factor for lung and many other cancers. But having a risk factor—or even several risk factors—for cancer does not necessarily mean that a person will get the disease. Some women who have many risk factors never get breast cancer, and many women who have no apparent risk factors (aside from being a woman) still get breast cancer. Even when a woman with breast cancer has a specific risk factor, often there is no way to know whether this risk factor actually caused her cancer.

Some of the risk factors that increase a woman's chance of breast cancer are known, whereas others have not been proven. There are also different kinds of risk factors. Some, like a person's age or race, cannot be changed. Others are linked to cancer-causing factors

---

DNA and Breast Cancer: Inherited and Acquired Changes

Scientists are making significant progress in understanding how certain changes in DNA can cause normal breast cells to become cancerous. DNA is the chemical that carries instructions for nearly everything our cells do. We usually resemble our parents because they are the source of our DNA. However, DNA affects more than our outward appearance.

Some genes (parts of DNA) contain instructions for controlling when cells grow, divide, and die. Certain genes that promote cell division are called oncogenes. Genes that slow down cell division, or cause cells to die at the right time, are called tumor suppressor genes. Cancer can be caused by DNA mutations that "turn on" oncogenes or "turn off" tumor suppressor genes. Certain inherited DNA changes can cause some cancers to occur frequently and are responsible for cancers that run in some families.

Most DNA mutations related to breast cancer, however, are not inherited; these changes occur during a woman's lifetime. Acquired mutations of oncogenes and/or tumor suppressor genes might result from radiation or exposure to cancer-causing chemicals. So far, though, studies have not identified any dietary substances or environmental chemicals that are likely to cause these mutations. We do know some risk factors linked to breast cancer (such as taking certain hormones) that may cause some of these mutations. Still, the causes of most acquired mutations remain unknown.

---

in the environment. Still other risk factors are related to personal behaviors, such as smoking, drinking, and diet. Some factors are actually linked to a lower risk of breast cancer; for example, physical activity can actually lower risk. And some factors influence risk more than others, as in the case of increasing age, which affects risk more than reproductive history. A woman's risk of breast cancer changes over time.

Risk Factors that Cannot Be Changed

Some risk factors cannot be changed. Being a woman and growing older are two risk factors you cannot avoid. Your body and your family history determine more unchangeable risk factors.

Gender

Simply being a woman is the main risk factor for breast cancer. Breast cancer can occur in men, but the disease is one hundred times more common among women. This is likely because men have less of the female hormones estrogen and progesterone, which can promote breast cancer cell growth. The American Cancer Society estimates that about two thousand new cases of invasive breast cancer are diagnosed among men in the United States each year. To learn more about breast cancer in men, contact the American Cancer Society at 800-227-2345 or www.cancer.org.

Aging

A woman's risk of breast cancer increases with age. About one in eight invasive breast cancers occurs in women younger than forty-five, whereas about two of three invasive breast cancers are found in women aged fifty-five or older.

Family History of Breast Cancer

Breast cancer risk is higher among women whose close blood relatives have also had breast cancer. Blood relatives can be from the mother's or the father's side of the family. Having one first-degree female relative (mother, sister, or daughter) with breast cancer approximately doubles a woman's breast cancer risk, and having two first-degree relatives increases her risk threefold.

Although the exact risk is not known, women with a history of breast cancer in a father or brother are also at increased risk for breast cancer. Altogether, less than 15 percent of women with breast cancer have had a family member with this disease. Therefore, more than 85 percent of women with breast cancer *do not* have a family history of this disease.

Estimated New Female Breast Cancer Cases and Deaths by Age, US, 2011*

Age	In Situ Cases	Invasive Cases	Deaths
Under 40	1,780	11,330	1,160
Under 50	14,240	50,430	5,240
50-64	23,360	81,970	11,620
65+	20,050	98.080	22,660
All ages	**57,650**	**230,480**	**39,520**

*Rounding to the nearest 10.
Source: Total estimated cases are based on 1995-2007 incidence rates from 46 states as reported by the North American Association for Central Cancer Registries. Total estimated deaths are based on data from US Mortality Data, 1969-2007, National Center fot Health Statistics, Centers for Disease Control and Prevention.

American Cancer Society, Surveillance Research, 2011

Genetic Risk Factors

About 5 to 10 percent of breast cancers are thought to be hereditary, resulting directly from gene defects, or mutations, inherited from a parent. The most common causes of hereditary breast cancer are inherited mutations in the *BRCA1* and *BRCA2* genes. *BRCA1* and *BRCA2* are human genes that belong to a class of genes known as tumor suppressors. Normally, these genes help prevent cancer by making proteins that keep cells from growing abnormally. People who have inherited a mutated gene from either parent are at much higher risk for breast cancer.

Early research studies found a lifetime risk of breast cancer as high as 80 percent for members of some families with *BRCA1* mutations. Later studies found somewhat lower risks, with a risk of breast cancer by age 70 estimated at 55 to 65 percent for women with *BRCA1* mutations and at about 45 percent for women with *BRCA2* mutations. In women born with one of these gene mutations, breast cancer tends to develop earlier and is found more often in both breasts, compared with women who lack these mutations. Women with these inherited mutations are also at increased risk for other cancers, particularly ovarian cancer. Men who inherit these mutations also have an increased risk of breast cancer and other cancers.

In the United States, BRCA mutations are most common in Jewish women of Ashkenazi (Central and Eastern European) origin, with about 2.5 percent of these women being a carrier for a mutation. In contrast, they are found in only one of every four hundred women (or 0.25 percent) in the US general population. Three specific mutations known as "founder mutations" account for most of the BRCA mutations found in Ashkenazi Jews.

They are called founder mutations because each one is thought to have been present in a single or small number of ancestors. Other founder mutations have been found in other groups, such as the populations of Iceland and Japan.

Some women have changes in a BRCA gene that is not clearly a mutation, meaning it is not known to cause cancer. Mutations linked to cancer are known as germline deleterious mutations. Changes that have not been linked to cancer are often called variants of uncertain significance. These changes are studied to see whether a link to cancer emerges.

Changes in other genes: Other gene mutations can also lead to inherited breast cancers. The following gene mutations are much rarer than BRCA mutations and often do not increase the risk of breast cancer as much. They are not frequent causes of inherited breast cancer.

- ***ATM:*** The *ATM* gene normally helps repair damaged DNA. Inheriting two abnormal copies of this gene causes the disease ataxia-telangiectasia, an immunodeficiency disorder. Inheriting one mutated copy of this gene has been linked to a high rate of breast cancer in some families.
- ***TP53:*** Inherited mutations of *TP53*, the tumor suppressor gene for the p53 protein, cause Li-Fraumeni syndrome. People with this syndrome have an increased risk of breast cancer and several other cancers, such as leukemia, brain tumors, and sarcomas (cancers of bones or connective tissue). This gene mutation is a rare cause of breast cancer.
- ***CHEK2:*** Li-Fraumeni syndrome can also be caused by inherited mutations in the *CHEK2* gene. Even when a mutation in this gene does not cause this syndrome, it can still increase a woman's breast cancer risk about twofold.
- ***PTEN:*** The *PTEN* gene normally helps regulate cell growth. Inherited mutations in this gene can cause Cowden syndrome, a rare disorder in which people are at increased risk for both benign and malignant breast tumors, as well as growths in the digestive tract, thyroid, uterus, and ovaries. Defects in this gene can also cause Bannayan-Riley-Ruvalcaba syndrome, which is not linked to breast cancer risk.
- ***CDH1:*** Inherited mutations in the *CDH1* gene cause hereditary diffuse gastric cancer, a syndrome in which a rare type of stomach cancer develops at an early age. Women with mutations in this gene also have an increased risk of invasive lobular carcinoma.

- **STK11:** Defects in the *STK11* gene can lead to Peutz-Jeghers syndrome. People with this syndrome develop pigmented spots on their lips and in their mouths, polyps in the urinary and gastrointestinal tracts, and are at increased risk for many types of cancer, including breast cancer.

Gene testing: Genetic tests can be done to look for mutations in the *BRCA1* and *BRCA2* genes (or, less commonly, in other genes, such as *PTEN* or *TP53*). Although testing can be helpful in some situations, the advantages and disadvantages of genetic testing must be considered carefully. The American Cancer Society strongly recommends that *before* proceeding with plans for genetic testing, women talk with a genetic counselor, nurse, or doctor who is qualified to interpret and explain the results. It is very important to understand and weigh the benefits and risks of these tests carefully before doing them. Many women may have relatives with breast cancer, but, in most cases, this is not the result of an inherited gene mutation. The results are often not clear cut, as in the case of variants of uncertain significance, in which the association with disease risk is not clear.

Experts agree that genetic testing should only be done when there is a reasonable suspicion that a mutation may be present. A genetic counselor (or other professional) can estimate the chance that a mutation is present based on a woman's personal and family history. Based on that history, a genetic counselor can also recommend who in the family is most likely to have a mutation, and therefore who should be tested first. Testing can have a wide range of consequences that need to be considered. Genetic testing is also expensive, and it is not covered by all insurance plans.

Women who are found to have inherited genetic mutations that increase breast cancer risk can take steps to reduce this risk, including taking medication or having risk-reduction surgery. These women can also carefully monitor changes in their breasts to detect cancer at earlier, more treatable stages. For women who already have breast cancer, knowing about a mutation can affect treatment decisions. These decisions can include whether to choose mastectomy or breast-conserving surgery or whether to have risk-reduction surgery, such as removing the ovaries and fallopian tubes (a bilateral salpingo-oophorectomy) or having the healthy breast removed (a prophylactic mastectomy).

Personal History of Breast Cancer

A woman with cancer in one breast has a three- to fourfold increased risk of a new cancer developing in the other breast. Treatment for the initial cancer can often decrease the risk of cancer developing in the opposite breast. A cancer in the opposite breast is different from a return of the first cancer.

Race and Ethnicity

For all ages combined, white women in the United States are slightly more likely to have breast cancer than are African American women. However, African American women are more likely to die of breast cancer. In women under age forty-five, breast cancer is more common in African American women, and African American women are more likely to be diagnosed with larger tumors and later-stage breast cancer.

Overall, the risk of breast cancer is highest among white women, followed in order of decreasing risk by African American, Asian, Hispanic, and Native American women.

Dense Breast Tissue

Women with denser breast tissue (as seen on a mammogram) have more glandular tissue and less fatty tissue and are at higher risk for breast cancer than women with less dense breast tissue. Dense breast tissue can also make it harder for doctors to spot problems on mammograms.

Lobular Carcinoma In Situ

Breast Cancer and Ethnicity

Breast cancer affects different groups of American women in different ways. For example, although white women are slightly more likely to get breast cancer than are African American women, African American women are more likely to die of this cancer. Asian, Hispanic, and Native American women are at lower risk for both developing and dying of breast cancer. What accounts for these differences? In most cases, doctors are not sure.

Social factors such as diet and lifestyle might play a role. For instance, the recent increase in breast cancer incidence in Asian American women is commonly attributed to the adoption of a Western lifestyle, which includes behaviors that put women at higher risk for breast cancer occurrence. These behaviors include delaying childbirth beyond the age of thirty, becoming overweight, not exercising enough, and drinking alcohol.

Characteristics of the tumors themselves can also differ by racial background. For example, African American women have a higher rate of breast cancer before menopause than do white women. In addition, African American women are more than twice as likely as white women to have estrogen receptor–negative and progesterone receptor–negative tumors, which tend to be more aggressive. Researchers are working to learn more about these differences and what might cause them.

In lobular carcinoma in situ (LCIS), cells that look like cancer cells are growing in the lobules (milk-producing glands) of the breast, but they do not grow through the walls of the lobules. Women with this condition have an eight- to tenfold increased risk of invasive cancer developing in either breast. For this reason, women with LCIS should make sure they have regular mammograms and doctor visits.

Certain Benign Breast Conditions

Women with certain benign breast conditions can have an increased risk of breast cancer. Some of these conditions are more closely linked to breast cancer risk than others. Doctors often divide benign breast conditions into three general groups, depending on how they affect breast cancer risk. All of these benign breast conditions are described in more detail in appendix C.

Nonproliferative lesions: These conditions are not associated with overgrowth of breast tissue. They either do not affect breast cancer risk or increase it only slightly.

Some nonproliferative lesions can be diagnosed without a biopsy. These include mastitis (inflammation of the breast), fibrosis (fibrous tissue), and simple cysts (fluid-filled sacs). Some other nonproliferative lesions will require a biopsy for diagnosis:
- mild hyperplasia
- adenosis
- duct ectasia
- periductal fibrosis
- benign phyllodes tumors
- single papillomas
- fat necrosis
- squamous metaplasia
- apocrine metaplasia
- epithelial-related calcifications
- other benign tumors:
  - lipoma
  - hamartoma
  - hemangioma
  - neurofibroma
  - adenomyoepithelioma

Proliferative lesions: With proliferative lesions, there is excessive growth of cells in the ducts or lobules of the breast tissue. They appear to raise a woman's risk of breast cancer slightly (up to two times the normal risk). They require a biopsy for diagnosis. There are two subgroups of proliferative lesions: proliferative lesions without atypia and proliferative lesions with atypia. Proliferative lesions without atypia include the following types:

- usual ductal hyperplasia without atypia
- fibroadenomas
- sclerosing adenosis
- several papillomas (called papillomatosis)
- radial scar

Proliferative lesions with atypia include the following types:
- atypical ductal hyperplasia (ADH)
- atypical lobular hyperplasia (ALH)

Women with a family history of breast cancer and either hyperplasia or atypical hyperplasia have an even higher risk of breast cancer.

For more information on noncancerous breast conditions, see pages 435–440. More information is also available by contacting the American Cancer Society at 800-227-2345 or www.cancer.org.

Previous Chest Irradiation

Women who have had radiation therapy to the chest during childhood or young adulthood as treatment for another cancer (such as Hodgkin disease or non-Hodgkin lymphoma) have a significantly higher risk of breast cancer. This increased risk varies according to the woman's age at the time of her radiation treatment. The risk of breast cancer developing after chest radiation is highest if radiation was given during adolescence, when the breasts are developing. If chemotherapy was also given, it might have stopped ovarian hormone production for some time, lowering the woman's risk. Radiation treatment after age forty does not seem to increase breast cancer risk.

Menstrual Periods

Women who have had more menstrual cycles because they started menstruating at an early age (before twelve) or who went through menopause at a late age (after fifty-five) have a slightly higher risk of breast cancer. This increased risk may be related to a higher lifetime exposure to the hormones estrogen and progesterone.

The Meaning Behind the Numbers

WHAT ARE STATISTICS?

Statistics refers to the science of using numbers to describe or better understand our world. In the case of breast cancer research, scientists use statistics to help them understand the relationship between disease and such factors as lifestyle, age, gender, and environment.

WHAT DO INCIDENCE AND MORTALITY MEAN IN STATISTICAL TERMS?

Incidence refers to the number or rate of new cases of cancer diagnosed during a specific time period. Mortality refers to the number or rate of deaths attributed to a particular type of cancer in a population during a specific time period.

WHY ARE RATES, RATHER THAN REAL NUMBERS, USED TO EXPLAIN CANCER OCCURRENCE?

By studying rates rather than simply reporting the number of cases, scientists can more realistically compare the occurrence of disease over time or in different populations. Rates are calculated from the number of deaths or cases reported over a particular time period and population data for the same period. Rates help scientists understand changes in patterns of a disease. For example, breast cancer mortality rates are beginning to decline in some groups of women, reflecting increased use of early detection methods and improved treatments.

WHAT DOES "LIFETIME RISK OF BREAST CANCER" MEAN?

Lifetime risk is an estimate of the probability of cancer developing from birth until death. The calculation incorporates two basic measures: the rate of newly diagnosed cancers in each age group and the mortality rate from all causes of death in each age group. The method takes into account that a person might die of some other cause. Risks are calculated over five-year age intervals to approximate a lifetime measure. If different organizations use different age cut-off points, then different lifetime risk estimates will emerge for the same disease. For example, one organization might say that a woman's lifetime risk of breast cancer developing is one in eight, but another will report this risk as one in nine. Most often, estimates of lifetime risk are actually averages—they can tell us about how many people in a large group can be expected to get cancer, but they do not tell us the risk for any one person. Within that large group will be people with higher risk and people with lower risk.

Diethylstilbestrol Exposure

From the 1940s through the 1960s, some pregnant women were given the drug diethyl-stilbestrol (DES) because it was believed to lower the chances of miscarriage. These women have a slightly increased risk of breast cancer. Women whose mothers took DES during pregnancy might also have a slightly higher risk of breast cancer. For more information on DES exposure, contact the American Cancer Society at 800-227-2345 or www.cancer.org.

Lifestyle-Related Factors and Breast Cancer Risk

Some breast cancer risk factors are related to lifestyle choices and can be avoided. Although there are several lifestyle-related risk factors for breast cancer, none are responsible for a significant number of cases of the disease. There is no certain way to prevent breast cancer. Nonetheless, avoiding or controlling some of the following risk factors (when it is practical to do so) may decrease a woman's chances of breast cancer.

Recent Oral Contraceptive Use

Women using oral contraceptives (birth control pills) have a slightly higher risk of breast cancer than women who have never used them. This risk seems to return to normal over time once the pills are stopped. Women who have not used oral contraceptives for more than ten years do not appear to have any increased breast cancer risk. When thinking about using oral contraceptives, women should discuss their other risk factors for breast cancer with their medical team.

Hormone Therapy After Menopause

Hormone therapy with estrogen (sometimes with progesterone) has been used for many years to help relieve symptoms of menopause and prevent osteoporosis (the thinning of the bones and loss of bone density). Earlier studies suggested it might have other health benefits, too, but these benefits have not been found in more recent, better-designed studies. This treatment goes by many names, such as postmenopausal hormone therapy, hormone replacement therapy, and menopausal hormone therapy.

There are two main types of hormone therapy (HT). For women who still have a uterus, doctors generally prescribe both estrogen and progesterone, which is known as combined HT. Because estrogen alone can increase the risk of uterine cancer, progesterone is added to help prevent this side effect. For women whose uterus has been removed by hysterectomy, estrogen alone can be prescribed. This treatment is commonly known as estrogen replacement therapy (ERT) or just estrogen therapy (ET).

Combined hormone therapy: Using combined HT after menopause increases a woman's risk of breast cancer and increases her risk of dying of the disease. These increases in risk can be seen with as little as two years of hormone therapy use. Combined hormone therapy also increases the likelihood that breast cancer will be found at a more advanced stage, possibly because hormone therapy increases breast density, thereby reducing the effectiveness of mammograms. However, the increased risks from combined hormone therapy seem to apply only to current and recent users of this therapy. A woman's breast cancer risk appears to return to that of the general population within five years of stopping combined hormone therapy.

The word bioidentical is sometimes used to describe versions of estrogen and progesterone with the same chemical structure as those found naturally in people. The use of these hormones has been marketed as a safe way to treat the symptoms of menopause. It is important to realize that there is no evidence that "bioidentical" or "natural" hormones are safer or more effective than synthetic versions, although there have been few studies comparing them. The use of these bioidentical hormones should be assumed to have the same health risks as any other type of hormone therapy.

Estrogen therapy (ET): The use of estrogen alone after menopause does not appear to increase the risk of breast cancer. In fact, some research has suggested that women who have had their uteruses removed and who take estrogen alone actually have a lower risk of breast cancer. However, these women do have more problems with strokes and blood clots. Some studies also have shown that long-term use (more than ten years) of estrogen therapy increases the risk of cancer.

At this time, there appear to be few strong reasons to use postmenopausal hormone therapy (either combined HT or ET), other than possibly for the short-term relief of menopausal symptoms. Along with increasing the risk of breast cancer, combined HT also appears to increase the risk of heart disease, blood clots, and strokes. Hormone therapy does lower the risk of colorectal cancer and osteoporosis, but this benefit must be weighed against the possible harms of hormone therapy, especially since there are other effective ways to prevent and treat osteoporosis. Although estrogen therapy does not appear to increase the risk of breast cancer, it does increase the risk of blood clots and strokes and may increase the risk of ovarian cancer.

The decision to use hormone therapy after menopause should be made after weighing the possible risks and benefits, based on the severity of the woman's menopausal symptoms and her other risk factors for breast cancer, heart disease, and osteoporosis. If a woman and her doctor decide to try hormone therapy to treat menopausal symptoms, it is usually best to use it at the lowest dose needed and for as short a time as possible.

Reproductive History

Women who have had no pregnancies or who had their first child after age thirty have a slightly higher breast cancer risk. Having many pregnancies and becoming pregnant at a young age reduce breast cancer risk. Pregnancy reduces a woman's total number of lifetime menstrual cycles, which might be the reason for this effect on risk.

Breastfeeding

Some studies suggest that breastfeeding may lower breast cancer risk slightly, especially if breastfeeding is continued for one and one-half to two years. But this has been a difficult area of study, especially in countries such as the United States, where breastfeeding for this long is uncommon. One large study found that for every year a woman breastfeeds, she lowers her risk of breast cancer by just over 4 percent. One explanation for this effect is that breastfeeding often delays the resumption of menses after pregnancy. This reduces a woman's total number of lifetime menstrual cycles.

Alcohol

The use of alcohol is clearly linked to an increased risk of breast cancer. The risk increases with the amount of alcohol consumed. Compared with nondrinkers, women who consume one alcoholic drink per day have a very small increase in risk. Those who have two to five drinks daily have about one and one-half times the risk of women who do not drink alcohol. Excessive alcohol use is also known to increase the risk of several other types of cancer.

Obesity and Weight Gain

Obesity refers to having an abnormally high proportion of body fat. (Overweight means an excess of body weight compared with set standards, whereas obesity is determined by excess body fat, not just excess weight.) Being overweight or obese has been found to increase breast cancer risk, especially for women after menopause. Before menopause, a woman's ovaries produce most of her estrogen, and fat tissue produces a small amount of estrogen. After menopause (when the ovaries stop making estrogen), most of a woman's estrogen comes from fat tissue. Having more fat tissue after menopause can raise estrogen levels and increase the risk of breast cancer. Women who are overweight also tend to have higher blood insulin levels. Higher insulin levels have been linked to some types of cancer, including breast cancer.

The connection between weight and breast cancer risk is complex. For example, the risk appears to be higher for women who gained weight as an adult but may not be higher for those who have been overweight since childhood. Excess fat in the waist area also may affect risk more than the same amount of fat in the hips and thighs. Researchers believe that fat cells in various parts of the body have subtle differences that may explain this.

The American Cancer Society recommends that women achieve and maintain a healthy weight throughout their lives, using the key strategies of getting regular physical activity and limiting intake of high-calorie foods and drinks.

Physical Activity

Evidence suggests that physical activity in the form of exercise reduces breast cancer risk. The main question is how much exercise is needed to reduce risk. In one analysis from the Women's Health Initiative (WHI) study, postmenopausal women who walked briskly as little as one and one-quarter to two and one-half hours per week had an 18 percent lower risk of breast cancer. Walking ten hours a week reduced the risk a little more.

Factors Whose Impact Is Uncertain or Controversial

There are some factors whose impact on breast cancer is not yet fully known or understood. For other factors, such as secondhand smoke, there is some controversy around the possible link to breast cancer risk.

Diet and Vitamin Intake

Many studies have looked for a link between certain diets and breast cancer risk, but the results have been conflicting. Some studies have indicated that diet might play a role, whereas others have found no evidence that diet influences breast cancer risk. Studies have looked at the amount of fat in the diet, intake of fruits and vegetables, and intake of meat, but no clear link to breast cancer risk has been found. Studies have also looked at vitamin levels, again with inconsistent results. Some studies have actually found an increased risk of breast cancer in women with higher levels of certain nutrients. To date, no study has shown that taking vitamins reduces breast cancer risk. Based on current evidence, a diet that balances caloric intake with energy expended and that is low in fat, low in red meat and processed meat, and high in fruits and vegetables might offer health benefits, including reducing cancer risk.

Most studies have found that breast cancer is less common in countries where the typical diet is low in total fat, low in polyunsaturated fat, and low in saturated fat. On the other hand, many studies of women in the United States have not found breast cancer risk to be related to dietary fat intake. Researchers are still not sure how to explain this apparent disagreement. It might be at least partly due to the effect of diet on body weight. Studies comparing diet and breast cancer risk in various countries are complicated by other differences, such as activity level, intake of other nutrients, and genetic factors that might also change breast cancer risk.

More research is needed to better understand the effects of different types of fat in the diet on breast cancer risk. Fat is a major source of calories, and excess calories can lead to weight gain. High-fat diets can lead to being overweight or obese, which is a risk factor for breast cancer developing after menopause. A high-fat diet has also been shown to influence the risk of several other types of cancer, and intake of certain types of fat is clearly related to heart disease risk.

The American Cancer Society recommends eating a healthy diet with an emphasis on plant sources. This includes eating at least two and one-half cups of vegetables and fruits each day, choosing whole grains over those that are refined, and limiting consumption of processed and red meats.

Environmental Contaminants or Pollutants

How do the substances in our environment influence breast cancer risk? A great deal of research has been done to try to answer this question, and more is under way. Of special interest are compounds in the environment that have been found in laboratory studies to have estrogen-like properties, which could in theory affect breast cancer risk. For example, substances found in some plastics (such as Bisphenol-A, or BPA), certain cosmetics and personal care products, pesticides (such as DDT), and polychlorinated biphenyls, or PCBs, seem to have such properties.

This issue understandably invokes a great deal of public concern, but research does not show a clear link between breast cancer risk and exposure to these substances. Studying such effects in people is difficult. More research is needed to better define the possible health effects of these and similar substances.

Induced Abortion

Several studies have provided very strong data that neither induced abortions nor spontaneous abortions (miscarriages) have an overall effect on the risk of breast cancer.

Tobacco Smoke

Most studies have found no link between cigarette smoking and breast cancer. Some studies have suggested smoking increases breast cancer risk, but this notion remains controversial.

An active focus of research is whether secondhand smoke increases the risk of breast cancer. Both mainstream and secondhand smoke contain chemicals that, in high concentrations, cause breast cancer in rodents. Chemicals in tobacco smoke reach breast tissue and are found in breast milk.

The evidence on secondhand smoke and breast cancer risk in human studies is controversial, at least in part because smokers have not been shown to be at increased risk. One possible explanation for this is that tobacco smoke might have different effects on breast cancer risk in smokers versus those who are just exposed to smoke.

A report from the California Environmental Protection Agency in 2005 concluded that the evidence about secondhand smoke and breast cancer is "consistent with a causal association" in younger, mainly premenopausal women. The 2006 US Surgeon General's report, *The Health Consequences of Involuntary Exposure to Tobacco Smoke*, concluded that "suggestive but not sufficient" evidence exists for a link. In any case, this possible link to breast cancer is yet another reason to avoid secondhand smoke.

Night Work

Several studies have suggested that women who work at night—for example, nurses working a night shift—might have an increased risk of breast cancer. This is a recent finding, and more studies are looking at this issue. Some researchers think the effect might be due to changes in levels of melatonin, a hormone whose production is affected by the body's exposure to light, but other hormones are also being studied.

Myths About Breast Cancer Risk

Some of the following factors are rumored to affect breast cancer risk, but no scientific or clinical evidence supports these claims.

Antiperspirants

The use of antiperspirants or deodorants does not cause breast cancer, contrary to Internet and e-mail rumors that have suggested as much. The claims that chemicals in underarm antiperspirants are absorbed through the skin, interfere with lymph circulation, and cause toxins to accumulate in the breast, eventually leading to breast cancer, are not consistent with the way antiperspirants work, the lymph drainage of the breast, or scientific concepts of how cancer is formed.

There is very little evidence to support this rumor. One small study found trace levels of parabens, which are used as preservatives in antiperspirants and other products and have weak estrogen-like properties, in a small sample of breast cancer tumors. But this study did not look at whether parabens caused the tumors, nor did it identify deodorants or antiperspirants as the source of the parabens. Although parabens are used in many cosmetic, food, and pharmaceutical products, most major brands of deodorants and antiperspirants in the United States do not currently contain parabens. This was also a preliminary finding, and more research is needed to determine what effect, if any, parabens may have on breast cancer risk. So far, no study has shown that parabens cause breast cancer.

No published scientific reports have shown a link between breast cancer and antiperspirants. A large study looking at possible causes of breast cancer found no increase in breast cancer in women who used underarm antiperspirants and/or shaved their underarms. Chemicals in such products are tested thoroughly to assure their safety.

Underwire Bras

Internet and e-mail rumors have suggested that underwire bras cause breast cancer by obstructing lymph flow. There is no scientific or clinical basis for this claim. Women who do not wear underwire bras regularly are more likely to be thinner or have less dense breasts, which would probably contribute to any perceived difference in risk.

Breast Implants

Several studies have found that breast implants do not increase breast cancer risk. Breast implants can cause scar tissue to form in the breast, making it harder to feel tumors. Implants can also make it harder to see breast tissue on standard mammograms, but additional methods can be used for complete examinations of breast tissue.

CHAPTER 3

Your Breast Cancer Workup

If you had a breast lump or abnormal mammogram finding, you will need a thorough workup. This can include a medical history, physical examination, imaging tests, and biopsy or other laboratory tests. You may have already had some of these procedures. Exactly which tests are helpful will depend on the type of cancer found and how far it has spread. This chapter summarizes the types of tests your medical team might suggest.

Doctor Visit and Examination

Often, the first step for someone who has a new breast lump, symptom, or change on a mammogram is to meet with her doctor. The doctor will review your medical history, asking questions about any symptoms and about factors that might relate to breast cancer risk. One important question, for example, is whether there is a family history of cancer. Before your visit, you might want to research your maternal (mother's side) and paternal (father's side) medical histories for any cancers, particularly any breast or ovarian cancers. Both sides of the family are important when determining your risk of having such cancer-related gene mutations as the *BRCA* gene. Your physical examination should include a general examination of your body and careful examination of your breasts and the lymph nodes under your arms. Your doctor will look for the following physical signs:

- any breast changes, including changes in texture, size, and relationship to skin and chest muscles
- any changes in the nipple or skin of the breast
- any evidence of lumps or masses in the breast

• lumps or bumps under the armpit or above the collarbone (which could be caused by enlarged lymph nodes from breast cancer metastasis)

The doctor will also perform a general examination of other organs to check for obvious spread of breast cancer and to help evaluate your general health.

Breast Imaging Tests

After completing your physical examination and taking your medical history, your doctor will recommend that you have breast imaging studies, such as a diagnostic mammogram, breast ultrasound, and/or MRI.

Mammograms

A mammogram is an x-ray of the breast. Breast x-rays have been done for more than seventy years, but the modern mammogram has only existed since 1969. That was the first year x-ray units specifically for breast imaging were available. Modern mammogram equipment designed for breast x-rays uses very low levels of radiation, usually a dose of about 0.1 to 0.2 rads per picture (a rad is a measure of radiation dose). Strict guidelines ensure that mammogram equipment is safe and uses the lowest dose of radiation possible. Many people are concerned about exposure to x-rays, but the level of radiation used in modern mammograms does not significantly increase the risk of breast cancer.

Whereas screening mammograms are used to look for breast disease in women who do not have symptoms, diagnostic mammograms are used to diagnose breast disease in women who have breast symptoms or an abnormal result on a screening mammogram. Symptoms such as a breast lump, spontaneous nipple discharge, or other changes in the breast might lead to your doctor ordering a diagnostic mammogram. A diagnostic mammogram includes more images of the area of concern to give more information about the size and character of the area. In some cases, special images known as cone or spot views with magnification are used to make a small area of abnormal breast tissue easier to evaluate.

Digital Mammograms

A digital mammogram (also known as a full-field digital mammogram, or FFDM) is like a standard mammogram in that x-rays are used to produce an image of your breast. The differences are in the way the image is recorded, viewed by the doctor, and stored. Standard mammograms are recorded on large sheets of photographic film. Digital mammograms are recorded and stored on a computer. After the examination, the doctor can look at them on a computer screen and adjust the image size, brightness, or contrast to see certain areas more clearly. Digital images can also be sent electronically to another site for a remote consultation with breast specialists. Not all centers offer the digital option, but it is becoming more widely available.

What a Mammogram Shows

The doctor reading the films will look for several types of changes, some of which might be caused by cancer.

Calcifications are tiny mineral deposits within the breast tissue, which look like small white spots on the mammogram films. They might or might not be caused by cancer. There are two types of calcifications: macrocalcifications and microcalcifications.

Macrocalcifications are larger calcium deposits that are most likely caused by aging of the breast arteries, old injuries, or inflammation. These deposits are related to non-cancerous conditions and do not require a biopsy (in which tissue is extracted for closer examination). Macrocalcifications are found in about half of women over age fifty, and in about one in ten women under fifty.

Microcalcifications are tiny specks of calcium in the breast. They can appear alone or in clusters. Microcalcifications, although of more concern than larger calcium deposits on a mammogram, usually do not mean that cancer is present. The shape and layout of microcalcifications help the doctor judge how likely it is that cancer is present. If the calcifications look suspicious, a biopsy will be done.

A mass, with or without calcifications, is another important change that can be seen on mammograms. Masses can be many things, including cysts (noncancerous, fluid-filled sacs) and noncancerous solid tumors (such as fibroadenomas), but they can also be cancer.

A cyst and a tumor can feel alike on a physical examination. They can also look the same on a mammogram. To confirm that a mass is really a cyst, a breast ultrasound is often done. Another option is to remove the fluid from the cyst with a thin, hollow needle.

If a mass is not a simple cyst (that is, if it is at least partly solid, known as a complex cyst), then you might need to have more imaging tests. A biopsy will usually need to be performed on a mass that is not a simple cyst. Some masses can be watched with periodic mammograms. The size, shape, and margins (edges) of the mass help the radiologist determine whether cancer is present.

Having your previous mammograms available for the radiologist is very important. Your past mammograms can be helpful in showing whether a mass or calcification has changed over time. If a mass or calcification has not changed for many years, this would mean that it is probably a benign condition and a biopsy is not needed.

Limitations of Mammograms

Mammograms will not find all breast cancers. They are best used to find tumors that cannot be felt. In someone with a lump in her breast, a mammogram can be a way to look more closely at the area containing the lump. It also can find other areas in the breast that should be examined more closely through biopsy—in which a small amount of tissue is removed and looked at under a microscope. But if a lump is present, a normal mammogram does not mean that you do not have breast cancer. If you have a breast lump, you should talk to your doctor about having a biopsy performed—even if your mammogram result is normal.

A mammogram also cannot prove that an abnormal area is cancer. To confirm whether cancer is present, a biopsy must be performed.

Mammograms are not as effective in younger women, usually because their breasts are dense and can hide a tumor. This may also be true for pregnant women and women who are breastfeeding. Since mammograms are not usually done in pregnant women and most breast cancers occur in older women, this is usually not a major problem.

What to Expect When You Have a Mammogram

- To have a mammogram, you must undress above the waist. The facility will give you a wrap to wear.
- A technologist will be there to position your breasts for the mammogram. Most technologists are women. You and the technologist will be the only ones in the room during the mammogram.
- To get a high-quality mammogram picture with excellent image quality, it is necessary to flatten the breast slightly. The technologist will place the breast on the mammogram machine's lower plate, which is made of metal and has a drawer to hold the x-ray film or the camera to produce a digital image. The upper plate, made of plastic, is lowered to compress the breast for a few seconds while the technician takes a picture. The whole procedure takes about twenty minutes. The actual breast compression only lasts a few seconds.

- You will feel some discomfort when your breasts are compressed, and compression can be painful for some women. Try not to schedule a mammogram when your breasts are likely to be tender, as they may be just before or during your period.
- Mammogram facilities are now required to send your results to you within thirty days. Generally, you will be contacted within five working days if there is a problem.
- Being called back for more testing does not mean that you have cancer. In fact, less than 10 percent of women who are called back for more tests are found to have breast cancer. Being called back occurs fairly often, and it usually just means an additional image or an ultrasound needs to be done to look at an area more closely. Callbacks are more common for first mammograms (or when there is no previous mammogram to look at) and in mammograms done in women who have not gone through menopause. They may be slightly less common with digital mammograms.

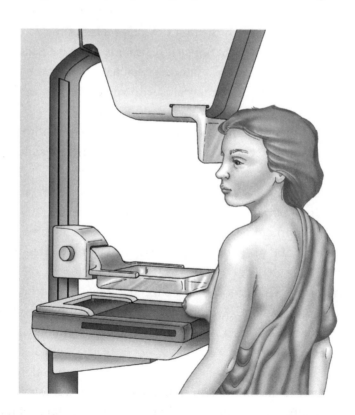

© Sam and Amy Collins

During a mammogram, the breast is pressed between the x-ray plate and the upper plastic plate to spread out the breast tissue.

Tips for Having a Mammogram

The following are useful suggestions for making sure you receive a quality mammogram:

- Discuss any new findings or problems in your breasts with your doctor or nurse before having a mammogram.
- If it is not posted visibly near the receptionist's desk, ask to see the US Food and Drug Administration (FDA) certificate that is issued to all facilities that offer mammography. The FDA requires that all facilities meet high professional standards of safety and quality in order to be a provider of mammography services. A facility cannot provide mammography without certification.
- Use a facility that either specializes in mammography or does many mammograms a day.
- If you are satisfied that the facility is of high quality, continue to go there on a regular basis so that your mammograms can be compared from year to year.
- If you are going to a facility for the first time, take a list of the dates of previous mammograms, biopsies, or other breast treatments you have had, as well as information about where they were done. If you have had mammograms done at another facility, take those mammograms with you to the new facility (or have them sent there) so they can be compared to the new ones.
- On the day of the mammogram, do not wear deodorant or antiperspirant. Some of these contain substances that can appear on the x-ray film as white spots and could interfere with the reading of the mammogram.
- You may find it easier to wear a skirt or pants rather than a dress, so that you will only need to remove your blouse for the examination.
- Schedule your mammogram when your breasts are not tender or swollen to help reduce discomfort and to ensure a good picture. Try to avoid the week before your period.
- Tell the technologist who is doing the mammogram about any breast symptoms or problems you are having. Be prepared to describe any medical history that could affect your breast cancer risk—such as surgery, hormone use, or family or personal history of breast cancer.

If you do not hear from your doctor within ten days, do not assume that your mammogram was normal. Call your doctor or the facility to request your results.

Breast Ultrasound

Ultrasound, also known as sonography, uses sound waves to outline a part of the body. For this test, a small, microphone-like instrument called a transducer is placed on the skin, which is often first lubricated with ultrasound gel. It emits sound waves and picks up the echoes as they bounce off body tissues. The echoes are converted by a computer into a black-and-white image that is displayed on the computer screen. This test is painless and does not expose you to radiation.

Ultrasound is widely available and can be a valuable tool to use along with mammography. Usually, breast ultrasound is used to look at a specific area of concern found on the mammogram. It is especially useful in distinguishing between cysts and solid masses.

Breast Magnetic Resonance Imaging

Magnetic resonance imaging (MRI) scans use radio waves and strong magnets instead of x-rays to take pictures of parts of the body. The energy from the radio waves is absorbed and then released in patterns formed by the type of body tissue and by the presence of certain diseases. A computer translates these patterns into a very detailed image of parts of the body. For breast MRI, a contrast medium, or liquid containing a metal called gadolinium, is often injected into a vein before or during the scan to show details more clearly.

MRI machines are quite common, but they must be specially adapted to be effective for breast imaging. MRI scans of the breast should be done only on these specially adapted machines, and the imaging facility should have the capability to perform MRI–guided breast biopsy, if necessary.

MRI scans can take a long time—often up to an hour. The woman must lie inside a narrow tube, face down on a platform specially designed for the procedure. The platform has openings for each breast that allow them to be imaged without compression. The platform contains the sensors needed to capture the MRI image. It is important to remain very still throughout the examination.

MRI can be helpful in looking at a breast mass or mammogram abnormality. In some cases, breast MRI can help define the size and extent of cancer within the breast tissue. It can be useful in younger women, whose dense breast tissue can make it more difficult to find tumors through mammography. Breast MRI may be used after breast cancer is found, to help view the tumor better and to be sure there are no other tumors in the same breast. It can also be used to look at the other breast, although so far this has not been found to be helpful in finding more cancers.

Breast MRI is recommended to screen women at high risk for breast cancer, such as those with a BRCA mutation. However, MRIs are extremely sensitive and can pick up lesions in the breast that will never cause any harm. This can sometimes result in further workup and biopsies that are not really necessary. For this reason, and because they are much more expensive than mammograms, breast MRIs are not routinely recommended for every woman.

Breast MRI

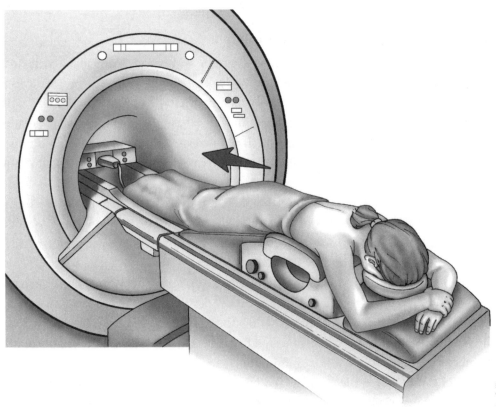

© Sam and Amy Collins

During a breast MRI, the patient lies face down on a padded table with hollow depressions for the breasts. The table then slides into the MRI machine.

Ductogram

Rarely, a ductogram, also called a galactogram, is used to look for the cause of nipple discharge. In this test, a very small plastic tube is placed into the opening of the duct in the nipple. A small amount of contrast medium is injected, which outlines the shape of the duct on an x-ray image. It will show whether there is a mass inside the duct.

Breast Biopsy

If a woman or her doctor finds a suspicious breast lump, or if imaging studies show a worrisome area, the woman must have a biopsy to determine whether cancer is present. In this procedure, a sample of tissue is removed for examination under the microscope. A biopsy is the only way to know whether an abnormal area of tissue is cancer.

There are several different types of breast biopsies. Biopsy can be done by a needle, or it can require a surgical procedure. Each type of biopsy has advantages and disadvantages, and the best type of biopsy for each situation depends on the patient. Needle biopsy is generally preferred over surgical biopsy as the first step in making a cancer diagnosis. A needle biopsy is far less invasive than a surgical biopsy and yields a diagnosis more rapidly and with less discomfort. In addition, it gives the woman an opportunity to discuss treatment options with her doctor before any surgery is performed. There is no danger that needle biopsy itself will cause the breast cancer to spread. Some patients will still require surgical biopsy, however, either as a first procedure or to remove all or part of a lump for microscopic examination after a needle biopsy has been performed. Surgery for breast cancer is discussed in detail in chapter 8.

Needle Biopsy

Two types of needle biopsies are used to diagnose breast cancer: fine needle aspiration and core needle biopsy.

Fine Needle Aspiration

Fine needle aspiration (FNA) uses a very thin needle and a syringe to withdraw a small amount of fluid and very small pieces of tissue from the tumor mass. The doctor can guide the needle into the suspicious area while feeling it. If the tumor is too deep inside the body to be felt, the doctor may use ultrasound or computed tomography (CT) to watch the needle on a screen while guiding it into the abnormal area. If the abnormal area is a cyst, FNA might be used to remove a sample of fluid.

The main advantage of FNA is that it does not require an incision. It is the easiest type of biopsy to have, but it has some disadvantages. It can sometimes miss a cancer if the needle is not placed precisely among the cancer cells. And, even if cancer cells are found, it is usually impossible to determine whether the cancer is invasive. Often, not enough cancer cells are removed to be able to perform some of the other laboratory tests that are routinely done on breast cancer specimens. A trained cytopathologist (a pathologist who is expert at examining cells rather than pieces of breast tissue) should interpret the FNA findings. If the FNA biopsy does not provide a clear diagnosis or the doctor is still suspicious, a second biopsy or a different type of biopsy should be done.

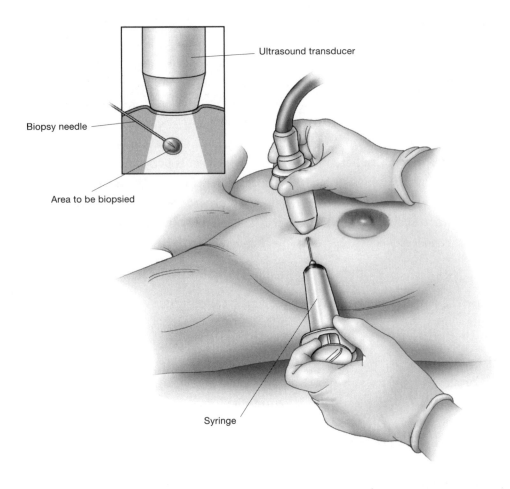

Fine needle aspiration using ultrasound

© Sam and Amy Collins

Core Needle Biopsy

Core needle biopsy uses a larger needle that is designed to remove a small cylinder, or core, of tissue. Several cores are often removed. The core needle biopsy is done by using local anesthesia in the doctor's office, clinic, or breast imaging center. Because it removes larger pieces of tissue, a core needle biopsy is more likely than an FNA to provide a clear diagnosis, although it can still miss some cancers.

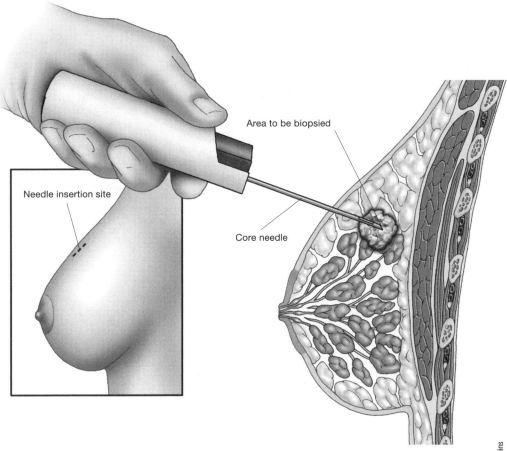

During a core needle biopsy, a needle is used to remove a small core of tissue. An imaging technique, such as ultrasound, may be used if the area of concern cannot be easily felt.

If a lump cannot be felt easily and can be seen only by use of mammography, ultrasound, or MRI, the doctor can use one of these imaging techniques to guide the needle during the biopsy. The mammogram-directed technique is called stereotactic core needle biopsy. In this procedure, digital mammogram images help the doctor map the exact location of the breast lump and guide the tip of the needle to the right spot. Ultrasound images can be used in the same way. The choice between a mammogram-directed stereotactic needle biopsy and ultrasound-guided biopsy depends on the type of breast change and the experience and preference of the doctor.

Stereotactic needle biopsy

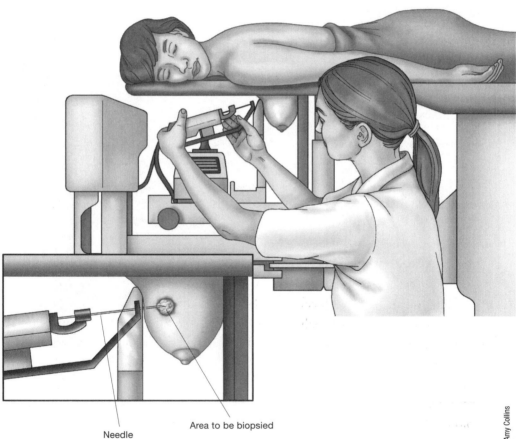

Needle

Area to be biopsied

© Sam and Amy Collins

During a stereotactic needle biopsy, the patient lies on a table with an opening for the breast. Before the biopsy needle is inserted, the breast is compressed between two plates, just as in a standard mammogram.

American Cancer Society

Image-guided biopsies can also be performed with a vacuum-assisted biopsy device. This type of biopsy is done with systems such as the Mammotome or ATEC (Automated Tissue Excision and Collection). For this procedure, the skin is numbed and a small incision (about a quarter of an inch) is made. A hollow probe is inserted through the incision into the abnormal area of breast tissue. The probe can be guided into place by using x-rays or ultrasound (or MRI, in the ATEC system). A cylinder of tissue is then sucked into the probe through a hole in its side, and a rotating knife within the probe cuts the tissue sample from the rest of the breast. Several samples can be taken through the same incision. Vacuum-assisted biopsies are done as outpatient procedures. No stitches are needed, and scarring is minimal. This method usually removes more tissue than a standard core needle biopsy.

Surgical Biopsy

Sometimes, surgery is needed to remove all or part of the lump for microscopic examination. This is referred to as a surgical or open biopsy. Usually, this is an excisional biopsy, in which the surgeon removes the entire mass or abnormal area and a surrounding margin of normal-appearing breast tissue. If the mass is too large to be easily removed, an incisional biopsy might be done instead. In an incisional biopsy, only part of the mass is removed. In rare cases, an incisional biopsy can be done in the doctor's office, but it is more commonly done in a hospital's outpatient department under local anesthesia (the patient is awake, but the breast is numbed). Both excisional and incisional biopsies can be performed under intravenous sedation with local anesthesia, or under general anesthesia (the patient is asleep).

If the area needing biopsy cannot be felt, a mammogram might be used to place a wire into the correct area to guide the surgeon. This technique is called wire localization. After numbing the area with a local anesthetic, the radiologist or surgeon uses x-ray images to guide a small hollow needle to the abnormal spot in the breast. A thin wire is inserted through the center of the needle and into the suspicious area, after which the needle is removed. The patient is then taken to the operating room, where the wire will be used to guide the surgeon to the right spot.

Excisional or incisional biopsies are more involved than an FNA biopsy or a core needle biopsy. They typically require several stitches and might leave a scar. Core needle biopsy is usually enough to make a diagnosis, but sometimes an open biopsy is needed when the lesion is in a location that is difficult to reach or when a core biopsy is not conclusive.

All biopsies can cause bleeding and may lead to swelling, which can make it seem like the breast lump is larger after the biopsy. This is generally nothing to worry about, and the bleeding and bruising resolve quickly in most cases.

Tests of Biopsy Samples

The biopsy samples of breast tissues are examined in the laboratory to determine whether cancer is present, its type, and other characteristics. Sometimes, these tests are not done until the entire tumor is removed, either by lumpectomy or mastectomy. The laboratory may also be able to perform tests that can help determine how quickly the cancer is likely to grow and, to some extent, what treatments are likely to be effective. This process can take several days and usually cannot be rushed. Your doctor should give you your results. You also can request a copy of your pathology report and ask to have it explained to you. See pages 78–83 for an example of a pathology report from a biopsy.

Pathology Second Opinions

Many people do not realize that they can get a second opinion on the pathology of their tissue. If you do wish to get a second opinion, talk with your doctor. You will need to request the slides from the pathologist who initially examined the sample. Many National Cancer Institute–designated facilities offer second opinion pathology services. Check with your insurance first to determine whether this service is covered. For more on second opinions, see page 109.

Cancer Type

The tissue is first looked at under a microscope to determine whether it is a carcinoma or some other type of cancer, such as a sarcoma. If there is enough tissue, the pathologist might be able to determine whether the cancer is invasive or in situ. The biopsy is also used to determine the cancer's type, such as invasive ductal carcinoma or invasive lobular carcinoma.

Tumor Grade

The pathologist also assigns a grade to the cancer, which is based on how closely the biopsy sample resembles normal breast tissue. The grade helps predict a woman's prognosis. In general, a lower-grade number indicates a slower-growing cancer that is less likely to spread, while a higher number indicates a faster-growing cancer that is more likely to spread. The tumor grade is one of the factors considered when determining the need for further treatment after surgery.

Histologic tumor grade (also called the Bloom-Richardson grade, Scarff-Bloom-Richardson grade, or Elston-Ellis grade) is based on the arrangement of the cells in relation to each other: whether they form tubules, how closely they resemble normal breast cells, and how many of the cancer cells are in the process of dividing (the mitotic count). This system of grading is used for invasive cancers, but it is not used for in situ cancers.

- **Grade 1** (well-differentiated) cancers have relatively normal-looking cells that do not appear to be growing rapidly and are arranged in small tubules. Grade 1 tumors are generally considered the least aggressive.
- **Grade 2** (moderately differentiated) cancers have cells that look more abnormal and are slightly faster growing.
- **Grade 3** (poorly differentiated) cancers lack normal features and tend to grow and spread most aggressively.

Ductal carcinoma in situ (DCIS) is sometimes given a nuclear grade, which refers to the size and shape of the nucleus in the tumor cells and the percentage of cells that are dividing. The presence or absence of dead or degenerating cancer cells, or necrosis, is also noted. When the cells die, they break down and can produce a whitish substance, called comedo necrosis. Necrosis can indicate a more aggressive cancer. Other factors important in determining the prognosis for DCIS include the surgical margin (how close the cancer is to the edge of the specimen) and the size (amount of breast tissue affected by DCIS). In situ cancers that are larger, have a high nuclear grade, areas of necrosis, or cancer at or near the edge of the sample are more likely to come back after treatment.

Hormone Receptors

Receptors are proteins on the outside surfaces of cells. Certain substances that circulate in the blood, such as hormones, attach to particular receptors. Normal breast cells and some breast cancer cells have receptors to which estrogen and progesterone attach. These two hormones often help breast cancer cells grow.

An important step in evaluating a breast cancer is to test a portion of the cancer removed during the biopsy or surgery to see whether it has estrogen or progesterone receptors. Cancer cells can contain neither, one, or both of these receptors. Breast cancers that contain either one of these receptors are called hormone receptor–positive, those with receptors for estrogen are referred to as ER–positive (or ER+) cancers, and those containing receptors for progesterone are called PR–positive (or PR+) cancers.

Cancers that are hormone receptor–positive tend to grow more slowly and are much more likely to respond to hormone therapy than cancers that lack these receptors.

All breast cancers should be tested for these hormone receptors at the time of breast biopsy or surgery. About two of three breast cancers contain at least one of these receptors. This percentage is higher in older women than in younger ones.

HER2/NEU

About one in five breast cancers has too much of a growth-promoting protein called HER2/neu (often just shortened to HER2). The *HER2/neu* gene instructs the cells to make this protein. Tumors with high levels of HER2/neu are referred to as HER2-positive.

Women with HER2-positive breast cancers have too many copies of the *HER2/neu* gene, resulting in greater than normal amounts of the HER2/neu protein. These cancers tend to grow and spread more aggressively than other breast cancers.

All invasive breast cancers are tested for HER2. The two main tests for HER2 are immunohistochemistry and fluorescence in situ hybridization.

Immunohistochemistry: In an immunohistochemistry (IHC) test, special antibodies that identify the HER2/neu protein are applied to the tissue sample, which causes cells to change color if many copies are present. This color change can be seen under a microscope. The test results are reported as 0, 1+, 2+, or 3+. If the results are 0 or 1+, the cancer is considered HER2-negative. People with HER2-negative tumors are not treated with drugs that target HER2. If the test comes back 3+, the cancer is HER2-positive. Patients with HER2-positive tumors may be treated with drugs such as trastuzumab, which target HER2. When the result is 2+, the HER2 status of the tumor is not clear.

What Is Triple-Negative Breast Cancer?

The term triple-negative breast cancer is used to describe breast cancers (usually invasive ductal carcinomas) whose cells lack receptors for estrogen or progesterone and are HER2-negative. Breast cancers with these characteristics are more common in younger women and in African American women. Triple-negative breast cancers tend to grow and spread more quickly than most other types of breast cancer. Because the tumor cells lack hormone receptors and are not HER2-positive, neither hormone-based therapy nor drugs that target HER2 are effective against these cancers. Chemotherapy can still be used to treat these cancers, and studies are ongoing to try to find the best drugs to fight triple-negative breast cancer.

This usually leads to testing the tumor with fluorescence in situ hybridization (described next).

Fluorescence in situ hybridization: The fluorescence in situ hybridization (FISH) test uses fluorescent pieces of DNA that specifically stick to copies of the *HER2/neu* gene in cells, which can then be counted under a special microscope. Many breast cancer specialists believe the FISH test is more accurate than the IHC test. However, it is also more expensive, and it takes longer to get the results. The IHC test is often used first.

A newer type of test, known as chromogenic in situ hybridization (CISH), works similarly to FISH, by using small DNA probes to count the number of *HER2/neu* genes in breast cancer cells. This test looks for color changes, not fluorescence, and it does not require a special microscope, which may make it less expensive. Right now, it is not used as much as IHC or FISH.

Tests of Ploidy and Cell Proliferation Rate

The ploidy of cancer cells refers to the amount of DNA they contain. If the cells contain a normal amount of DNA, they are said to be diploid. If the amount is abnormal, then the cells are described as aneuploid. Tests of ploidy can help determine prognosis, but they rarely change treatment and are considered optional. They are not usually recommended as part of a routine breast cancer workup.

The S-phase fraction (SPF) is the percentage of cells in a sample that are replicating (copying) their DNA. DNA replication means that the cell is getting ready to divide into two new cells. The rate of cancer cell division can also be estimated by a Ki-67 test. If the SPF or Ki-67 labeling index is high, it means that the cancer cells are dividing more rapidly, which indicates a more aggressive cancer.

Tests of Gene Patterns

Researchers have found that looking at the patterns of different genes at the same time (sometimes referred to as gene expression profiling) can help predict whether an early-stage breast cancer is likely to come back after initial treatment. Two such tests, which look at different sets of genes, are now available: the Oncotype DX and the MammaPrint.

Oncotype DX: The Oncotype DX test may be helpful when deciding whether treatment with chemotherapy after surgery (called adjuvant chemotherapy) might be useful in women with certain early-stage breast cancers that usually have a low chance of coming back (stage I or II estrogen receptor–positive breast cancers without lymph node involvement). It can also be helpful for patients whose cancer is more advanced.

The test looks at a set of twenty-one genes in cells from tumor samples to determine a "recurrence score," which is a number between zero and one hundred:

- Women with a recurrence score of seventeen or below have a low risk of recurrence (cancer coming back after treatment).
- Those with a score of eighteen to thirty are at intermediate risk.
- Women with a score of thirty-one or more are at high risk.

The test estimates risk, but it cannot tell for certain whether a woman's cancer will come back or whether she will benefit from chemotherapy. It provides one piece of information (out of many) that can help guide women and their doctors when deciding whether more treatment might be useful. Generally, a recurrence score of thirty-one or greater means that the cancer is more likely to come back after treatment and that the patient might benefit from such treatment as chemotherapy.

MammaPrint: The MammaPrint test can be used to help determine the likelihood that certain early-stage (stage I or II) breast cancers will recur in a distant part of the body after initial treatment. It can be used for either ER–negative or ER–positive tumors.

This test looks at the activity of seventy different genes to determine the risk of recurrence. The result can help doctors decide whether additional treatment might be needed.

Usefulness of these tests: Although some doctors are using these gene pattern tests (along with other information) to help make decisions about offering chemotherapy, others are waiting for more research to show that they are helpful. Large clinical trials of these tests are under way. In the meantime, women interested in gene pattern tests should discuss with their doctors whether the tests might be useful for them.

Other Tests After Cancer Has Been Diagnosed

If your biopsy results show that you have breast cancer, your doctor might order other tests to find out whether your cancer has spread and to help determine your best treatment options. The decision as to which tests are done will be based on the extent of the cancer and the results of your medical history and physical examination. Tests that might be done are listed on pages 53–56.

Chest X-ray

Before surgery, women with breast cancer often have a chest x-ray done to make sure that the breast cancer has not spread to the lungs.

Bone Scan

A bone scan can help show whether cancer has metastasized to the bones. Bone scans can be more useful than standard x-rays because they can show all of the bones at the same time.

For this test, a small amount of low-level radioactive material is injected into a vein. Over the course of a couple of hours, the substance settles in areas of bone change throughout the entire skeleton. You then lie on a table for about thirty minutes while a special camera detects the radioactivity and creates a picture of your skeleton.

Areas of bone change attract the radioactive material, appearing as "hot spots" on the skeleton. These areas can suggest the presence of metastatic cancer, but arthritis or other bone diseases can also cause the same pattern. To distinguish between these conditions, your medical team might use other imaging tests, such as simple x-rays, CT scans, or MRI scans, to get a better look at the areas that appear as hot spots, or they might take biopsy samples of the bone.

A bone scan is not needed for most cases of early-stage breast cancer, but it might be ordered if you have signs or symptoms of cancer metastasis to the bone, such as bone pain or changes on certain blood tests. This test is often ordered in patients with known metastases to check the bones for cancer spread. Other than the needle stick to inject the radioactive material, a bone scan is painless.

Computed Tomography

The computed tomography (CT) scan is an x-ray test that produces detailed cross-sectional images of your body. Instead of taking one picture, like a regular x-ray, a CT scanner takes many pictures as it rotates around you while you lie on a table. A computer then combines these pictures into images of slices of the part of your body being studied.

Before any pictures are taken, you might be asked to drink one to two pints of a liquid called oral contrast material. This helps outline the intestine so that healthy tissues are not mistaken for tumors. You might also receive an intravenous (IV) line through which a different kind of contrast is injected. The IV contrast helps better outline structures in your body. The injection might cause some flushing (a feeling of warmth, especially in the face). Some people are allergic to the IV contrast and get hives. Rarely, more serious reactions can occur, such as trouble breathing or low blood pressure. Medicine can be given to prevent and treat allergic reactions. Be sure to tell the doctor if you have ever had a reaction to any contrast material used for x-rays or if you are allergic to shellfish.

A CT scan takes longer than a regular x-ray. You need to lie still on a table while the scan is done. During the test, the table moves in and out of the scanner, a ring-shaped machine that completely surrounds the table. You might feel a bit confined during the scan.

In women with breast cancer, a CT scan is used most often to look at the organs of the chest and abdomen when there are indications the cancer may have spread to other organs. It is not needed in most cases of early-stage breast cancer.

CT–Guided Needle Biopsy

If an abnormality is seen on a CT scan but it is not clear whether it is cancer, the suspicious area may need to be biopsied. The biopsy can be done by using the CT scan to precisely guide the biopsy needle into the suspicious area. For this procedure, you remain on the CT scanning table while a radiologist advances a biopsy needle through the skin and toward the location of the mass. CT scans are repeated until the doctors are sure that the needle is within the mass. A fine needle biopsy sample (a tiny fragment of tissue) or a core needle biopsy sample (a thin cylinder of tissue about ½-inch long and less than ⅛-inch in diameter) is then removed and sent to be examined under a microscope. CT–guided needle biopsy is not used for biopsies of breast tumors, but it may be used to take a biopsy from a suspected area of cancer metastasis, such as the liver.

Magnetic Resonance Imaging

Magnetic resonance imaging (MRI) scans use radio waves and magnets to produce detailed images of internal organs without the need for x-rays. Breast MRI can be useful in some women who have cancer or are suspected to have cancer. Otherwise, MRI is most useful in looking at the brain and spinal cord in women with symptoms suggesting their cancer has spread. It is also helpful in looking at bones, because it can find things that might not be seen on regular x-rays. It might be used when a patient is having symptoms such as pain but regular x-rays are not showing abnormalities. MRI is not needed for most cases of early-stage breast cancer.

There are some differences between using MRI to look at the breast and using it to look at other areas of the body. First, when MRI is used to look at other areas of the body, you will lie face up in the machine. Second, the contrast material called gadolinium is not always needed to look at other areas of the body. You may have the option of having the scan in a less-confining machine, known as an "open" MRI machine. The images from an open machine are not always as good, though, so this may not be an option.

Positron Emission Tomography / Computed Tomography

A positron emission tomography/computed tomography scan combines a positron emission tomography (PET) scan with a computed tomography (CT) scan. In a PET scan, radioactive glucose (sugar) is injected into the patient's vein to look for cancer cells. Because cancers use glucose at a higher rate than normal tissues, the radioactivity will tend to concentrate in the cancer. A scanner can spot the radioactive deposits. PET scans can be helpful for spotting small collections of cancer cells, and they can find areas where the cancer has spread in the body. The picture from a PET scan is not as finely detailed as images from CT or MRI scans. Some machines combine the PET scan with a CT scan, allowing correlation of any abnormal areas seen on PET with the CT images. PET or PET/CT is not needed for early-stage breast cancer, but PET/CT scans can be very helpful when cancer in the breast has grown into the skin or nearby structures (called locally advanced disease), especially with inflammatory breast cancer.

Blood Tests

Some blood tests are needed to prepare for surgery, to screen for evidence of cancer metastasis, and to plan treatment after surgery.

Complete Blood Count

A complete blood count (CBC) determines whether the blood has the correct types and numbers of blood cells. Abnormal test results can reveal other health problems (such as anemia) and can indicate that the cancer has spread to the bone marrow. If you receive chemotherapy, doctors will repeat this test before each cycle, because chemotherapy affects the blood-forming cells of the bone marrow.

Blood Chemical and Enzyme Tests

Blood chemical and enzyme tests are done in women with invasive breast cancer and are not needed for in situ cancer. Abnormal results on these tests might mean that the cancer has spread to the bones or liver. If these test results are abnormal, your doctor might order other tests, such as bone scans or CT scans, to look for cancer metastasis.

Tumor Marker Testing

If your doctor suspects that your cancer is advanced, he or she might test your blood for certain chemicals, called tumor markers, that are released from cancer cells. Some tumor markers that are used include CA-15-3, CA 27-29, and CEA. In some women, the blood levels of these substances go up when the cancer has spread to bones or other organs, such as the liver. These levels are not elevated in all women with breast cancer, so testing them is not always helpful. If a tumor marker is elevated before treatment, it is often checked again after treatment. This level should go down as the amount of cancer in the body decreases. These tests can allow your doctor to monitor the progress of your treatment without having to do imaging tests, such as CT scans. Tumor marker testing is not needed for women with early-stage breast cancer.

PART TWO

Preparing for Treatment

The last section explained the basics of breast cancer, breast cancer risk, and some of the tests and procedures you may experience during your journey with this disease. In this section, we take a step forward into what happens next, after diagnosis.

A diagnosis of breast cancer raises many feelings and concerns. It affects people in different ways—physically, mentally, emotionally, and spiritually. And it affects not only the woman herself but also those close to her—her family and friends. For parents of young children, a breast cancer diagnosis can be particularly frightening. In addition to coping with this change yourself, you will want to help your children cope, too.

You might feel pressured to make a decision about treatment right away. If you feel rushed, keep in mind that your cancer took time to reach the stage it's in now. In most cases, it is wise to spend some time collecting information, assembling and talking with your medical team, and researching your choices. Ask your team how much time you can reasonably take to explore your treatment options.

In the following chapters, we will help you understand what your diagnosis means, how you can begin to cope, and how to navigate the medical system.

CHAPTER 4

Understanding Your Diagnosis

Before you can move forward in your cancer treatment, you will need to understand what your breast cancer diagnosis means. What kind of breast cancer do you have? What is your prognosis? What meaning does all this have for you?

This chapter is meant to help you understand the results of your diagnostic tests and pathology report. This understanding can help you put your prognosis in perspective and look toward what your future may hold.

The Biopsy Pathology Report

Any time a procedure is done to remove tissue from your body—such as a biopsy or surgery—that tissue is examined and a pathology report is created. The pathology report contains the diagnosis and other information that will help determine treatment options. It is created by a pathologist, a doctor who diagnoses and classifies your cancer by using laboratory tests, such as examination of tissue, fluid, and cells under a microscope. The pathologist helps determine the exact cell type and extent of your cancer.

All women who receive a cancer diagnosis will have had a biopsy, and your doctor will use the pathology report from that procedure to determine the next steps in your treatment. If your breast cancer is treated with surgery, you will also have a pathology report from that operation. The pathology report from surgery will be more detailed and will include more information. See chapter 8 for more information about the surgery pathology report.

The pathology report is often quite long and complex and is typically divided into numerous subheadings. The doctor will review the results with you and can give you a copy of the report if you ask. A sample biopsy pathology report is included at the end of this chapter, and a sample surgical pathology report is included at the end of chapter 8.

Patient, Doctor, and Specimen Identification

This section includes your name, medical record number issued by the hospital, the date of the biopsy or surgery, and the unique number of the specimen assigned by the laboratory.

Diagnosis

The most important part of the pathology report is the final diagnosis. In essence, it is the "bottom line" of the testing process. A doctor relies upon this final diagnosis in recommending an appropriate treatment plan. If the diagnosis is cancer, this section will indicate the exact type of cancer and may include the cancer's grade (explained on pages 48–49).

Clinical Information

The next portion of the report often contains information about you provided by the doctor who removed the tissue sample. This information might include pertinent medical history and special requests for the pathologist. For example, if a lymph node sample is taken from a patient who already has cancer in another organ, the doctor will indicate the type of the original cancer. This information can guide the pathologist's selection of tests to determine whether any cancer in that lymph node metastasized from the prior cancer or is a new cancer that developed in the lymph node.

Gross Description

The next part of the report is called the gross description. The medical meaning of gross refers to features that can be identified without a microscope simply by measuring, looking at, or feeling the tissue. For a small biopsy sample, this description would be a few sentences describing its size, color, and consistency. This section also records the number of tissue-containing samples submitted for processing.

Larger biopsy or tissue specimens—for example, from a mastectomy for breast cancer—will have much longer descriptions, including the sizes of the breast and the cancer, how close the cancer is to the nearest surgical margin (edge of the tissue specimen), how many lymph nodes were removed, and the appearance of the noncancerous breast tissue. The report includes a description of the exact location where tissue was removed.

For cell samples (called cytologic specimens), the gross description is very short and usually indicates the number of slides or smears made by the doctor.

Microscopic Description

This description records what the pathologist saw under the microscope. It typically includes the appearance of the cancer cells, how they are arranged together, and how much the cancer penetrates nearby tissues in the specimen. For typical cases of common cancers, or for benign tissues, the report might not include a microscopic description. Results of any additional studies are included in the microscopic description or in a separate section.

Special Tests or Markers

The pathologist may have done tests to look for special proteins, genes, or to determine how fast the cells are growing. For breast cancer, this often includes tests to see whether the tumor is hormone receptor–positive or hormone receptor–negative and an immunohistochemistry test to see whether the cancer is HER2-positive. The Ki-67 and S-phase fraction tests show how fast the cancer is growing. The results of such tests are reported in this section.

Comment

After the final diagnosis is made, the pathologist might list additional information for the medical team taking care of the patient. The comment section is often used to clarify a concern or make recommendations for further testing.

Summary

Some pathology reports for cancer contain a summary of findings most relevant to making treatment decisions.

Understanding Your Pathology Report

The pathologist will look at the tissue removed during your biopsy or surgery to determine whether cancer is present. The pathology report will state whether the cancer is invasive (infiltrating)—that is, if it has grown outside the area where it started and into surrounding tissue. Remember, noninvasive (in situ) cancers stay inside the milk ducts or lobules of the breast, whereas invasive cancers break through into other parts of the breast and may eventually spread to other parts of the body through the bloodstream or lymphatic system.

Your pathology report will also include information about whether your cancer is likely to be aggressive. This assessment is based on what usually happens with cells that look like the ones taken from the biopsy sample. Cancer cells that look most like normal cells are called well-differentiated, grade 1, or low-grade and tend to be less aggressive. Cells that look a little more abnormal are called moderately differentiated, grade 2, or intermediate-grade. The most abnormal cells are called poorly differentiated, grade 3, or high-grade, and they are considered the most aggressive.

When cancer is removed from the breast, the surgeon tries to remove the entire tumor with an extra margin of normal tissue to be sure that all of the cancerous tissue has been removed. If the margins are clear of cancer, the report might read, "the margins are uninvolved by the tumor" or "the margins are negative." The report may include the distance from the tumor to the margin, which is helpful in deciding whether additional surgery is necessary. Even if the margins are clear, it is best to have them also be a certain width to minimize the chance that cancer has been left behind (and could later grow back). If margins are not clean, the report might say, "the margins are involved by the tumor" or "the margins are positive for tumor." Positive margins might mean that some cancer has been left behind and that more surgery is needed. If a margin is positive, the report will state which margin contains cancer, to help guide the surgeon if more surgery is needed.

Breast Cancer Staging

Staging is the process of gathering information from certain examinations and diagnostic tests to determine how widespread the cancer is. The stage is based on whether the cancer is invasive or noninvasive, the size of the tumor, how many lymph nodes are involved, and whether it has spread to other parts of the body. The stage of a cancer is one of the most important factors in selecting treatment options and determining prognosis.

Tests done for staging depend on your medical history and results of the physical examination and biopsy, and may include such imaging tests as chest x-ray, mammograms of both breasts, bone scans, computed tomography (CT) scans, magnetic resonance imaging (MRI) scans, and positron emission tomography (PET) scans. Blood tests may also be performed to evaluate your overall health and help detect whether the cancer has spread to certain organs, but these tests do not directly affect staging.

The American Joint Committee on Cancer (AJCC) TNM System

A staging system is a standardized way in which the cancer care team describes how far the cancer has spread. The system most often used to describe the growth and spread of breast cancer is the TNM staging system, also known as the American Joint Committee on Cancer (AJCC) system.

The stage of a breast cancer can be based either on the results of physical examination, biopsy, and imaging tests (called the clinical stage) or on the results of these tests plus the results of surgery (called the pathologic stage). The staging described here is the pathologic stage, which includes the findings after surgery, when the pathologist has looked at the breast mass and nearby lymph nodes. Pathologic staging is likely to be more accurate than clinical staging, as it allows the doctor to get a firsthand impression of the extent of the cancer. Clinical staging is used most often to decide on initial treatment, that is, to determine whether surgery should be used as the first treatment or whether chemotherapy or hormone therapy should be given first.

In TNM staging, information about the tumor (T), nearby lymph nodes (N), and distant organ metastases (M) is combined, and a stage is assigned to specific TNM groupings. T stands for the size of the cancer, N stands for spread to nearby lymph nodes, and M stands for metastasis (spread to distant places in the body). If the T and N categories are based on clinical staging, the letter "c" is placed in front. If they are based on pathologic staging, a letter "p" may be used. The T, N, and M groupings are described using numbers from 0 to 4, and the stage of the cancer is described by using the number 0 or the Roman numerals I through IV.

Primary Tumor (T) Categories

The letter T followed by a number from 0 to 4 describes the tumor's size and spread to the skin or chest wall under the breast. Higher T numbers indicate a larger tumor and/or more extensive spread to tissues near the breast.

TX: Primary tumor cannot be assessed (this is only used if breast cancer spread is found in someone whose breasts were already removed).

T0: No evidence of primary tumor.

Tis: Carcinoma in situ (noninvasive breast cancer). This includes DCIS, LCIS, and Paget disease of the nipple with no associated tumor mass.

T1 (includes T1a, T1b, and T1c): The cancer is 2 cm across (about ⅘ of an inch) or smaller.

T2: The cancer is more than 2 cm but not more than 5 cm (two inches) across.

T3: The cancer is more than 5 cm across.

T4: The cancer is any size and has spread to the chest wall or the skin. This includes inflammatory breast cancer.

Tumor sizes

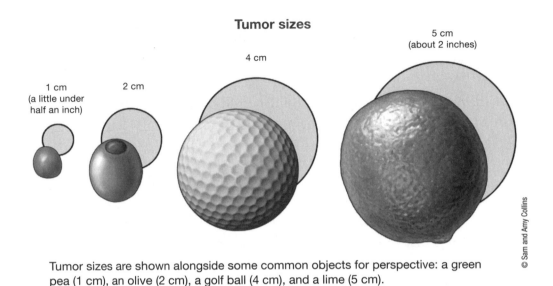

5 cm
(about 2 inches)

4 cm

1 cm
(a little under
half an inch)

2 cm

© Sam and Amy Collins

Tumor sizes are shown alongside some common objects for perspective: a green pea (1 cm), an olive (2 cm), a golf ball (4 cm), and a lime (5 cm).

N Categories

The letter N followed by a number from 0 to 3 indicates whether the cancer has spread to lymph nodes near the breast and, if so, how much. Lymph node staging for breast cancer has changed over time as technology has evolved. Earlier methods were useful in finding large deposits of cancer cells in the lymph nodes but could miss microscopic areas of cancer spread. Over time, newer methods have made it possible to find smaller and smaller deposits of cancer cells. Experts have not been sure what to do with the new information. Do tiny deposits of cancer cells affect outlook the same way that larger deposits do? How much cancer in the lymph node is needed to see a change in prognosis or treatment?

These questions are still being studied, but for now, a deposit of cancer cells must contain at least two hundred cells or be at least 0.2 mm across (less than 1/100 of an inch) for it to change the N stage. An area of cancer metastasis in a lymph node that is smaller than 0.2 mm (or less than two hundred cells) does not change the stage, but it is recorded with abbreviations that reflect the way the area of metastasis was detected. For example, the abbreviation "i+" means that cancer cells were seen only when a special stain, called immunohistochemistry, was used. The abbreviation "mol+" is used when cancer is found through a technique called PCR. (PCR and immunohistochemistry are not routinely used to look at lymph nodes in breast cancer.) These very tiny areas are sometimes called isolated tumor cells. If the area of cancer metastasis in the lymph node is at least 0.2 mm across (or two hundred cells), but still not larger than 2 mm, it is called a

Breast Cancer Staging Groups			
Stage	**T**	**N**	**M**
Stage 0	Tis	N0	M0
Stage IA	T1	N0	M0
Stage IB	T0	N1mi	M0
	T1	N1mi	M0
Stage IIA	T0	N1	M0
	T1	N1	M0
	T2	N0	M0
Stage IIB	T2	N1	M0
	T3	N0	M0
Stage IIIA	T0	N2	M0
	T1	N2	M0
	T2	N2	M0
	T3	N1	M0
	T3	N2	M0
Stage IIIB	T4	N0	M0
	T4	N1	M0
	T4	N2	M0
Stage IIIC	Any T	N3	M0
Stage IV	Any T	Any N	M1

Used with the permission of the American Joint Committee on Cancer (AJCC), Chicago, Illinois. The original source for this material is the *AJCC Cancer Staging Manual*, Seventh Edition (2010) published by Springer Science and Business Media LLC, www.springer.com, pg. 349.

micrometastasis. Micrometastases may affect outcome and are counted only if no larger areas of cancer spread are present. Areas of cancer spread larger than 2 mm are known to affect outcome and do change overall stage. These larger areas are sometimes called macrometastases, but they may just be called metastases.

NX: Nearby lymph nodes cannot be assessed (for example, if they have been removed previously).

N0: Cancer has not spread to nearby lymph nodes.

N0(i+): Tiny amounts of cancer are found in the axillary lymph nodes by using special stains. The area of cancer spread contains less than two hundred cells and is smaller than 0.2 mm.

N0(mol+): Cancer cells cannot be seen in the axillary lymph nodes (even using special stains), but traces of cancer cells are detected using a test called PCR.

N1: Cancer has spread to one to three axillary lymph node(s), and/or tiny amounts of cancer are found in the internal mammary lymph nodes on sentinel lymph node biopsy.

> **N1mi:** Micrometastases (tiny areas of cancer spread) are found in lymph nodes under the arm. The areas of cancer metastasis in the lymph nodes are 2 mm or less across (but at least 200 cancer cells or 0.2 mm across).

> **N1a:** Cancer has spread to one to three lymph nodes under the arm with at least one area of metastasis larger than 2 mm.

> **N1b:** Cancer has spread to internal mammary lymph nodes, but this metastasis was found only on sentinel lymph node biopsy (it did not cause the lymph nodes to become enlarged).

> **N1c:** Both N1a and N1b apply.

N2: Cancer has spread to four to nine lymph nodes under the arm, or cancer has enlarged the internal mammary lymph nodes (either N2a or N2b, but not both).

> **N2a:** Cancer has spread to four to nine lymph nodes under the arm, with at least one area of metastasis larger than 2 mm.

> **N2b:** Cancer has spread to one or more internal mammary lymph nodes, causing them to become enlarged.

N3: Any of the following:

> **N3a:**
> - Cancer has spread to ten or more underarm lymph nodes, with at least one area of metastasis greater than 2 mm, OR
> - Cancer has spread to the lymph nodes under the clavicle, with at least one area of metastasis greater than 2 mm.

> **N3b:**
> - Cancer is found in at least one axillary lymph node (with at least one area of metastasis greater than 2 mm) and has enlarged the internal mammary lymph nodes, OR
> - Cancer involves four or more axillary lymph nodes (with at least one area of metastasis greater than 2 mm), and tiny amounts of cancer are found in internal mammary lymph nodes on sentinel lymph node biopsy.

N3c: Cancer has spread to the lymph nodes above the clavicle with at least one area of metastasis larger than 2 mm.

M Categories

The letter M followed by a 0 or 1 indicates whether the cancer has spread to distant organs (for example, the lungs or bones).

M0: No distant spread of cancer is found on x-rays (or other imaging tests) or by physical examination.

cM0(i +): Small numbers of cancer cells are found in blood or bone marrow (found only by special tests), or tiny areas of metastasis (no larger than 0.2 mm) are found in lymph nodes away from the breast.

M1: Cancer spread to distant organs is present. The most common sites are the bones, lung, brain, and liver.

Summary of Breast Cancer Stages

Once your T, N, and M categories have been determined, this information is combined in a process called stage grouping to determine the disease stage. The stage of invasive cancer is expressed in Roman numerals from stage I (the least advanced stage) to stage IV (the most advanced stage). Noninvasive cancer is listed as stage 0.

STAGE 0: Tis, N0, M0

Ductal carcinoma in situ (DCIS) is the earliest form of breast cancer. In DCIS, cancer cells are still within a duct and have not invaded the surrounding fatty breast tissue. Lobular carcinoma in situ (LCIS), also called lobular neoplasia, is sometimes classified as stage 0 breast cancer, but most oncologists believe it is not a true breast cancer. In LCIS, abnormal cells grow within the lobules but do not grow through the lobule walls. Most breast cancer specialists think that LCIS itself does not usually become invasive cancer, but that women with LCIS are at increased risk for invasive breast cancer later. This later cancer may be either invasive ductal or invasive lobular. Paget disease of the nipple (without an underlying tumor mass) is most commonly also stage 0. In all of these cases, the cancer has not spread to lymph nodes or distant sites.

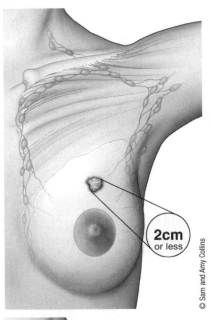

STAGE IA

The tumor is 2 cm (about ⅘ of an inch) across or less (T1) and has not spread to lymph nodes (N0) or distant sites (M0).

© Sam and Amy Collins

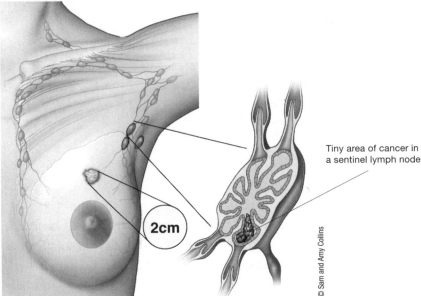

Tiny area of cancer in a sentinel lymph node

© Sam and Amy Collins

STAGE IB

The tumor is 2 cm across or smaller (T1) or is not found (T0). Micrometastases are found in one to three axillary lymph nodes (the cancer in the lymph nodes is greater than 0.2 mm across and/or more than 200 cells, but is not larger than 2 mm)(N1mi). The cancer has not spread to distant sites (M0).

STAGE IIA

One of the following applies:

1. T0 or T1, N1 (but not N1mi), M0: The tumor is 2 cm across or smaller or is not found (T1 or T0) and either:
    - it has spread to one to three axillary lymph nodes, with the cancer in the lymph nodes larger than 2 mm (N1a), OR
    - tiny amounts of cancer are found in the internal mammary lymph nodes on sentinel lymph node biopsy (N1b), OR
    - it has spread to one to three lymph nodes under the arm and to the internal mammary lymph nodes (found on sentinel lymph node biopsy) (N1c).

    The cancer has not spread to distant sites (M0).

OR

2. T2, N0, M0: The tumor is more than 2 cm across but less than 5 cm across (T2) and has not spread to the lymph nodes (N0). The cancer has not spread to distant sites (M0).

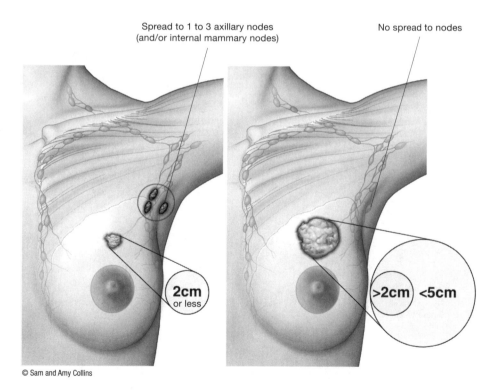

© Sam and Amy Collins

STAGE IIB

One of the following applies:

1. T2, N1, M0: The tumor is more than 2 cm but less than 5 cm across (T2). It has spread to one to three axillary lymph nodes and/or tiny amounts of cancer are found in the internal mammary lymph nodes on sentinel lymph node biopsy (N1). The cancer has not spread to distant sites (M0).

OR

2. T3, N0, M0: The tumor is more than 5 cm across but does not grow into the chest wall or skin and has not spread to the lymph nodes (T3, N0). The cancer has not spread to distant sites (M0).

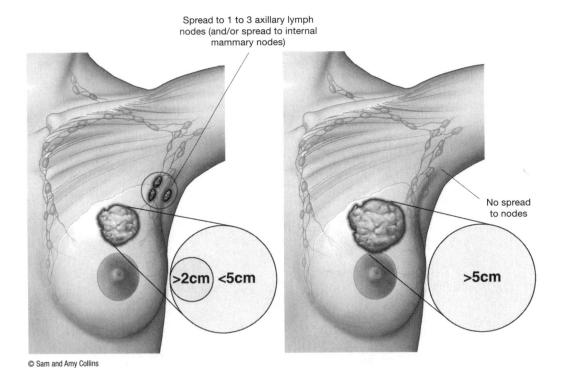

Spread to 1 to 3 axillary lymph nodes (and/or spread to internal mammary nodes)

No spread to nodes

>2cm <5cm

>5cm

© Sam and Amy Collins

STAGE IIIA

One of the following applies:

1. T0 to T2, N2, M0: The tumor is not more than 5 cm across (or cannot be found) (T0 to T2). It has spread to four to nine axillary lymph nodes (N1), or it has enlarged the internal mammary lymph nodes (N2). The cancer has not spread to distant sites (M0).

OR

2. T3, N1 or N2, M0: The tumor is larger than 5 cm across but does not grow into the chest wall or skin (T3). It has spread to one to nine axillary nodes, or to the internal mammary nodes (N1 or N2). The cancer has not spread to distant sites (M0).

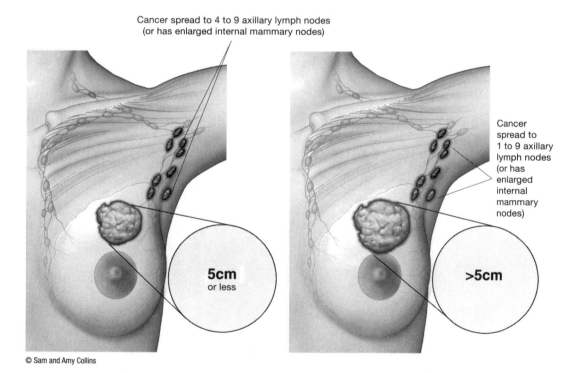

Cancer spread to 4 to 9 axillary lymph nodes (or has enlarged internal mammary nodes)

5cm or less

Cancer spread to 1 to 9 axillary lymph nodes (or has enlarged internal mammary nodes)

>5cm

© Sam and Amy Collins

STAGE IIIB: T4, N0 to N2, M0

The tumor has grown into the chest wall or skin (T4), and one of the following applies:

- It has not spread to the lymph nodes (N0).
- It has spread to one to three axillary lymph nodes and/or tiny amounts of cancer are found in internal mammary lymph nodes on sentinel lymph node biopsy (N1).
- It has spread to four to nine axillary lymph nodes, or it has enlarged the internal mammary lymph nodes (N2).

The cancer has not spread to distant sites (M0).

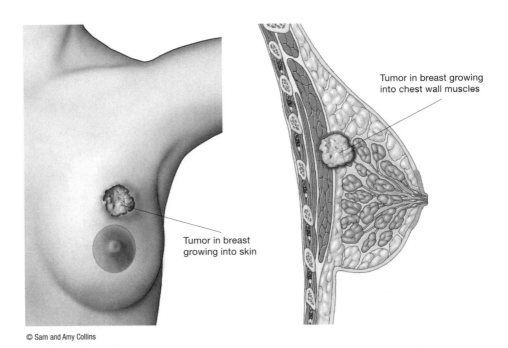

Tumor in breast growing into chest wall muscles

Tumor in breast growing into skin

© Sam and Amy Collins

Inflammatory breast cancer is classified as T4 and is at least stage IIIB when it is diagnosed. If it has spread to many nearby lymph nodes (N3), it may be stage IIIC. If it has spread to distant lymph nodes or organs (M1), it is stage IV. (See page 13 for an illustration of inflammatory breast cancer.)

Stage IIIC: Any T, N3, M0

The tumor is any size (or cannot be found), and one of the following applies:
- Cancer has spread to ten or more axillary lymph nodes (N3).
- Cancer has spread to the lymph nodes under the clavicle (collarbone) (N3).
- Cancer has spread to the lymph nodes above the clavicle (N3).
- Cancer involves axillary lymph nodes and has enlarged the internal mammary lymph nodes (N3).
- Cancer has spread to four or more axillary lymph nodes, and tiny amounts of cancer are found in the internal mammary lymph nodes on sentinel lymph node biopsy (N3).

The cancer has not spread to distant sites (M0).

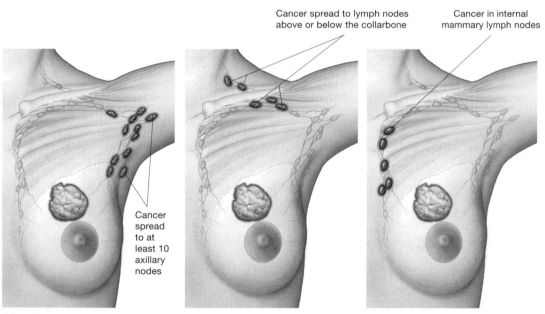

Cancer spread to lymph nodes above or below the collarbone

Cancer in internal mammary lymph nodes

Cancer spread to at least 10 axillary nodes

© Sam and Amy Collins

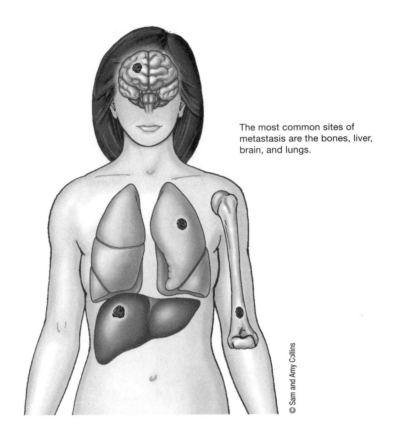

The most common sites of metastasis are the bones, liver, brain, and lungs.

© Sam and Amy Collins

STAGE IV: any T, any N, M1:

The cancer can be any size (any T) and may or may not have spread to nearby lymph nodes (any N). It has spread to distant organs or to lymph nodes far from the breast (M1). The most common sites of metastasis are the bones, liver, brain, and lungs.

Understanding Your Prognosis

One of the first things women worry about after receiving a cancer diagnosis is whether they will get better. It is natural to be concerned about your future.

You and your medical team are armed with more medical advancements and knowledge than ever before to help you overcome breast cancer, and your chances of surviving breast cancer are better than they have ever been. Researchers are finding better ways to detect and treat cancer, and the chance of recovery continues to improve. The earlier a cancer is found and treatment is begun, the better the chance of a cure.

Questions to Ask Your Medical Team About Your Diagnosis

- **What is the exact type** of my breast cancer? How common is that type of breast cancer?
- **Has the cancer spread** beyond where it started?
- **How much experience do you have** treating this type of cancer?
- **Would you explain** my pathology report?
- **What is the stage of** my cancer? What does that mean in my case?
- **How does the stage of my cancer** affect my treatment options?
- **Should I get** a second opinion? How do I do that?
- **What is your opinion** of my prognosis? What are my chances of survival, based on my cancer as you see it?
- **Did a pathologist** experienced in diagnosing breast cancer review my slides?
- **Should someone else**—a second pathologist, for example—look at my slides?
- **Were estrogen and progesterone** receptor tests performed on my tumor?
- **Was HER2/neu testing** performed on my tumor?
- **Were any other tests done** on my biopsy sample?
- **What other tests** will I need to undergo?

A prognosis is a prediction of the probable course and outcome of a disease and an indication of the likelihood of recovery from that disease. When doctors discuss a person's prognosis, they are projecting what is likely to occur for that individual. If a cancer is likely to respond well to treatment, the doctor may say that the person has a good or favorable prognosis. If a doctor expects that a cancer may be difficult to control, the person with cancer may be said to have a poor or unfavorable prognosis.

A particular prognosis does not necessarily indicate what is going to happen in your case. A person's cancer prognosis is determined by many factors, including the type of cancer, its stage, and its grade. Other factors that also can affect a prognosis include a person's age, general health, and the effectiveness of treatment. And ongoing cancer research continues to yield new developments in cancer treatment that can improve prognosis.

Doctors use statistics to help estimate prognosis. It can be upsetting to see your prognosis reflected by a number or percentage. But just because the statistics don't look promising does not mean that those odds will apply to you. Statistics are averages based on large numbers of people. They include those who did not receive the best care, those who had other medical problems, those who did not take care of themselves, and those who refused treatment altogether. The numbers cannot be used to predict what will happen to a particular person, because no two individuals are alike. Your body is as unique as your personality and your fingerprints. No one can say precisely how you will respond to cancer or treatment, and even your doctor may not know exactly what will happen. You may have special strengths, such as a history of excellent nutrition and physical activity, a strong family support system, or a deep faith, which could make a difference in how you respond to cancer treatment.

Survival Statistics

Survival statistics indicate how many people with a certain type and stage of cancer survive for a certain amount of time after diagnosis. The most common measure used is the five-year survival rate. The five-year survival rate refers to the percentage of people with cancer who live at least five years after their cancer is diagnosed. Many people live much longer than five years after diagnosis, but five-year rates are used as a standard. It is also important to keep in mind that people with cancer can die of other things, and these five-year survival rates count deaths from all causes (not just cancer).

In order to get five-year survival rates, doctors have to look at people who were treated at least five years ago. Improvements in treatment since then may result in a more favorable outlook for people now being diagnosed with breast cancer.

Survival rates are often based on previous outcomes of large numbers of people who had the disease, but they cannot predict what will happen in any particular person's case. Many other factors may affect a person's outlook, such as her age and general health, whether the tumor is hormone receptor–positive or –negative, and how well the cancer responds to treatment. Your doctor can tell you how the numbers below may apply to you, as he or she is familiar with the aspects of your particular situation.

Some people cope better when they know the survival rates for their cancer type and stage; for others, the statistics for their cancer can cause fear or confusion. You should decide for yourself whether you wish to read further and see the survival statistics for breast cancer. Keep in mind that a prognosis can change over time if the cancer progresses or treatment is effective. Requesting prognostic information is a personal decision. It is up to you to decide how much information you want, how to cope with it, and what decisions you make next.

The numbers below come from the National Cancer Data Base and are based on people whose breast cancer was diagnosed in 2001 and 2002.

Survival at Five Years According to Stage of Breast Cancer

Stage	Survival Rate
0	93%
I	88%
IIA	81%
IIB	74%
IIIA	67%
IIIB	41%*
IIIC	49%*
IV	15%

*These numbers are correct as written (stage IIIB shows worse survival than stage IIIC).
Used with the permission of the American Joint Committee on Cancer (AJCC), Chicago, Illinois. The original source for this material is the *AJCC Cancer Staging Manual*, Seventh Edition (2010) published by Springer Science and Business Media LLC, www.springer.com, pg. 358.

Sample Biopsy Report (with Explanatory Comments)

SURGICAL PATHOLOGY REPORT

Patient: Margaret Wilson
Hospital #YYYYYY
Birth date: NN/NN/NNNN (Age: #)
Sex: F
Submitted by: Charlotte Hill, MD

Specimen # XXXXXX
Obtained on: (date)
Received on: (date)
Reported on: (date)
Department: Surgery

DIAGNOSIS:
BREAST, RIGHT, CORE BIOPSIES:
• INFILTRATING DUCTAL CARCINOMA, GRADE III.
• DUCTAL CARCINOMA IN SITU, INTERMEDIATE GRADE.
• ANGIOLYMPHATIC INVASION AND PERINEURAL INVASION ARE IDENTIFIED
• MICROCALCIFICATIONS ASSOCIATED WITH INFILTRATING CARCINOMA.

SPECIMEN:
Right breast, three 14-gauge cores.

CLINICAL HISTORY/OPERATIVE FINDINGS:
Ultrasound-guided core biopsy. IDC.

GROSS DESCRIPTION:
The specimen is received in formalin and is labeled with the patient's name and medical record number designated "right." It consists of three cylindrical core needle biopsy samples ranging in length from 1.0 to 1.5 cm. The specimen is submitted entirely and wrapped in lens paper in cassette "1A." Cassette in formalin at 2:45 p.m.

This information is essential in assuring that your report doesn't get confused with that of another patient with a similar or identical name and that it gets delivered to your doctor. Every specimen is given a pathology number, which is often based on the year and the number of the specimen in that year.

This is the most important section of the report—its "bottom line."
This indicates the type of cancer (infiltrating ductal) and its grade (grade III). Angiolymphatic invasion means that the cancer is growing into blood or lymph vessels. Perineural invasion means that the cancer is growing along nerves. Microcalcifications were found in the area of invasive cancer. If this biopsy was done because of calcifications on a mammogram, finding the calcification in the biopsy samples helps the doctor know that the correct areas were biopsied. Ductal carcinoma in situ was also found.

This information identifies how many biopsy samples were obtained and from where they were taken. This is especially important for patients who have samples taken from more than one area during the same operation.

This information helps the pathologist and surgeon to consider the microscopic findings in the context of your medical situation.

This section describes the number of specimens received and their approximate size. Doctors use the metric system in describing the size of samples—1 cm is a little less than half an inch. This section also describes the basic processing of the tissue and which parts were placed in small containers (called cassettes) during processing.

Sample Biopsy Report (with Explanatory Comments) (continued)

MICROSCOPIC DESCRIPTION:
Microscopic examination performed.

SPECIAL STAINS:

ERQ (88360)	DONE
PRQ (88360)	DONE
HERCEPQ (88360)	DONE
MIB1Q (88360)	DONE
FISH	DONE
FISH	DONE

SPECIAL PROCEDURES

BLOCK:
1A
SPECIMEN TYPE:
Fixed Paraffin Sections

ESTROGEN RECEPTOR / PROGESTERONE RECEPTOR
Cancer Prognostic Panel
Immunohistochemistry with ChromaVision ACIS
Quantitation Image Analysis

Test Name Assay Type	Staining Intensity Average	Percent Positive (%)	Result
Estrogen Receptor	2+	17	Positive
Progesterone Receptor	3+	89	Positive
HER2	2.0		Equivocal/2+ (FISH ordered)
Ki-67 (MIB-1)	3+	17	Intermediate

REFERENCE RANGES

Test Name	NEGATIVE/ LOW	EQUIVOCAL/ INTERMEDIATE	POSITIVE/HIGH
Estrogen Receptor	< 1%		=/> 1%
Progesterone Receptor	< 1%		=/> 1%
HER2	< 1.8 (1+)	=/> 1.8 - < 2.2 (2+)	>/= 2.2 (3+)
Ki-67	< 10%	=/>10% to </= 20%	> 20%
p53	< 10%		=/> 10%

If the appearance of this cancer under the microscope was in any way unusual, the pathologist would have added its description here. Some pathologists briefly describe all cancers. Others describe only the unusual ones. If no description is added by the pathologist, the laboratory's computer system automatically adds, "Microscopic examination performed" to confirm that the pathologist really checked the sample under the microscope.

This lists the special stains used to examine the tissue. The results are listed separately in the next section.

This section lists the results of the special stains. The tumor is positive for estrogen and progesterone receptors. The immunohistochemistry (IHC) test for HER2 showed 2+, which is "equivocal" (not definite either way). As a result, a FISH test for HER2 will be done. A Ki-67 test also was done, which estimates how fast the cancer cells are dividing. If it is high (> 20 percent), it means that the cancer cells are dividing more rapidly, a sign of a more aggressive cancer.

A list of reference ranges for the special stains is given below the results. This lets you see the criteria for what is considered "positive" or high for each test.

Sample Biopsy Report (with Explanatory Comments) (continued)

ER: DAKO ID5, ENVISION +, ANTIGEN RETRIEVAL
PR: DAKO PgR 636, ENVISION +, ANTIGEN RETRIEVAL
HER2: HERCEPTEST, DAKO CYTOMATION, FDA APPROVED
Ki-67: DAKO, MIB-1, ENVISION +, ANTIGEN RETRIEVAL
P53: DAKO, DO-7, ENVISION +, ANTIGEN RETRIEVAL

COMMENT:

Formalin-fixed, deparaffinized sections were incubated with the above panel of monoclonal and/or polyclonal antibodies. Localization is via an avidin biotin, streptavidin biotin, or peroxidase-labeled polymer immunoperoxidase method with or without the use of heat-induced epitope-retrieval techniques. Positive and negative control slides were reviewed and showed appropriate results.

The results of these tests should not be used as the sole basis for diagnosis and/or treatment. The results may prove useful when used in conjunction with other diagnostic procedures and clinical evaluations. Use of these results, in this manner, can be considered to fall within the scope of the practice of medicine.

FLUORESCENCE IN SITU HYBRIDIZATION

SPECIMEN:

Right breast, core biopsies.

CLINICAL HISTORY/REFERRING DIAGNOSIS:

Infiltrating ductal carcinoma.

GROSS DESCRIPTION:

Paraffin block, labeled 1A.
TEST PERFORMED/PROBES USED:
HER2/neu gene locus-specific probe (17q11.2-q12)
Chromosome 17 alpha satellite DNA-specific probe (17p11.1- q11.1)

RESULTS:

POSITIVE for HER2/neu gene amplification
nuc ish 17p11.1-q11.1(D17Z1 x 1.7),17q11.2-q12(HER2 x 4.8)[30]

INTERPRETATION:

Fluorescence in situ hybridization was performed using the above listed DNA probes (PathVysion, Abbott Molecular, Inc.). The probes were simultaneously hybridized to a section of the formalin-fixed, paraffin-embedded tissue submitted for evaluation.

Of 30 interphase nuclei analyzed, the ratio of HER2 fluorescent signals to chromosome 17 centromere signals was 3.8, which indicates amplification of HER-2/neu gene (values > 2.2 are considered positive for amplification). Positive and negative controls were appropriate. Correlation with clinical and other laboratory parameters is suggested.

COMMENT:

The results of this test should not be used alone as the sole basis for diagnosis and/or treatment. These results may, however, prove useful when used in conjunction with other diagnostic procedures and clinical evaluations. Use of these results, in this manner, can be considered to fall within the scope of practice of medicine. This test was developed and its performance characteristics determined by the _____Medical Laboratories. It has been cleared or approved by the US Food and Drug Administration.

The name of each specific assay is listed, often including the name of the company making the test. A description of the specific procedures followed to do the special stains is also listed.

Because the cancer was 2+ for HER2 by IHC, the cancer was sent for further HER2 testing with fluorescence in situ hybridization (FISH). The results were positive—meaning that the HER2 gene is amplified. This means that the patient may benefit from treatment with drugs that target HER2, such as trastuzumab (Herceptin) and lapatinib (Tykerb).

CHAPTER 5

Coping with Your Diagnosis and Moving Forward

When you heard the words "you" and "breast cancer" in the same sentence, you may have panicked, thinking, *Is this a mistake? Do I really have cancer? How is this possible?* As the words "breast cancer" echoed through your brain, you may have wondered, *Will I die? Will I lose my breast? Will I be in pain?*

It is natural to be upset and anxious about how cancer will affect your life, and it is normal to have trouble accepting and coping with the diagnosis. You might feel shock, anger, fear, denial, frustration, loss of control, confusion, and grief. You might be anxious about your self-image, future priorities, and sexuality; you might worry about your family, your career, medical bills, and the possibility of dying. You may feel numb. This chapter is designed to show you how you can move forward and take control of what's happening. You can begin to manage your cancer and cancer treatment.

Moving Forward After Diagnosis

Today, most women who receive a diagnosis of breast cancer can look forward to a healthy future. After the initial shock of diagnosis, most women find that with time they can continue with their normal lives. They learn to adapt and go on with their work, activities, and social relationships.

However, the time between diagnosis and the start of treatment can be confusing, overwhelming, and stressful. Challenges will include deciding the following: Whom can you count on to help you through all of this? How will you manage all of the details and new information? How will you use information to make decisions?

Making Informed Decisions

If you have just received a breast cancer diagnosis, you are probably coming to terms with what the diagnosis means for you, your life, and your loved ones. On top of this, you're expected to investigate treatment options and make life-changing decisions. You might have information thrust upon you from many directions from well-meaning individuals, including doctors, friends, family, coworkers, and even other women dealing with breast cancer.

The thought of researching your options for breast cancer treatment—and reflecting on what you want and need—can be overwhelming at first. But it can also be empowering. Spending time looking at your choices can be important in helping you face your cancer and helping you play an active role in your situation.

Most medical professionals agree that you should learn as much as you can before making decisions. It might be tempting to sign a consent form and "get rid of this thing," but making informed decisions takes time. It involves education, understanding, and being at peace with choices that will affect you for the rest of your life. Taking a few days or even a few weeks to think about your options will allow you to make an informed choice you feel comfortable with, and, in most cases, it will not endanger your overall outcome. Most experts agree that for most women, taking a few weeks to get a second opinion or make decisions about treatment does not create dangerous delays. Talk to your doctor about how quickly you need to act.

Steps to Take After Diagnosis

Consider the following suggestions after receiving a diagnosis of breast cancer:

- **Reach out** to your family, friends, and others. Rely on them in times of crisis for whatever support you need. You've helped others in the past; now ask for and accept their help.
- **Take the time you need** to make decisions. There is usually no need to rush into treatment.
- **Inform yourself.** Take charge of your treatment decisions. Learn all you can about breast cancer and your treatment options. Contact the American Cancer Society (800-227-2345 or www.cancer.org) for more information.
- **Prepare questions** for your medical team, and don't be afraid to ask them. Then make sure you understand the answers you get.
- **Be good to yourself**—physically and emotionally. Draw on your own personal strengths. Each step of the journey can make you more aware of just how strong you can be.

With new treatment options and a better understanding of the disease, you can be informed and involved. You can play a valuable role in your treatment and healing. You have some time—time to educate yourself about this disease, time to talk to others who have been through it, time to explore your treatment options, time to organize your thoughts, and time to find the right medical team for you.

Educate Yourself

Learning as much as you can about breast cancer and your treatment options is a helpful and constructive way to come to terms with your situation. The women who are happiest with their treatment results are often those who were satisfied with the information they received before they made their treatment decision. Gather information and ask questions. This will help you make informed decisions that are best for you.

When you are looking for information about any type of cancer, you first need to know exactly what type of cancer you have. Talk with your medical team. Ask them for information about your specific type of cancer, including the cell type and the stage of your cancer. This information is helpful because your cancer treatment will be designed for just you, and knowing these specifics will help you find the best information for your situation.

The amount of information available can be overwhelming, and not all of that information, particularly on the Internet, is helpful or accurate. Bad information can hurt you when it comes to cancer. Knowing where information is coming from can be useful because it may give you some insight into why the individual or organization is providing that information. In the United States, the most reliable sources of health information tend to be government agencies, hospitals, universities, and major public health and health advocacy organizations, such as the American Cancer Society. These groups use current information that is reviewed by noted experts and updated often. Talk to your doctors about any information you find to learn whether and how it applies to you. *Remember that general information cannot take the place of medical advice from your doctor or medical team.* Also remember that you do not have to know every detail, ask all the right questions, and make all the decisions on your own. It is possible to gather too much information and end up feeling swamped and overloaded.

To review breast cancer information, get news on the latest treatment options and clinical trials, speak to an oncology nurse, or find out about free programs and support services, contact the American Cancer Society at 800-227-2345 or www.cancer.org. The National Cancer Institute is also a good source of information (800-422-6237 and www.cancer.gov). For a more complete list of cancer information sources, refer to the resource guide in the back of this book.

Getting the Support You Need

Dealing with the emotions triggered by your cancer diagnosis is as important to your comfort and recovery as managing physical symptoms. How you feel can affect how you look at yourself, how you view life, and the decisions you make about treatment. A positive attitude can certainly improve the quality of your life. But it is natural to feel sad, stressed, or unsure sometimes, and it is important to acknowledge and deal with these painful feelings. Facing these feelings can help you move forward.

Do not be surprised if you feel grief. Research has shown that grief is a process with distinct stages, and it might come and go throughout your cancer experience. Grieving leads to healing and might involve such feelings as shock, denial, bargaining, guilt, anger, and depression. Be patient with yourself. You will not feel physically or emotionally balanced right away, and there might be times that you feel like you are losing the balance you have found. Take the time you need to come to terms with your situation. When you are ready, challenge yourself to accept these feelings and move past them. You will find that your strength and hope are still there, ready to pull you through.

Your spouse or partner may be your most important source of support. But some women find that their partner reacts to their breast cancer diagnosis by withdrawing. They may think the person with cancer will feel even more burdened if they share their fears or sadness. But when partners try to protect each other, both suffer in silence. No couple gets through a cancer diagnosis and treatment without some anxiety and grief. It is important to discuss those fears with one another so that you can shoulder the load together, rather than alone.

It is important for your mental health that you find someone you can talk to. Consider talking with someone who will listen and let you sort out your thoughts without offering advice. You might feel too distant from your loved ones to talk to them about your deepest emotions right now. You are in a situation they can't really understand.

You may find it helpful to talk with a professional counselor who has experience working with people affected by cancer. These professionals are unbiased people who can listen to you, offer coping strategies, and help you find solutions to the problems you're facing. Through counseling, you can gradually feel more in control of your situation.

Another option that works for many women is a support group of other women who are dealing with breast cancer. Valuable support for many women comes from the community of women who have "been there"—women who have themselves been through breast cancer. More than 2.5 million people who have had breast cancer currently live in the United States. People who have firsthand knowledge of what you are going through can be great sources of emotional strength, encouragement, and information. Reaching out to others and receiving reassurance can help you feel connected to others at a time when you might feel quite isolated and afraid. In forming a support system, you will also be more likely to keep a realistic perspective as you progress through treatment and recovery. See the sidebar below for information on American Cancer Society programs for people going through cancer.

Talking to other women about their breast cancer experience can give you insight, knowledge, and hope. While no two people's life or cancer experience will be just the same, other women who have or have had cancer may understand your feelings and your concerns in a way that others cannot. You can speak to other women about the emotional aspects of breast cancer or the best place to explore prosthesis options. You can talk about cancer's effects on your family, your outlook on life, and your sense of self-worth. Other women with breast cancer can relate to your feelings and can tell you

American Cancer Society Support Programs

The American Cancer Society Cancer Survivors Network[SM] **(CSN)** is an online community created by and for cancer survivors and caregivers. It's a safe and welcoming place to find and connect with others like you to share cancer-related stories, support, and practical tips. CSN has many interactive features such as discussion boards, chat rooms, blogs, and secure internal CSN e-mail. Members can also create their own personal pages and contribute photos, poems, audio, video, resources, and more. CSN membership is free and available around the clock.

Another program that is helpful for many women is the American Cancer Society's **Reach To Recovery®**. Specially trained volunteer breast cancer survivors offer information and support to others facing diagnosis or treatment. Support is given individually, either face-to-face or on the phone. This program has been supporting women and men with breast cancer for more than forty years.

Contact the American Cancer Society at 800-227-2345 or www.cancer.org, or talk to your doctor, nurse, or social worker to get a list of support groups in your area. Additional resources that might be useful are listed in the back of this book.

how they coped with their own feelings, or they can just listen as you express yours. You can share information you have learned about the disease and treatment options so that you can help someone else, or you can seek others' advice. Maybe you just want to sit in and listen. You can participate in support groups in whichever ways you feel comfortable and that work best for you.

How you get support is your choice. Think about what you need most, and then think about who can help fill those needs. Breast cancer can be emotionally and physically draining. It is okay to admit that you do not have all the answers and that you cannot do everything. Ask others to step in when you need and want help.

Support for Younger Women

Even though breast cancer in younger women is statistically rare (only about one in eight invasive breast cancers occurs in women under age forty-five), this provides no solace to the young women with this disease. Although women who develop breast cancer at such young ages share some concerns with women whose cancers are diagnosed at older ages (such as survival, treatment decisions, and body image), they also have unique concerns. For example, younger women tend to be more concerned with such issues as fertility, breast cancer during pregnancy, premature menopause, and sexual functioning. They might need more information on juggling work and family responsibilities and dealing with financial burdens caused by cancer.

Because most breast cancers are diagnosed in women older than fifty, younger women might feel that many breast cancer support groups are not for them. Young women with breast cancer can get support and information specifically for younger women from the Young Survival Coalition and Stupid Cancer (formerly called The I'm Too Young for This! Cancer Foundation). These organizations offer support, provide community events, and work to end isolation and improve quality of life for young adults (fifteen to thirty-nine years old) affected by cancer. See the resource guide for more information about these and other support organizations.

Support for Women Who Are Pregnant

Breast cancer occurs in about one in three thousand women who are pregnant in the United States, making it the most common cancer in pregnant and postpartum women. One positive note for women with breast cancer who are pregnant: the cancer itself does not seem to affect the baby's development. Also, the cancer cannot be passed along to your baby during the pregnancy. Pregnancy might make it harder to find, diagnose, and treat breast cancer, but most studies have shown that the outcomes are about the same among pregnant women and women who are not pregnant with breast cancer found at the same stage. If you are pregnant, talk to your doctor about treatment options that will maximize your chances for a healthy baby and healthy recovery from breast cancer.

Women who are pregnant when their breast cancer is diagnosed can find support and talk with other women in similar situations by contacting Hope for Two: The Pregnant with Cancer Network. See page 457 for more information.

Talking to Friends and Family

Only you know the right time and the right words to use to tell your family and friends about your diagnosis. Sharing this experience with loved ones gives them a chance to offer their support. Your honesty and openness can help open new lines of communication and make relationships stronger and better.

Start by making a list of people that you want to talk to in person. Then you can make another list of less close friends that another friend or family member may contact with the news.

Be Good to Yourself

Look for signs of the progress you are making. Maybe you called and talked to a Reach To Recovery volunteer, or maybe you've finally read through all of the information the nurse gave you. Reaching each milestone along this journey is cause for celebration. Reward yourself for being brave and facing a difficult situation. Pamper yourself even if you don't feel brave. Surround yourself with people who will support you, make you feel better, and will do things for or with you. Avoid people who upset or discourage you.

Before you talk to others about your illness, think about your own feelings, your reasons for telling others, and what you expect of them. Be ready for a wide range of reactions. When you share information about your diagnosis, your family and friends will have many different feelings. They also will need support at this time. They might be able to express their feelings to you, or they may try to hide them.

Each person reacts and copes differently when they learn someone close to them has cancer. You may notice changes in how people act around you after you tell them the news. People may feel uncomfortable because they do not know what to say or how to act. This situation is new for you and for them, too. They may feel sad and uncomfortable and may be afraid of upsetting you. They might be frightened by the possibility of losing you. Sometimes people find it easier to say nothing because they are afraid of saying the wrong thing. Some friends may act awkward and distant, while others will continue to be themselves. Some may ask too many questions or be overly helpful. It will take time for everyone to get more comfortable talking about it.

You may have friends or family members who say unhelpful things, such as telling you to "cheer up" or that "God never gives us more than we can handle" when you talk to them about your sadness, worries, or fears. It is okay to ask them gently whether they would be willing just to listen, without judgment or giving advice (unless you ask for it). Do not allow yourself to be discouraged by people who are uncomfortable with your feelings. Some people are unable to listen because of their own experiences or feelings. That has nothing to do with you. You may have to accept that some people are not the best sources of support. Others may handle it better.

It can be emotionally exhausting to repeat the details of your illness to everyone who is concerned about you. You might want to ask a family member or friend to be your spokesperson. There are also websites designed for people dealing with serious illnesses where friends and family can get updates (such as CaringBridge.org). Having a friend or family member take on the task of regularly updating the site is especially helpful. As another option, some people send out group e-mails every few days to update their concerned friends whenever something changes.

For Parents: Helping Children Understand a Cancer Diagnosis*

Cancer is often called a "family disease" because your illness will have an impact on your entire family. Do not keep your cancer diagnosis a secret from your children. Some parents think that they can protect their children from this difficult truth, but it is far better to share information honestly—to talk with them about the diagnosis and what it means for your family. Trying to protect children from the truth can do far more harm than good. Children whose parents are honest with them and share information as appropriate generally experience less anxiety.

Children often pick up on the anxiety and worry of their parents. They also have vivid imaginations and tend to imagine the worst. Even if you do not talk openly about your cancer diagnosis, they will likely sense that something is wrong. Without honest explanations, children usually draw their own conclusions. Your children may incorrectly determine that your silence means that whatever is happening is too terrible to share. Another risk of keeping cancer a secret is that children will sense that you are trying to hide something. They might end up feeling isolated and uncertain about

*Much of the information in this section was adapted from *Cancer in Our Family: Helping Children Cope with a Parent's Illness, Second Edition* (Atlanta: American Cancer Society; 2013), written by Sue P. Heiney, PhD, RD, FAAN, and Joan F. Hermann, MSW.

whether they can trust the information you do share with them. It is impossible to shield children from all of the stressful parts of life, and following the natural desire to protect them will usually not make things more pleasant or secure in the long run.

Talking to Children About Cancer

The first and most important step in helping children deal with your cancer diagnosis is to offer appropriate information about your breast cancer right from the start. If possible, you should be the first one to tell your children you have breast cancer. If they hear about it from someone else—for example, a curious neighbor or a classmate who has heard other people talking—it can damage their trust in you. The discussion should come before you start treatment. Have this discussion in a quiet place where you will not be interrupted. Make sure to leave plenty of time for your children to ask questions and express their feelings.

First, try to explain your cancer diagnosis and prepare your children for the ways in which they will be affected. Your children will be better able to cope with these changes when they are prepared ahead of time. It is best to communicate information about cancer honestly, in a way that allows each child to understand, ask questions, and have a role in what's happening in his or her life. With that in mind, be truthful with your children about cancer and its effects, but only to the extent that is appropriate for each child's age and ability to understand.

All children need to know the following basic information: the name of the cancer (you may simply tell them "breast cancer"), the part(s) of the body where the cancer is located, how the cancer will be treated, and how family life will be affected by the disease and treatment. Your children also need reassurance. Remind them that they are safe, secure, and loved. Though treatment may cause you to be absent from time to time and could require that they be left in the care of others, reassure your children that you are not abandoning them. Tell them that their needs will be met no matter what happens.

Don't avoid such hard questions as, "Will you die?" Answer these kinds of questions honestly but as optimistically as the situation allows. For example, you might say, "This is a serious illness, but I am getting the best possible treatment, and the doctor thinks I'm doing very well." When optimism seems unrealistic, parents need to acknowledge how hard it is to live with uncertainty and emphasize their determination to face whatever happens together as a family.

Keep in mind that talking with children about cancer should not be a one-time event; it is a process that should continue over time. If the cancer goes into an extended remission or continues as a chronic problem, children will need updates tailored to their own changing emotional and developmental needs.

What to Tell Children

Knowing about cancer and what to expect during treatment can help your children feel more in control. When talking to your children about cancer, communicate the following:

- **They did not cause your cancer,** and it is not their fault that you got sick.
- **You may feel sick or upset** because of the cancer and its treatment, not because of anything they have done.
- **Cancer is complex.** There are more than one hundred different kinds of cancer, and different cancers have different treatments.
- **Cancer is not contagious;** people cannot transmit it to one another.
- **Cancer is not a death sentence.** More people are cured by today's treatments, and new treatments are in development.
- **Family routines may change,** but reassure your children that their needs will be met. Children should be encouraged to continue the activities that are important to them.

Be as honest and sensitive as you can, and use a straightforward approach. Try to answer questions as clearly and openly as you can. Try not to hide your feelings from your children. Lead by example; share your feelings and admit your fears, within reason. Try to give your children a balanced perspective—cancer is a serious illness, but not a hopeless one.

Consider Your Child's Developmental Stage

Deciding what and how much to share about your cancer diagnosis will depend largely on the age and developmental stage of the child. Factors such as the child's personality, the way information is presented, and the specific circumstances of your family will also affect how your children will react to this news.

Do not make assumptions about how much your children understand. Cancer and cancer treatment can be very difficult to explain to children. After your discussion, ask your children to restate in their own words what they understand about the cancer. That way you can correct any misunderstandings and gauge the extent of their grasp of the situation.

Talking to young children (up to age eight): When talking to young children, use simple, age-appropriate language. Start by asking what they understand or think about the illness. From the ages of two to seven, children think concretely, so simple, specific terms must be used when talking about illness. For example, "Mommy is sick and her medicine is making her hair fall out." Explain to young children that cancer is a sickness that happens inside the body—in this case, the breast. Showing them the location of the cancer will make it even more concrete. Using books or dolls or drawing pictures can help, too. Tell them you will be getting treatment to make the cancer go away. Tell them that if you do not get medicine or treatment, the cancer might grow bigger and spread to other parts of your body, so that is why you must get treatment now.

As much as possible, explain the effects of the illness and the side effects of the treatment—such as any changes to your body as a result of surgery, catheters (what they are and why they're necessary), tiredness, hair loss, weight loss, skin changes, and mood swings—so that the children are not left to fantasize about why these things are happening. Remember that children are familiar with being sick, but be careful about saying things such as, "It's like when you had a sore throat and had to go to the doctor." These types of statements can cause young children to think that the next time their throat hurts, it means they might have cancer.

Talking to older children (eight and older): Older children are able to understand complex explanations and will need more detailed information about your situation. They might be interested in seeing pictures of cancer cells or learning more about cancer. Explain to older children that cancer cells are cells that grow in the body that do not belong there. Something has gone wrong with these cells, and they keep growing and dividing rapidly instead of dying as they should. Eventually, cancer cells can lump together and form a tumor.

You can explain to older children that cancer treatment works by attacking the cells in the body that divide rapidly. Side effects can occur because other healthy cells in the body also divide rapidly and can be affected by the treatment. Prepare your children for any side effects you expect. For example, if your treatment involves chemotherapy and hair loss is expected, you can explain beforehand that the medicine may make your hair fall out. These discussions should prepare your children for the changes they will see in you during treatment. It is also important to reassure your children, regardless of age, that they did not cause your cancer, and it is no one's fault that you got sick.

Children's Reactions

Children may exhibit a variety of reactions to your cancer diagnosis. Shock, distress, denial, fear, anxiety, anger—these are all normal reactions. But children often have a hard time expressing their feelings, so it is important to pay attention to the child's behavior for clues as to how that child is feeling. A child who is very dependent may become more dependent or clingy. A quiet child may become even more quiet and withdrawn. Not all children react to a family crisis by acting out. Encourage your children to share their feelings with you. Help them sort out their feelings, and if reactions are extreme or long lasting, professional help may be needed.

How your children react to your cancer diagnosis will very much depend on how you and other adults are handling the crisis. Children often interpret what is happening in the world around them by watching their parents. While this responsibility may feel like an added burden, your example can help your children develop effective tools for coping with other stressful situations down the road. Some families even grow closer as a result of having a loved one with cancer.

Young children's possible reactions: Young children have less capacity to understand how their lives will be affected by a cancer diagnosis. Their responses are typically more self-centered, and their concerns relate to how the news directly affects them. The initial news might not seem to make a big impact on a young child, but you may see a more noticeable effect after treatment begins and actual changes—such as time apart because of treatment—begin to take place.

Young children regularly engage in "magical thinking"—meaning that they believe they can make all kinds of things happen. They might also believe that bad things have occurred because they have been angry with their mom or dad. Small children see themselves as the center of the universe and often think that bad things happen because they were naughty. So when a parent receives a cancer diagnosis, children often feel guilty and think they are to blame. At some point, most children believe that something they did or did not do could have caused their parent's illness. Children usually will not express this fear, however, so bring up the issue yourself and reassure them about it. You might say something such as, "The doctors have told us that no one can cause someone else to get cancer—none of us did anything that made me get breast cancer."

Young children also worry that cancer is contagious and that they or their other parent will get cancer. It is a good idea to correct these ideas before children experience anxiety or become distressed. Explain that cancer is a different kind of illness; your children do not have to worry that someone "gave" you cancer or that they will get cancer from you. Reassure your children by saying that it would also be very unusual for their other parent to get sick.

Another worry your child might have is that everyone who has cancer dies because of it. You might want to tell your children that, years ago, people with cancer often did die because doctors did not know much about how to find it early or treat it effectively. The outlook for many people with cancer today is much more hopeful.

Older children's possible reactions: Older children can have a range of complicated reactions to a parent's cancer. At this age, they are beginning to understand death as a permanent state. Many children feel scared and unsure about the future and might feel alone and abandoned. If other family members have died of cancer in the past, children this age might assume that death will happen again in this instance. Explain to older children that there are many kinds of cancer and many kinds of treatment. All people respond differently to treatment and have different outcomes. Older children may still struggle with issues of guilt. Be sure to remind them that it is no one's fault that you have cancer.

Adolescent Daughters of Mothers with Breast Cancer

Adolescence can be a trying time for mothers and daughters. Communication can be strained, and the stress of cancer treatment and the changes it can cause in the family can add to that strain. Adolescent girls may feel uncomfortable talking about breast cancer at the same time that they are undergoing breast development.

A diagnosis of breast cancer may cause you to worry about your daughter's risk later on in life. If you are concerned about your daughter's risk of breast cancer, it's a good idea to discuss your concerns with your doctor. If he or she thinks your family history suggests a genetic breast cancer, then a thorough breast cancer risk assessment may be suggested so you and your family can learn more about any potential risk for your daughter. Chances are your daughter's risk is only slightly increased from that of other women.

Make sure your daughter is instructed in breast self-examination as she nears the end of adolescence. Regular breast cancer screening should be followed unless it is determined that she is at higher risk for breast cancer. See appendix A for the American Cancer Society's recommendations for screening and early detection. For more information about breast cancer risk assessment, contact us at 800-227-2345 or on the web at www.cancer.org.

Teens in particular can feel ambivalent about a sick parent, wanting to help but feeling angry and guilty about wanting to escape. Their reactions can be especially difficult if they were not getting along with the parent before the illness. Teens are also aware of cancer news in the media, might have friends who have dealt with cancer in their families, and are mature enough to think of the future in more concrete terms. Older children and teens sometimes feel overwhelmed by the parent's pain and their own helplessness in dealing with it. As a result, some may become withdrawn, while others might become anxiously overinvolved in the parent's care. You may see behavior changes. Some act out aggressively and destructively or abandon their social outlets; others begin to have problems in school. Some children and teens even develop headaches, rashes, and other psychosomatic problems.

Because teens can better understand what is happening, it can be tempting to share almost everything with them. Try not to overload your teenager. Try to balance the support you need from your children while maintaining their academic, extracurricular, and social lives. Parents can help promote healthy teen development by allowing them to continue normal activities as much as possible. Since older children and teens can be very sensitive to feeling and being different from their peers, minimizing the differences caused by the illness will make it easier for them to cope. Children this age need time and energy for schoolwork and friends. Staying in contact with friends might not seem like a priority to parents, but these relationships are very important for adolescents and can offer your child a much-needed outlet.

Helping Children Cope

Here are some things you can do to help your children cope with changes caused by your cancer diagnosis and treatment:

- For young children, extra attention might be all they need to adjust to the situation. Talk to them, try to get them to tell you about their feelings, and always express your love. Children, especially very young ones, need continuous reassurance that they will be safe, secure, and loved.
- Before starting cancer treatment, prepare your children, especially young ones, for the times you will need to be away from home. Give them a brief explanation about what to expect when you come back home. Because cancer and its treatment can require frequent absences, your children, at times, may need to be left in the care of others. Reassure your children that they are not being abandoned—that they will always be taken care of, no matter what happens.

- Tell your children's teachers and school guidance counselors about your illness so that they can watch for problems that might crop up in school.
- Develop a support network for your children. Seek help from social workers at your hospital, treatment center, or through other support groups. Having additional support can relieve the pressure when your own capacity to cope with your children's reactions and needs is limited. Ask about support groups specifically for children of parents with cancer. Do not be afraid to call upon friends and relatives to help.
- Children thrive on routine—it helps them feel safe. Let them know that their daily needs will still be met and activities will not stop: they can still have their favorite sandwiches for lunch, go to their sports and activities, and play with friends. Consistent routines are important for giving children the security they need to stay on track. Teens in particular need to spend time with their peers and have their privacy respected.
- Continue to set limits on negative behaviors. Discipline might be difficult to enforce when children act out or behave badly as a way of coping with the stresses of a family illness. But a breakdown in rules can actually add to their feelings of insecurity. Tell your children that you love them but will not accept destructive or bad behavior.
- Ask your children for their input when resolving some of the home management issues that come up when dealing with your illness. Involving children in this process can give them a much-needed sense of competence. Give children manageable tasks and let them help you. These "special jobs" allow children to feel more in control and give support to you and to the family. By involving your children in these ways, you are acknowledging their valuable role as members of the family.

Recognizing Signs of Problems

Be alert for signs of problems at home or in school. Your children may have some of the following reactions to your cancer diagnosis:

- Young children can regress, meaning they can become babyish in their behaviors or return to behaviors they had previously outgrown. For example, they might wet the bed, act clingy, or have tantrums. School-age children may resist going to school, have problems with schoolwork, or develop difficulties in relationships with siblings and peers. Children of all ages may have nightmares or trouble sleeping, lose their appetite, develop physical complaints, become unusually quiet or fearful, or begin to fail at tasks at which they are usually successful.

- Children who were having problems in school before the cancer diagnosis will probably have increased difficulties afterwards. Counseling may be needed to help them manage their distress and avoid problems with schoolwork and peer relationships. Sometimes a child's withdrawal from peer relationships is a sign of depression.
- Any major changes in behavior that persist for more than a couple of weeks are warning signs that your child is having problems. If he or she starts talking about wanting to die or suddenly gives away favorite possessions, seek help from a mental health professional right away.
- Because children come to rely so much on their parents, they may react strongly or even angrily if a parent cries or otherwise seems fragile. Children may not seem as sympathetic or supportive as you might wish. They may be angry with you and critical of your changed appearance and failure to attend to their needs.

When to Get Professional Help

It may be difficult to determine when your children need additional help coping with your cancer diagnosis. Changes in behavior can provide clues into how a child is coping. The biggest factors to consider when evaluating behavior changes are the degree and duration of that symptom or behavior. Extreme changes in behavior that last longer than a day or two may be cause for concern. Several subtle behavior changes together may be just as concerning as one big change. Symptoms lasting weeks may be signs that professional help may be needed.

Older children and teenagers are better at hiding their feelings, and their behavior may not always be a good indicator as to how they are coping. Encourage older children to discuss their feelings openly. Support groups for adolescents and teens can help connect them with others who are in similar situations. If your child is very depressed or starts talking about suicide, contact a mental health professional immediately.

CHAPTER 6

Making the Medical System Work for You

Navigating the medical system can be confusing and overwhelming, especially after receiving a breast cancer diagnosis. Information gathering and effective communication are key to understanding your choices and being an active participant throughout your breast cancer treatment.

In this chapter, we will discuss the types of health care professionals you may see over the course of your treatment, as well as choosing a doctor and treatment facility, getting a second opinion, understanding your rights as a patient, designating a primary caregiver, and maintaining your medical information. With knowledge and planning, you can partner with your medical team to ensure you get the best care available.

Your Medical Team

Having a qualified and supportive medical team can increase your chances for a positive treatment experience and recovery. Before starting your treatment, it helps to understand the roles of different health professionals that you might need.

Who Your Medical Team Is and What It Does

To be an active member of your medical team, it helps to be clear about the roles of the medical professionals and support staff who will coordinate and provide your care. These people will help you make decisions, be in charge of any necessary surgery, guide your treatment, and help you manage any problems that come up. They will also answer questions and help you meet your general health needs. Knowing where to turn for certain types of information will help you play an active role in your care.

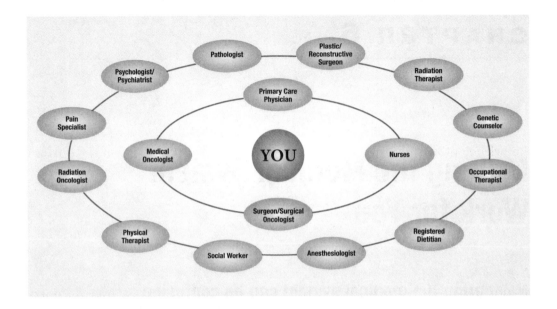

One person on your medical team will take the lead in coordinating your care. You may be able to help determine who this person is if you wish. Your primary care doctor has probably known you longer and better than the other caregivers, so he or she may be your strongest ally. You might prefer to have your surgeon or medical oncologist oversee all aspects of your treatment. It should be made clear to all team members who is in charge, and that person should inform the others of your progress. The alphabetical list below describes some of the medical professionals you might meet and what they do.

Anesthesiologist

Before surgery, you will meet with the anesthesiologist. An anesthesiologist is a medical doctor who gives you anesthesia (drugs or gases) to put you to sleep before surgery and to prevent or relieve pain during and after surgery.

Genetic Counselor

A genetic counselor is a health care professional trained to help people through the process of genetic testing. A genetic counselor can explain the available tests to you, discuss the pros and cons, and address any concerns you may have. This counselor can arrange for genetic testing and then help interpret results. A certified genetic counselor has at least a master's degree and has passed both a general competency examination and a specialty genetic counseling examination.

Medical Oncologist

A medical oncologist is the doctor you will see after your cancer diagnosis. He or she might have been recommended by your primary care physician or family doctor. The oncologist is a cancer expert who understands specific types of cancer and their treatments and who helps people with cancer make decisions about the best course of treatment. The oncologist will interact with you and your family and will have thorough knowledge of the information in your medical files, such as test results, pathology reports, and imaging scans. An oncologist prescribes chemotherapy, hormone therapy, and other drugs to treat your cancer and will refer you to other specialists. He or she will work closely with the other members of your medical team to ensure that you are getting the best treatment possible. The oncologist will also handle any medical issues that arise during cancer treatment and your long-term follow-up care. He or she can keep you informed about the latest treatments and resources.

Nurses

During your treatment, you will meet different types of nurses. A registered nurse (RN) has an associate's or bachelor's degree in nursing or has completed a hospital-based nursing program and, in either case, has passed a state licensing examination. Registered nurses can monitor your condition, give treatments, teach you about side effects, and help you adjust physically and emotionally to breast cancer. A nurse practitioner (NP) is an RN with a master's or doctoral degree who can diagnose and manage breast cancer care. Nurse practitioners share many tasks with your doctors, such as recording your medical history, doing physical examinations, tracking your response to treatment, and providing follow-up care. In most states, NPs can prescribe medicines under a doctor's supervision. A clinical nurse specialist (CNS) is a nurse who has a master's degree in a specific area, such as oncology, psychiatry, or critical care nursing. The CNS often lends expertise to staff and might provide special services to patients, such as educating them or their families and leading support groups. An oncology-certified nurse is a registered nurse who has in-depth knowledge of cancer care and who has passed a special certification examination. Oncology-certified nurses are found in all areas of oncology practice.

Occupational Therapist

An occupational therapist is a health care professional who helps restore self-care, work, or leisure skills. An occupational therapist generally has a four-year degree and is certified.

Pain Specialist

Pain specialists are doctors, nurses, and pharmacists who are experts in managing pain. They can help you find pain control methods that are effective and allow you to maintain your quality of life. Not all doctors and nurses are trained in pain care, so you may have to request a pain specialist if your pain relief needs are not being met.

Pathologist

Pathologists are medical doctors who are specially trained to diagnose disease by examining tissue and fluid samples under a microscope. They can determine the classification (cell type) and help determine the stage (extent) of the cancer. The pathologist writes the pathology report so that you and your medical team can decide on treatment options.

Physical Therapist

Physical therapists are trained health care professionals who help you with rehabilitation after surgery. They will teach you exercises and other stretching and strengthening techniques and might use massage or heat to help restore, maintain, or improve your body's strength, function, and flexibility. A physical therapist might also be consulted if you develop lymphedema (severe swelling) after surgery or radiation. Some physical therapists are certified as lymphedema specialists. These therapists have undergone further training in techniques to reduce or prevent lymphedema symptoms.

Plastic / Reconstructive Surgeon

Plastic or reconstructive surgeons are medical doctors who specialize in operations to restore the appearance of areas of the body affected by injury, disease, or treatments for cancer and other diseases. You might consult with such a surgeon before and/or after breast cancer surgery. Your plastic/reconstructive surgeon can perform breast reconstruction procedures either immediately after mastectomy or at a later time separate from the original cancer surgery.

Primary Care Physician

A primary care physician may be a general doctor, gynecologist, internist, or family practice doctor. This is often the doctor who examined you when, or if, you first reported symptoms of breast cancer. It may be the doctor who first discovered signs of breast cancer. This member of your treatment team will discuss your diagnosis with you, will be involved in your breast cancer care, and may be in charge of coordinating your treatment. Your primary care physician plays an important role in your medical team by providing details of your medical history to other members of the team. He or she will also refer you to cancer specialists and might be a key part of your long-term follow-up care.

Psychologist / Psychiatrist

A psychologist is a licensed mental health professional who may be part of your medical team. He or she provides counseling on emotional and psychological issues. A psychologist may have specialized training and experience in treating people with cancer. A psychiatrist is a medical doctor specializing in mental health and behavioral disorders. Psychiatrists provide counseling and can also prescribe medications.

Radiation Oncologist

Radiation oncologists are medical doctors who specialize in treating cancer with radiation (high-energy x-rays). They will help you make decisions about your radiation therapy and determine how much and what kind of radiation you should receive after surgery or to control advanced breast cancer. This member of your medical team evaluates you frequently during and after treatment. Radiation oncologists are assisted by radiation therapists during treatment and work with radiation physicists, experts trained to ensure that the right dose of radiation is delivered to you. The physicist is assisted by a dosimetrist, a technician who helps plan and calculate the dosage, number, and length of your radiation treatments.

Radiation Therapist

Radiation therapists are specially trained technicians who work with the equipment that delivers radiation therapy. They position you during treatments and administer the radiation therapy.

Registered Dietitian

A registered dietitian (RD) is specially trained to help you make healthy diet choices and maintain a healthy weight before, during, and after cancer treatment. A registered dietitian has at least a bachelor's degree and has passed a national competency examination.

Social Worker

Social workers are health care professionals with a bachelor's or master's degree in social work and, in most cases, are licensed or certified by the state in which they work. They are experts in coordinating and providing nonmedical care. Social workers are trained to help you and your family deal with a range of emotional and practical problems, such as finances, childcare, family concerns and relationships, transportation, and problems with the health care system. If the social worker is trained in cancer-related issues, he or she can counsel you about your fears, answer questions about diagnosis and treatment, and may lead cancer support groups. You might see your social worker either during a hospital stay or on an outpatient basis.

Surgeon / Surgical Oncologist

Surgeons are medical doctors who perform surgery. (A surgical oncologist specializes in using surgery to diagnose and treat cancer.) You will talk with your surgeon before and after you have a biopsy, lumpectomy, or other surgical procedure. The surgeon might first perform diagnostic surgery to determine the location or extent of your breast cancer, and then might remove tumors and surrounding tissue, if needed. Your surgeon will work closely with surgical nurses, the anesthesiologist, your medical oncologist, and your radiation oncologist. He or she will issue a surgical report to your primary care physician and/or your oncologist, which will help determine your treatment plan.

Finding a Doctor and Treatment Facility

The medical professional who diagnosed your breast cancer is not necessarily the one who should treat it. A doctor who has experience with cancer and its treatment will provide expertise and knowledge your primary care physician or gynecologist may not have. Choosing a doctor and treatment facility is a critical step in getting the best treatment possible. You want a doctor with excellent skills, but you also want someone with whom you feel comfortable. Your doctor should be a technical expert and a compassionate ally. Communication is an important part of your relationship with your doctor.

Some people choose a doctor first, whereas others seek out a treatment facility and look for a doctor that practices there. There is no "right" approach. If you have health insurance, your choice may be limited to doctors and treatment facilities that participate in your insurance plan. You also have the option of seeing a doctor outside your health care plan and paying the costs yourself, though this will not be feasible for all women.

The most important question to ask when choosing a doctor is whether the doctor is experienced in treating your specific kind of cancer. Doctors at large centers will have more experience diagnosing and treating cancer, and it is important that your doctor has specialized training and experience with your type of cancer.

If you are considering a certain doctor, ask about the number of procedures the doctor has performed and the number of people the doctor has treated for breast cancer. Ask about the doctor's patient load and the types of cancer he or she is experienced in treating. Find out which hospitals or treatment centers the doctor is affiliated with—ask yourself whether these are places you would want or be able to go for surgery or other care. A teaching affiliation, especially with a respected medical school, might indicate that the doctor is a respected leader in the field. Academic physicians who maintain practices often are in close touch with experts around the country and are usually well versed in the latest therapies. Medical doctors doing research have usually published their findings in medical journals, so you might look online for his or her published articles to learn more about the doctor's experience, philosophy, and approach.

The National Cancer Institute (NCI) maintains an online database of NCI-designated Cancer Centers, recognized for their scientific excellence. The database can be found at http://cancercenters.cancer.gov/cancer_centers/index.html. You can search for a treatment center by location or get a complete list. You can also find a treatment center using the NCI's Cancer Information Service, 800-4-CANCER (800-422-6237). Seeking treatment in an NCI-approved cancer center might be especially important if you have a particularly complex case.

There are other resources you can use to identify doctors who specialize in treating breast cancer:

- The American Board of Medical Specialties (ABMS) maintains a list of all board-certified doctors. If the doctor subscribes to the ABMS service, you can get information about his or her certification status and a list of certified specialists by geographic area. You can do this by checking in the *Official ABMS Directory of Board Certified Medical Specialists*® (carried by some libraries), calling 866-ASK-ABMS (866-275-2267), or visiting www.abms.org.
- The American Medical Association (AMA) has an online Doctor Finder database at www.ama-assn.org. It provides basic information on licensed doctors in the United States who are AMA members. Users can search for doctors by name or by medical specialty. You can get a variety of information, such as

contact information, medical school and residency training, and major professional activities.

If you are considering a certain treatment center, ask whether it is accredited by the Commission on Cancer (CoC) of the American College of Surgeons. You can check this yourself by visiting www.facs.org/cancer. If the center has been accredited by the CoC, you will know that it meets stringent standards and offers total cancer care, including lifetime follow-up care. You will also know that the center's ability to deliver quality cancer care is closely monitored by the CoC, whether you receive treatment in a large internationally known hospital or a small local setting.

At the very least, a hospital should be accredited by The Joint Commission. This accreditation and certification is recognized nationwide as a symbol of quality that reflects an organization's commitment to meeting certain performance standards. You can find out whether a treatment center is accredited online at the Commission's Quality Check at www.qualitycheck.org. Accredited hospitals are also listed in the *American Hospital Association Guide to the Health Care Field*, found in many public libraries. Surprisingly, about one hospital in five fails to earn Joint Commission accreditation. The extent and variety of services a facility offers is a key measure. The best hospitals offer these services, staff, and facilities:

- a postoperative recovery room
- an intensive care unit
- anesthesiologists
- a pathology laboratory, diagnostic laboratory, and blood bank
- around-the-clock staffing
- a tumor board
- social work services
- respiratory therapies, physical therapists, and rehabilitation services
- advanced diagnostic and therapeutic equipment (CT scans, radiation therapy, etc.)

Understanding the Terms

It can be helpful to know some of the terms used to describe doctors and their training and credentials. Specialists are doctors who completed their residency training in a specific area, such as medical oncology or plastic surgery, and have been board certified. Some doctors also choose to become subspecialists, which involves additional training in an area of a specialty. Board certification means that a medical doctor has been trained and has taken national certification examinations. Doctors can be board certified in more than one specialty.

Once you have identified the specialist you'd like to see, do not be surprised if it takes several weeks to get an appointment. Remember, you have time. Finding someone with an excellent reputation is worth the research and the wait.

Evaluating Doctors' Practices

When evaluating a doctor's practice, consider the issues listed here. Try to learn this information by talking to doctors, nurses, and other patients within the practice.

- Appointments should be easy to make.
- The office environment should be clean, comfortable, and convey a sense of both efficiency and concern.
- The doctor's staff should treat you with courtesy and respect.
- Waiting times should not be excessive.
- Examinations and conversations should take place in private without being rushed.
- Your doctor should be open to the contributions of other health care professionals, such as social workers, nurses, home care providers, or physical therapists. He or she should be willing to make referrals.
- Nurses and nurse assistants should take time to answer your questions, explain what's happening, and provide the information you need.
- Phone calls should be returned quickly.
- The results of laboratory tests should be reported promptly and copies mailed, if requested.

Getting a Second Opinion

Taking the time to get a second opinion—to ensure that your diagnosis is correct and your treatment plan is the best one for you—can be very valuable. Asking your doctor to refer you to another doctor for a second opinion does not mean that you do not respect your doctor's diagnosis and recommendations. Second opinions are done frequently, and your doctor should welcome the request. Your body and your life are in question, and it is understandable that you would want to have confirmation about the diagnosis and treatment plan. Your doctor may be able to help arrange an appointment with another specialist. Your insurance provider might pay for an additional opinion if you request it, and some insurance plans will require that you get a second opinion, especially if the doctor is recommending surgery.

Questions to Ask When Choosing a Doctor and a Hospital

WHAT IS YOUR EXPERIENCE AND TRAINING?

- Are you board certified?
- How long have you been in practice?
- What is your specialty? Do you have a subspecialty?
- What training have you had in treating breast cancer?
- How many women with breast cancer have you treated in the past year?
- Do you have experience treating my type of cancer?

WHAT CAN I EXPECT FROM OFFICE VISITS?

- What are your office hours? Can you be contacted outside those hours? How?
- Who sees your patients when you are on vacation?
- May I record our conversations so that I can review the details later?
- May I bring someone to my appointments to take notes?

WHAT ABOUT AFFILIATIONS AND REFERRALS?

- Are you or others in your practice involved in clinical trials of new treatments?
- What hospitals are you affiliated with?
- To which hospital do you prefer to admit your cancer patients? Why?
- What other types of doctors will be on my medical team? Could you tell me the names of specialists I should see? Will you handle the referrals to these specialists?
- Can you suggest a breast cancer specialist who can offer me a second opinion?

HOW WILL I STAY INFORMED?

- Which member of my medical team will be my main contact, and how do I get in touch with that person if I have questions or concerns?
- Is this person available to talk with my family about their concerns?
- May I have copies of correspondence, tests, and reports?

CAN I GET ADDITIONAL SUPPORT AND INFORMATION?

- Do you have information about breast cancer support groups?
- Do you have information about breast cancer that I can take home with me?
- Where can I find more information about breast cancer?

If you pursue a second opinion of your diagnosis, speak with the doctor or hospital to determine what materials they need. You may need to request the slides from the pathologist who examined the sample initially or take copies of any imaging tests or blood tests that have been done. Some doctors might ask to have this information ahead of time so they can review it and be prepared when meeting with you.

Set a deadline for yourself to meet with your first doctor so you can discuss the treatment options you've researched. Given the vast and sometimes conflicting information available, you can easily become consumed with doing more research and getting more medical opinions rather than evaluating the information you have gathered. Be careful not to fall into the trap of searching for someone to tell you what you want to hear. It is important that you make informed decisions, but not at the cost of putting off treatment altogether.

Participating in Your Medical Care

As you begin treatment, remember that you are an active member of your medical team. You can play an active role by talking openly with your medical team, keeping records of your medical information, and knowing and understanding your rights as a patient.

Understanding Your Rights as a Patient

According to the American Hospital Association's Patient's Bill of Rights, all patients have a right to considerate and respectful health care; understandable information about diagnosis, treatment, and prognosis; and the opportunity to discuss and make decisions about these things. As a patient, you also have the right to know the identity of those involved in your care, know the immediate and long-term financial impact of treatment choices, review your medical records, consent or decline to take part in clinical trials, and be told about hospital policies and practices that relate to patient care. In addition, you have the right to privacy, confidentiality, and continuity of care. If you feel that these rights are not being met, bring it to the attention of your medical team.

Designating Your Primary Caregiver

Few things are as important as participating fully in your medical treatment, but you can exhaust yourself if you try to do it alone. Having someone who is aware of everything that is going on and who can accompany you to appointments can relieve a great deal of your stress. Choose someone you trust completely to be your primary caregiver. It should be someone who listens well and will be available when you need help. Discuss your needs with this person and think of him or her as the partner accompanying you on your breast cancer journey.

The primary caregiver is often a spouse or partner, or it might be another family member or a close friend. Although many of your loved ones might be caring for you, your primary caregiver is the person who is "in the loop" and is as informed as you are throughout your cancer journey. Make sure the person you choose understands what you need from him or her.

Let your primary caregiver and members of your medical team know how you prefer to participate in making decisions and how much information you want to be given. Doctors differ in how much information they give to patients and their families, and patients differ in the amount of information they need or want. It is up to you to tell your doctor if he or she is giving you and your caregiver too much or too little information. Let your team know whether you would like them to keep your primary caregiver (or another person) informed about your illness and treatment. You may need to sign permission forms to allow your medical team to share health-related information with the people you designate.

Communicating with Your Medical Team

Tell your doctors and caregivers about any concerns you have so they can answer questions and help you find a solution. Only you know how you are feeling. Doctors, nurses, family members, and friends cannot meet your needs if you do not make them known.

It is not unusual to focus on the things that unnerve you most, such as the thought of losing your breast or a fear of recurrence. Talking about the things that worry you the most can help you deal with your concerns and put them in perspective.

Retaining Information

Keep track of the details your medical team provides, both for your own reference and to share with other members of your team so they can give you the best possible care. Large amounts of in-depth information about your health and your care will be exchanged during meetings with your medical team. Processing and documenting this information can be difficult. You may not be familiar with some of the terminology, and you may feel overwhelmed or anxious. It may help you to write down the name and position of each team member you deal with and detail the information he or she shares with you. Whenever you can, get information in writing rather than verbally, so you can refer to it later. As much as possible, bring your primary caregiver with you to the doctor's office. Support from your loved ones will not only help you communicate, it can also help lessen the stress of hearing information and making decisions alone.

It can also be helpful to use video or sound recording devices to record appointments with doctors. Recordings allow others to hear accurate details later, and it can also help reduce calls to the office to have information repeated or reworded. Ask to record important appointments for later review. If your doctors are uncomfortable allowing you to record your meetings, explain your reasons. If recording is not possible, ask another person to come to your appointment and take notes.

Making Sure You Understand

If you don't understand something, ask that it be repeated, rephrased, or explained. You might say, "I'm having trouble grasping what you said—would you mind telling me again? Could you put it another way?" Another tactic is to repeat what was said and ask for confirmation: "Let me see whether I have this right. You're saying that..."

Ask a lot of questions. Prepare a list of questions ahead of time, asking the most important ones first. This book contains many questions you might want to ask your medical team, and you will most likely have questions of your own. Also, bring in any information you want to discuss. Let your doctors know you expect to play an active role in your treatment decisions and that you are researching your options; show them that you are an educated patient and that you want them to be supportive partners.

Questions to Ask Yourself to Ensure Good Communication with Your Medical Team

- **How much information do I want to be told** about my diagnosis and health status?
- **How do I want my medical team** to communicate with me about these issues (for example, giving me the facts or breaking it to me gently)?
- **What conditions would I prefer** when talking with my doctor (quiet, no interruptions, having a recorder or personal advocate to capture information, etc.)?
- **What is most important to me** when I consider treatment options (I want to live longer, I want to minimize side effects, I want to avoid pain, etc.) and how can I communicate this to my treatment team?
- **Is there anything I can do** to make communication with my team easier?
- **How can I reach my doctor** in an emergency? After hours? On weekends or holidays?

Taking Enough Time

Arrange for office visits or phone calls that allow adequate time for discussions. Tell your doctor at the beginning of the visit if you have questions. If you still have questions at the end of the visit, say so and schedule another appointment or phone call to address them. Your doctor should take your questions seriously. He or she should be interested in your concerns and not make you feel rushed. If your doctor does not respond this way, bring it up at your next visit. Otherwise, you may begin to question your treatment plan and/or lose confidence in your doctor. Make sure that your doctor has answered all your concerns and questions, no matter how small. It might take more than one visit to discuss all your concerns, as new questions will likely come to mind.

Maintaining Your Medical Information

From the time you receive your breast cancer diagnosis, you will be communicating with your medical team and receiving and requesting medical information. Knowing the details about your cancer and treatment can help you cope. But it also means you will have a lot of information and paperwork to deal with.

One good way to organize your medical information is to use a three-ring binder with dividers, with information organized into the following categories:

1. **PERSONAL INFORMATION DIRECTORY.** This section should include the basics of your breast cancer diagnosis, as well as personal information, such as the following:
   - your date of birth and that of your partner or spouse
   - basic insurance information and contact number
   - work, home, and cell phone numbers
   - names and phone numbers of people to call in an emergency
   - names and phone numbers for babysitters or anyone you might need to contact quickly

   It should also include other details of your medical history (including noncancer-related details) in case you need it. See a sample on the next page.

2. **ONGOING TREATMENT LOG.** Doctors might need information about your cancer treatment to make decisions about how to treat any future health issues. Keeping this information organized can also help you if there are questions or concerns about health insurance

Sample Personal Information Directory

AMANDA BROWN • Date of Birth: 1/31/55

Insurance: Aetna • Group# 12345678 • ID# 12345678 • Contact: 800-000-0000

Allergies: penicillin

Medical History:

- Appendix removed 2/75 • History of high blood pressure
- Mother had postmenopausal breast cancer

Breast cancer diagnosis/treatment:

- Infiltrating ductal carcinoma, stage IIA, diagnosed in right breast 1/12/10
- Lumpectomy of right breast and 8 underarm lymph nodes, Northpoint Hospital, Dr. K. Webb, 1/18/10
- Chemotherapy course, Northpoint Treatment Center, Dr. J. Webster, Adriamycin and cyclophosphamide, 2/12, 3/5, 3/26, 4/16
- Radiation to start 5/7 and continue for 5 weeks

Amanda's medical team:

Dr. A. Smith, primary care physician: 404-555-3870

Dr. K. Webb, surgeon: 404-555-5798

Dr. J. Webster, medical oncologist: 404-555-5499

CONTACTS:

Bill Brown (husband), DOB 6/14/53

Amanda and Bill at home: 404-555-1234

Amanda at work: 404-555-3456

Bill at work: 404-555-6789

Amanda's cell: 404-555-1011

Bill's cell: 404-555-1213

Call in an emergency:

Daughter and son-in-law Jenny and Craig Smith at home: 404-555-9068

Craig at work: 404-555-6418

Craig's cell: 404-555-1598

Jenny's cell: 404-555-7986

Granddaughter Elizabeth's babysitter Sarah Long: 404-555-6520

Neighbor:

Frances Clarke at home: 404-555-9962; at work: 404-555-4518; cell: 404-555-8250

Brody the dog:

North Avenue Kennel: 404-555-4387

Treatment Log

Diagnosis: _Infiltrating ductal breast cancer, Stage IIA_

Diagnosis Date: _1/12/10_

Details from 1/12 needle biopsy (by Dr. J. Webster) pathology report: _____

Well-differentiated carcinoma (this means the cancer cells are relatively normal-looking cells

and do not appear to be growing rapidly; they are arranged in small tubules), also called Grade 1

Progesterone receptor negative, Estrogen receptor positive, HER2 negative

CT scan scheduled for 1/15. Karen at Dr. Webster's office talked to Pam at Aetna and

got okay for test. Lumpectomy scheduled for 1/18

1/18/10 Lumpectomy of right breast and 8 underarm lymph nodes removed by Dr. K. Webb

   -Tumor was 1.5 cm across

   -2 nodes showed tiny amount of cancer (called micrometastasis)

   -Called stage IIA

No cancer spread was found on the CT scan

Dr. Webster discussed treatment plan with me 1/20 in her office

   -Need to get chemo and radiation to be sure all cancer cells are killed

   -Will also start tamoxifen to block estrogen receptors on cancer cells, will be taking this

   for at least 5 years. (*Note: need to get prescription and talk to doc about side

   effects)

   -Nurse Pam to verify insurance coverage for treatment plan.

Chemotherapy Plan(s) & Date(s): _AC (Adriamycin and cyclophosphamide) every 3 weeks for_

4 total cycles. Start dates: 2/12, 3/5, 3/26, 4/16 then start radiation 5/4 and get it

every day for 5 weeks. With AC chemo drugs I will get Kytril and decadron to help prevent

nausea. Also will get prescription for Compazine 10 mg pills that I take every 4 hours if needed

to prevent nausea (*need to get this prescription filled before getting chemo). Karen getting

approval from insurance for meds.

or other benefit claims. Keep a detailed diary of events and information related to your treatment, listing the following information:

- dates and names of doctors and/or treatment center(s) visited
- the names of those in the office with whom you have had contact
- information given to you about your cancer diagnosis and your care

Note the dates and details of all procedures and treatments:

- the names and amounts (doses) of all chemotherapy and/or other drugs given
- the exact location of the radiation treatment field
- the total amount of radiation you received
- when treatments began and ended

A sample treatment log is on the previous page. You might also want to ask for a treatment summary after each treatment. This document will list all drugs and doses received. Keep these summaries with your records.

You can also record your symptoms and make notes about any problems or side effects you have. This will allow you to answer your doctors' questions about your treatment history and how you responded to treatment. See the sample side effect log on page 248.

3. **MEDICAL TEAM DIRECTORY.** Collect information from your medical team, making sure you know the names and all contact information of all of your doctors, past and present. You might use a plastic business card holder to organize the information. As you meet new members of your medical team, ask for their contact information to include in your file. Copy this information and submit it to your various doctors' offices and treatment centers to be put in your permanent file.

4. **INSURANCE INFORMATION.** File your insurance information in the binder so that it will be handy when you need it. Include these pieces of information:

- insurance policy number and the address and phone number of your insurance company
- names of those with whom you have had contact at the insurance company
- a copy of your health insurance policy and your benefit booklet
- copies of materials you received when you enrolled in the insurance plan and updates you have received since then

You will need a copy of your actual insurance policy so that you know what services and treatments are covered. Before treatment begins, review your policy carefully and take note of each aspect of your coverage. Make sure the information is clear to you. The worksheet on the next page can help you organize the information. Learning the details of your insurance plan and its provisions now will help you better plan for the coverage you can expect for your diagnosis and treatment. It will also give you an idea of what you might have to pay yourself.

Your insurance agent and benefits director are good sources of information, but if you have trouble understanding the information or want confirmation of information, call your state insurance commissioner's office for help. Be sure to ask your insurance carrier whether additional insurance is available to you. Your insurance plan might provide extra coverage under a "catastrophic illness" clause. Be sure to fill out all insurance paperwork before your treatment begins—otherwise, your insurance company might not pay for it.

Keep copies of all correspondence between you and your insurance company and Medicaid or Medicare. Whenever possible, communicate in writing, by fax, or by e-mail so you have a written record. But if you speak to a representative over the phone, be sure to write down the name and title of the person with whom you spoke, the date and time of the call, and a detailed summary of the conversation. Also, keep all bills, statements, explanations of benefits (EOBs), and payment records. Include specific information about the procedures, tests, and medicines that were paid for and those that were not.

5. **MEDICAL CONSULTATIONS, LETTERS, AND PHONE CALLS.** Include the following information:
   - any correspondence with doctors or other health care professionals regarding your illness and care
   - second-opinion conference summaries
   - a log of all health-related phone calls, including the names and titles of people with whom you spoke, the dates and times of calls, and a detailed summary of the conversations

6. **REPORTS.** In this section, include the following information:
   - pathology reports on all tissue samples
   - dated reports of blood work, mammograms, x-rays, bone scans, and any other tests that are done
   - operative reports from all surgeries

Insurance Coverage Worksheet

When evaluating your insurance policy, you'll want to find out the specific amounts and limits of your coverage. It might be helpful to jot down the details of your coverage below and refer to them when necessary. Ask as many questions as you need to be sure you understand your plan.

Yearly Deductible: How much of your own money must you spend on doctor bills before the health care plan begins to pay?

_____

_____

Annual Coinsurance Limit: What is the total amount you must pay during a calendar year, not counting the deductible, before the insurance company begins to pay expenses at 100 percent?

_____

_____

Copayment: How much would you need to pay (your copay) for each visit to an HMO or PPO doctor or therapist?

_____

_____

Choice of Medical Service Provider: Can you pick your own doctor, or must you choose someone who belongs to your insurance plan group?

_____

_____

Specific Illnesses Excluded: Are there any illnesses, such as cancer, that your policy won't cover?

_____

_____

Specific Treatments Excluded or Limited: Under what circumstances would you qualify for treatments—such as stem cell transplantation, treatment of infertility, chiropractic care, or physical therapy—that the policy limits or will not cover?

_____

_____

Hospital Costs Covered: What part of hospital costs will the policy cover?

_____

_____

Days of Hospital Coverage in a Year: If you need to be hospitalized, how many days of hospitalization will the insurance pay for each year?

_____

_____

Prescription Drugs: How much do you have to pay for prescription drugs?

_____

_____

Payment Limits*: Are there annual or lifetime limits on what your insurance will pay in benefits?

_____

_____

Home Health Care Visits: If a nurse needs to see you at home, how many visits will the policy pay for?

_____

_____

Mental Health Therapy: How many outpatient mental health visits will the policy cover per year?

_____

_____

_____

*Some parts of the 2010 Affordable Care Act will go into effect beginning January 2014, which may affect your coverage. Speak with your insurance provider for more information, or call the American Cancer Society at 800-227-2345.

7. **MEDICINES.** In this section, list the following information:
   - names and doses of prescribed medicines
   - dates they were prescribed
   - names of the doctors who prescribed each medicine
   - notes about when and how you should take them
   - description of what each medicine is meant to do
   - side effects, symptoms, or problems you should watch for, and when you should report them to the doctor
   - any vitamins, herbs, supplements, or over-the-counter medicines you're taking

8. **CALENDAR.** A one-year calendar on a single page allows you to see at a glance the overall progress of your treatment. It also shows you the bigger picture—for example, when your surgery, radiation, and/or chemotherapy treatments are—and it allows you to schedule vacations, business trips, and other events between treatments. (See sample calendar on the next page.)

9. **FOLLOW-UP CARE.** In this section, include all recommendations from your medical team about these aspects of your care:
   - frequency of checkups
   - tests that should be done at checkups
   - the schedule of follow-up care

10. **MAINTAINING YOUR HEALTH.** This is the place for information or tips about staying well or taking care of yourself before, during, and after treatment. Examples include ways to prevent the nausea that often results from chemotherapy and tips for caring for radiated skin. Also, keep such information as general wellness plans, diet suggestions, and exercise guidelines.

11. **POTENTIAL PROBLEMS.** Ask members of your medical team about short-term and long-term risks or problems that could result from your disease or treatment, such as lymphedema, changes in your blood cell counts, damage to healthy tissues in the area treated with radiation, damage to your organs or body systems, or increased cancer risk. Take notes about what you can do to prevent or be alert to these potential future health problems.

2010 Partial Year-at-a-Glance Calendar

January

S	M	T	W	TH	F	S
					1	2
3	4	5	6	⑦ 9am mammogram	8	9
10	11	⑫ 9am biopsy Dr. Webster	13	⑭ 2pm appt w/surgeon– Dr. Webb	⑮ 1pm CT scan–lab after for bloodwork	16
⑰ No food or drink after midnight ²⁴/₃₁	⑱ 7am Surgery Dr. Webb	⑳ 10am appt Dr. Webster 25	19 26	21 27	22 28	23 29	30

February

S	M	T	W	TH	F	S
1	2	③ 3pm appt for 2nd opinion Dr. Strom	4	5	6	
7	8	9	10	⑪ 10:30 appt w/radiation doc Dr. Ames	⑫ 1st chemo–Start Tamoxifen	13
14	15	16	17	18	19	20
21	22	23	24	25	26	27
28						

March

S	M	T	W	TH	F	S
	1	2	3	4	⑤ 2nd chemo	6
7	8	9	10	11	12	13
14	15	16	17	18	19	20
21	22	23	24	25	㉖ 3rd chemo	27
28	29	30	31			

April

S	M	T	W	TH	F	S
				1	2	3
4	5	6	7	8	9	10
11	12	13	14	15	⑯ 4th & last chemo	17
18	19	20	21	22	23	24
25	26	27	28	29	30	

May

S	M	T	W	TH	F	S
						1
2	3	4	5	6	⑦ start radiation	8
9	10	11	12	13	14	15
16	17	18	19	20	21	22
²³/₃₀	²⁴/₃₁	25	26	27	28	29

June

S	M	T	W	TH	F	S
	1	2	3	4	5	
6	7	8	9	⑩ Radiation done	11	12
13	14	15	16	17	18	19
20	21	22	23	24	25	26
27	28	29	30			

12. **COMMUNITY RESOURCES.** File the addresses, phone numbers, and websites of local and national organizations and other resources in this section. Include relevant news, advice, and tips you have received from these organizations and any materials you have printed out from the Internet. Refer to the resource guide in the back of this book for valuable resources for people with breast cancer and their loved ones.

13. **QUESTIONS.** Keep a record of the questions you have about your care and the answers you receive. Date each entry for future reference.

By keeping a comprehensive record of what happens during your cancer experience, you will be making sure that everyone involved in your treatment—including you—is as informed as possible. Having your own records allows you to review the information you have collected and make informed decisions about your care. Your interest and persistence also shows your medical team that you are a valuable team member who wants to be involved in the details of your care.

PART THREE

Treatment

More treatment choices exist today for breast cancer than ever before. The treatment choices available to you depend on the type of breast cancer you have, the stage of your cancer, and other factors, such as your age, health, and personal preferences.

You might feel overwhelmed by the thought of making such an important choice. Try to remember that this is your illness, your body, and your life. Only you and your medical team can choose the most appropriate way to treat your cancer.

Some women choose to be heavily involved in making decisions, whereas others prefer that their doctor choose their treatment plan. You may be tempted to choose a treatment method that worked for a friend or family member. But unless the other person's medical situation was exactly the same as yours, a different treatment option might better meet your needs. You might be tempted to rely on a "cure" you heard about in the media. These articles and stories usually mention research possibilities that will take years to be determined effective, if at all.

There are many possible types and combinations of treatment for breast cancer, including surgery, radiation, chemotherapy, targeted therapy, and hormone therapy. This section is designed to give you an overview of current treatments. In the following chapters, you'll find in-depth information about the latest therapies and treatment options, clinical trials, and complementary and alternative therapies. In addition, chapter 10 describes the most common treatment options based on your particular situation.

CHAPTER 7

Exploring Treatment Options

More treatment options exist for cancer than for many other illnesses, mostly due to ongoing advances in research and technology. Sometimes women are faced with many choices and can feel rushed into making decisions. But it takes time to weigh the risks and benefits of any decision, including this one. It is worth taking the time to understand your situation. Learn all you can about your cancer, your treatment options, and your health, in order to fight the cancer as well as you can.

Not so long ago, when a lump was found in a woman's breast, she signed a release form before she went into surgery for her biopsy. If the lump was found to be cancerous, the woman would wake up to find that her breast had been completely removed with a total mastectomy. Things have changed a lot since then. Today, there are many options to consider.

Each treatment option will have different advantages and disadvantages. Even though two therapies might offer equal opportunities for treating your cancer, they might have far different effects on your life. It will not necessarily be simple for you to determine which treatment is the best for you and your specific cancer. You'll want to weigh the risks and benefits of each option against your personal preferences, family demands, and career needs.

Making Informed Decisions About Treatment Choices

In order to make informed decisions about treatment, first decide what is most important to you—your priorities and needs. Are you striving for a longer life—without cancer? Keeping your breast? Maintaining some of your normal routines and way of life as you deal with treatment? What is the goal of treatment? To cure the cancer, to control the disease, to treat symptoms?

Try using the Treatment Worksheet on the next page to evaluate each treatment you are considering. Write down all the issues that come to mind for each treatment: how long it will take, what the side effects are, what the pros and cons might be, and anything else that comes to mind. Include as much information as you can.

As a starting point, ask yourself the following questions:

- What are the pros and cons of each treatment or procedure? Do I need more information about particular treatment options? How can I get that information?
- Considering all the advantages and disadvantages, which option seems to make the most sense to me for my particular breast cancer? Does my medical team agree?
- What will I need to do in my life to get through the treatment I have chosen (for example, get extra help at home or at work)?
- Who makes up my support team and how will they help me?
- What steps should I take before treatment begins?

Writing down the major points of information about treatment options might help you sort through your thoughts and feelings on each. If you are still having difficulty making up your mind, ask yourself: What's bothering me? Whom should I talk to?

Consulting Your Medical Team

In the last chapter, we discussed the various people who might be part of your medical team. Build a medical team you trust, and listen carefully to what they say. Before you decide on a treatment plan, make sure you have enough information to feel confident that the treatment plan you and your team are putting together is best for you. Take the time you need to consider all of your options before beginning treatment.

Your doctors might recommend one treatment or suggest multimodality therapy. Multimodality therapy is a combination of different treatments, each designed to play an important role in treating your cancer. In many cases, using multimodality therapy can increase the chances of curing your cancer.

Get as many details as possible about why your doctor or medical team is recommending certain treatments and how the treatment(s) would affect you. To decide on your treatment plan, you will need as balanced a view as possible. If possible, take your caregiver with you to your appointments—it can be hard to remember everything your

Treatment Worksheet

Treatment: _____

Length of Treatment: _____

Benefits: _____

_____

Short-Term Side Effects: _____

_____

Long-Term Side Effects: _____

_____

Preparations Needed Before Treatment: _____

_____

_____

Arrangements Needed During Treatment: _____

_____

_____

Day-to-Day Effects on My Life: _____

_____

_____

My Reservations or Fears: _____

_____

Probable Outcome: _____

_____

My Questions: _____

_____

_____

_____

Questions to Ask Your Medical Team About Your Treatment Options

- **What are my treatment options?**

- **What treatment plan do you recommend** and why? Do the members of my medical team agree on the details of the proposed plan?

- **How soon does my treatment** need to start?

- **What is the goal of this treatment plan?** Is it to cure the cancer, extend my life, or control my symptoms (or some combination of these)?

- **How successful is this treatment** for the type and stage of cancer I have?

- **How will you evaluate** how well this treatment is working?

- **What options will I have** if this treatment doesn't work?

- **What can you tell me about the safety** of this treatment?

- **What are the possible immediate,** short-term, and long-term side effects of the treatment? Can anything be done to prevent or lessen these side effects?

- **What side effects** should I report right away?

- **How will this treatment affect my life?** What changes should I expect to make in my work, family life, and leisure time?

- **Will any treatment have side effects** that can affect another treatment? For example, if I get radiation or chemotherapy first, will I have to delay surgery? For how long?

- **What is the timetable for treatments?** If I receive a combination of treatments, how long will I wait between them? How long will the whole plan take?

- **Will I have to stay in the hospital?** Can any of the treatments be done on an outpatient basis?

- **What will my energy level be like?**

- **Can I exercise?** Should I begin exercising?

- **Should I follow a special diet** or make other lifestyle changes?

- **Can I keep working during treatment?** Can I travel?

- **How much will my treatment cost?** Is my treatment plan covered by my insurance?

doctor says at each visit. In addition to preparing a list of questions to ask and taking notes, some people find it helpful to have someone else there to help take notes.

Your doctor is not your only source of information. Talk to nurses, other members of your medical team, and other specialists caring for you. Consider asking social workers or psychologists about both emotional and practical issues. A vital part of developing a treatment plan is to identify which members of the team can answer specific types of questions and how to reach them if needed.

Types of Treatment for Breast Cancer

Breast cancer can often be treated successfully, and women today have a variety of options. These are the main types of treatment for breast cancer:

- Surgery
- Radiation therapy
- Chemotherapy
- Hormone therapy
- Targeted therapy
- Bone-directed therapy (bisphosphonates and denosumab)

Treatments can be classified into broad groups, based on how they work and when they are used.

Treatment Options: Local Versus Systemic Treatments

Depending on your situation, your treatment may involve local treatments, such as surgery and radiation, and some type of systemic treatment, such as chemotherapy, targeted therapy, and/or hormone therapy. Local treatments aim to remove or destroy cancer cells in a particular place in the body. Systemic treatments reach and affect cells throughout your body. Often, two or more types of treatment are used in combination.

Systemic therapy given after surgery is called adjuvant therapy. The goal of this therapy is to kill any cancer cells that could remain after surgery. Even in the early stages of the disease, cancer cells can break away from the primary breast tumor and spread through the bloodstream. These cells usually do not cause symptoms you can feel, they do not show up on x-rays or CT scans, and they cannot be felt during a physical examination. But they can establish new tumors in other places in the body. Systemic therapy is also the main treatment for women with metastatic breast cancer.

Sometimes systemic therapy is given before surgery; this is called neoadjuvant therapy. Usually, doctors use neoadjuvant therapy to try to shrink the tumor enough to make surgical removal possible. This may allow some women with more advanced tumors to become candidates for surgery or allow women who would otherwise need a mastectomy to have breast-conserving surgery. Neoadjuvant therapy can also help your doctor determine how well the cancer is likely to respond to certain treatments (chemotherapy, targeted therapy, or hormone therapy) if they are needed after surgery.

Side Effects of Treatment

Most treatments for cancer come with some risk of side effects. Any treatment or drug powerful enough to kill cancer cells can be strong enough to affect your body in other ways. Talk to your doctor about the likelihood that you will have side effects. You will likely feel more in control if you know the potential side effects of the treatments you plan to undergo, you understand how common or uncommon they are, and you understand what can be done to control or prevent the side effects.

The next two chapters explore the main treatment options for breast cancer and touch on the potential side effects you might face. Chapter 13 explores side effects in more detail and includes ways to cope with these issues.

CHAPTER 8

Surgery

Most women with breast cancer will have some type of surgery.
The primary goal of breast cancer surgery is to remove the cancer from the breast and from the lymph nodes, if it has spread there. Depending on your situation, your doctor might recommend breast-conserving surgery (usually lumpectomy or partial mastectomy) or mastectomy (removal of the breast). You may also need to have lymph nodes near the breast removed. The surgery will also result in a pathology report. This report will contain more details, which can affect your treatment plan. The surgery pathology report is discussed on page 147.

Will I Lose My Breast?

Treatments for breast cancer have changed over time, and breast cancer treatment is more advanced than ever. Newer therapy techniques—including breast-conserving surgeries such as lumpectomy—mean that most women with breast cancer will not need to have their breast removed. They can often choose between breast-conserving surgery (almost always with radiation therapy) and mastectomy. Mastectomies are performed less often than in the past.

A woman's choice of treatment will be influenced by certain aspects of her cancer, her age, the image she has of herself and her body, her hopes and fears, and her current situation in life. For example, some women will select breast-conserving surgery and radiation therapy over mastectomy for cosmetic and body-image reasons. Radiation therapy to the breast is almost always recommended after breast-conserving surgery to help reduce the risk of the cancer coming back in the breast. Sometimes, radiation therapy is recommended even after mastectomy.

On the other hand, some women choose mastectomy (sometimes even choosing to have the unaffected breast removed also) because it gives them more peace of mind, regardless of the effect on their body image. Some women are more concerned about the effects of radiation therapy than body image. Some simply do not want (or are not able) to have daily radiation treatments. Some of these women choose to have breast reconstruction (either immediately or later) to minimize effects on body image.

Although losing a breast can be upsetting at first, you can learn to adjust to the change over time. Many women report that mastectomy did not change their lives to a great degree. Some have said that it is one body part they could learn to live without. Unlike arms, legs, or eyes, breasts are not needed to perform daily tasks or live well.

If you are facing mastectomy, remember that sophisticated breast reconstruction options are open to you if you so choose. Your plastic surgeon can often reconstruct your breast immediately after mastectomy, such that you wake up with the new breast in place. Some women choose to deal with breast reconstruction after their treatment is completed, and still others choose not to have reconstruction at all. These options are discussed later in chapter 15. The important thing to remember about breast reconstruction is that there are various options available to you, and it is your choice whether to pursue them.

Breast-Conserving Surgery

Breast-conserving surgery is sometimes called lumpectomy or partial or segmental mastectomy. In breast-conserving surgery, part of the affected breast is removed. How much is removed depends on the size and location of the tumor and other factors. In a lumpectomy or partial mastectomy, the surgeon removes the tumor and a small rim of normal tissue around it. A quadrantectomy is a less common surgery that removes a larger part of the breast—up to one quarter of it, with or without overlying skin. If cancer cells are found at or close to the margin—the edge of the tissue removed during biopsy or surgery—surgery can usually be done again to remove the remaining cancer and obtain a better margin.

In almost all cases of invasive breast cancer, radiation therapy is given after breast-conserving surgery. If radiation therapy is to be given after surgery, the surgeon may place small metallic clips inside the breast during surgery. These clips are visible on x-rays and are used to mark the area for the radiation treatments.

Some of the possible short-term side effects of breast-conserving surgery include pain, wound infection, temporary swelling, hematoma (accumulation of blood in the wound), and seroma (accumulation of clear fluid in the wound). The larger the portion

Lumpectomy/partial mastectomy

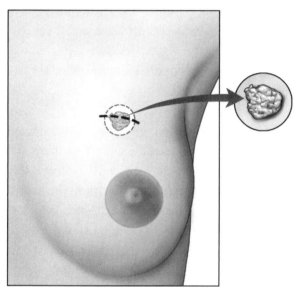 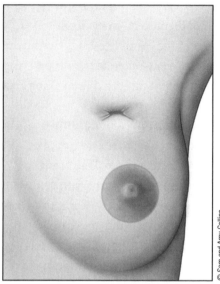

© Sam and Amy Collins

The tumor is removed with a rim of normal breast tissue.

Postoperative appearance depends on the amount of tissue removed, but there will be a small scar and often an indentation in the breast.

of breast tissue removed, the more likely it is that there will be a noticeable change in the shape of the breast afterward. If your breasts look very different in size after surgery, you may be able to have reconstructive surgery or have the unaffected breast reduced in size to make the breasts more alike. Sometimes this procedure can be done during the initial surgery. It is important to talk with your doctor and/or a plastic surgeon before surgery to get an idea of how your breasts are likely to look afterward and to learn what your options might be.

Breast-conserving surgery is an option for most, but not all, women with breast cancer. See the section "Choosing Between Breast-Conserving Surgery and Mastectomy" on page 137 for more information.

Mastectomy

Mastectomy is surgery to remove the entire breast, sometimes along with nearby tissues. There are different types of mastectomies.

Simple (Total) Mastectomy

In a simple, or total, mastectomy, the surgeon removes the entire breast but does not remove any lymph nodes from the underarm or muscle tissue from beneath the breast. Simple mastectomy is used to treat invasive or widespread noninvasive breast cancer. Sometimes both breasts are removed (a double mastectomy), especially as a preventive surgery in women at very high risk for breast cancer. Postoperative appearance is very similar to a modified radical mastectomy (see next page).

Skin-Sparing Mastectomy

A skin-sparing mastectomy is a newer variation of a simple mastectomy. It can be an option for women with smaller tumors who are considering having breast reconstruction at the same time as the surgery to remove the cancer. In a skin-sparing mastectomy, the breast tissue is removed as with simple mastectomy, but most of the skin over the breast (other than the nipple and areola) is left intact. Implants or tissues from other parts of the body are then used to reconstruct the breast. Many women prefer this approach because it usually results in less scar tissue and a reconstructed breast that seems more natural.

Nipple-Sparing Mastectomy

Another newer approach, known as a nipple-sparing mastectomy or areola-sparing mastectomy, may be an option for women who have smaller tumors that are far from the nipple and the skin of the breast. (Cancers that are larger or closer to the nipple are more likely to have cancer cells hidden in the nipple, which means a higher risk the cancer will come back.)

In a nipple-sparing mastectomy, the breast tissue is removed, but the breast skin and nipple and/or areola are left in place. In areola-sparing mastectomy, the nipple and its ducts may be removed while the circle of tissue around it is kept. As with skin-sparing mastectomy, nipple- and areola-sparing procedures require that breast reconstruction be done at the same time as the surgery to remove the cancer. The surgeon often removes the breast tissue beneath the nipple during the procedure to check for cancer cells. If cancer is found, the nipple must be removed. Even when no cancer is found under the nipple, some doctors give the nipple a dose of radiation during or after the surgery to reduce the risk of the cancer coming back, although this is not done everywhere.

Nipple- and areola-sparing procedures are more controversial, however, than some other types of mastectomy, and there are problems with nipple-sparing operations. Even when the nipple can be spared, it typically lacks feeling because the nerves to it have been

Modified radical mastectomy

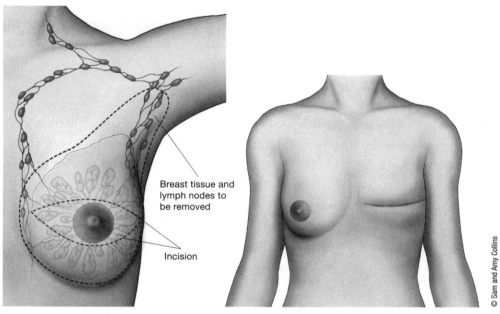

Breast tissue and lymph nodes to be removed

Incision

© Sam and Amy Collins

Postoperative appearance

cut. Afterward, the nipple does not have a good blood supply, so it can sometimes wither away or become deformed. In some cases, the nipple may look out of place later, particularly in women with larger breasts. This surgery leaves less visible scars, but if it is not done properly, it may leave some breast tissue behind. Because of this, some experts consider nipple-sparing surgery too risky to be a standard treatment for now. Doctors are working to try and improve the safety and outcomes of nipple-sparing surgeries.

Saving the nipple from the removed breast to use later (called nipple saving or nipple banking) is no longer favored by most surgeons. The tissue can be injured by the way it is stored or preserved, and there have been other problems with this surgery.

Modified Radical Mastectomy

In a modified radical mastectomy, the surgeon removes the entire breast, the lining over the chest muscles, and some axillary (underarm) lymph nodes. Surgery to remove the lymph nodes is discussed in the section "Lymph Node Surgery" on pages 138–142.

Radical Mastectomy

In a radical mastectomy, the entire breast, the axillary lymph nodes, and the chest wall muscles under the breast are removed. At one time this surgery was quite common, but doctors use it rarely now because modified radical mastectomy and breast-conserving surgeries, combined with such treatments as radiation and chemotherapy, have been shown to be as effective as radical mastectomy.

Possible Side Effects of Mastectomy

Aside from pain and changes to the breast's appearance, possible side effects of mastectomy include infection at the surgery site, hematoma (buildup of blood in the wound), and seroma (buildup of clear fluid in the wound). If axillary lymph nodes are also removed, other side effects can occur.

Radical mastectomy

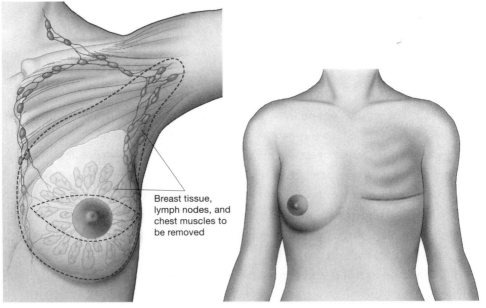

Breast tissue, lymph nodes, and chest muscles to be removed

© Sam and Amy Collins

Because the chest muscles are removed, the ribs are prominent after surgery.

Choosing Between Breast-Conserving Surgery and Mastectomy

Many women with early-stage, localized cancers can choose between breast-conserving surgery and mastectomy. When deciding between breast-conserving surgery and mastectomy, consider the pros and cons of each approach.

The main advantage of breast-conserving surgery is that a woman is able to keep most of her breast. A disadvantage is the usual need for several weeks of radiation therapy after the surgery. However, the need for radiation will depend on the situation: a small number of women who have breast-conserving surgery do not need radiation, whereas some women who have a mastectomy will need it after surgery.

You may have an initial gut preference for mastectomy as a way to get rid of the cancer. But neither option eliminates the possibility that the cancer will come back. In most cases, mastectomy does not give a woman a better chance of long-term survival or a better outcome from treatment.

Most women and their doctors prefer breast-conserving surgery and radiation therapy, but your choice will depend on several factors, including the following:
- how you feel about losing your breast
- how you feel about having radiation therapy
- how far you have to travel and how much time it would take to have radiation therapy
- whether you want to have surgery to reconstruct your breast after a mastectomy
- your preference for mastectomy as a way to "get rid of the cancer as quickly as possible"
- your fear of the cancer coming back

Breast-conserving surgery and radiation therapy may not be appropriate for these patients:
- women who have already had radiation therapy to the affected breast
- women with two or more areas of cancer in the same breast that are too far apart to be removed through one surgical incision without significantly changing the appearance of the breast
- women whose initial lumpectomy and repeat excision(s) have not completely removed the cancer (cancer cells are still seen at or near the surgical margins)
- women with serious connective tissue diseases such as scleroderma or lupus, which might make them especially sensitive to the side effects of radiation therapy
- women who would need to receive radiation therapy during pregnancy

- women with tumors larger than 5 cm (about two inches) across that did not shrink much with neoadjuvant chemotherapy
- women with inflammatory breast cancer
- women with cancers that are large relative to breast size

Other factors may need to be taken into account. For example, young women with breast cancer and known BRCA mutations are at high risk for second breast cancer occurrences. Some women in this situation have the other breast removed to reduce the risk of a second cancer, and so might choose to have the original cancer treated with mastectomy, too.

Questions to Ask Your Medical Team About Breast-Conserving Surgery or Mastectomy

- **What are the risks** and benefits of having lumpectomy or mastectomy?
- **Would one type of surgery** reduce the chances of cancer recurring more than the other?
- **How many lymph nodes,** if any, will be removed?
- **Will I need radiation therapy** or other treatments after surgery?
- **What side effects** should I expect from the surgery? What can be done to help with these side effects? What side effects should I report immediately?
- **Can you show me pictures** of completed procedures for each of the surgical options I'm considering?
- **How would I look after** mastectomy if my breast is not reconstructed?
- **If I choose mastectomy,** what are my reconstruction options?
- **If I choose not to have reconstruction,** what prostheses are options for me?

Lymph Node Surgery

Lymph nodes are small, bean-shaped collections of immune system tissue throughout the body that normally help fight infections. If breast cancer cells break away from the main tumor, they often travel first to nearby lymph nodes, especially those under the arm (the axillary lymph nodes).

It is important for a woman with breast cancer to know whether the cancer has spread to her lymph nodes. This is critical for women with invasive breast cancers, because it helps determine the stage of the cancer, which in turn affects treatment options and outcomes. If the lymph nodes are affected, the cancer cells are more likely to have spread to other parts of her body. Women with ductal carcinoma in situ or lobular carcinoma in situ often do not need lymph node testing, because the risk for spreading is low. If there is extensive ductal carcinoma in situ, lymph nodes may need to be tested.

Surgery to remove some of the underarm lymph nodes for examination under a microscope is the best way to determine whether the cancer has spread to the lymph nodes. But for some women, such as those who are elderly or who have other serious medical conditions, removing the lymph nodes might be considered optional. The lymph nodes under the arm can be removed in two ways: axillary lymph node dissection and sentinel lymph node biopsy.

Axillary Lymph Node Dissection

In an axillary lymph node dissection (ALND), a surgeon will remove between ten and twenty lymph nodes from the armpit (in clusters of lymph nodes, known as anatomic groups). This is usually done at the same time as the mastectomy or breast-conserving surgery, but it may

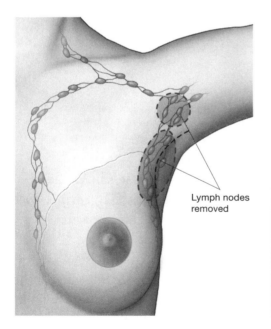

Lymph nodes removed

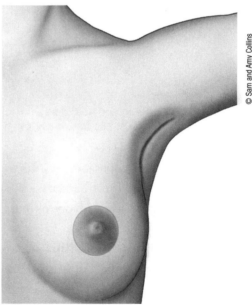

© Sam and Amy Collins

Postoperative appearance

Axillary lymph node dissection

Sentinel lymph node biopsy

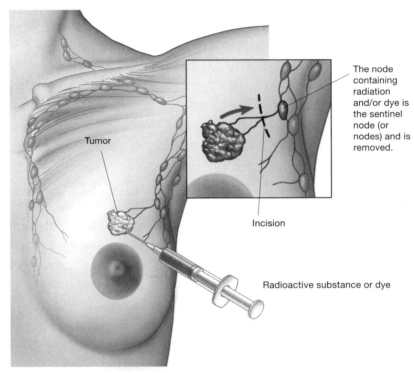

The node containing radiation and/or dye is the sentinel node (or nodes) and is removed.

Tumor

Incision

Radioactive substance or dye

© Sam and Amy Collins

During a sentinel lymph node biopsy, a radioactive substance and/or blue dye is injected into the tumor, near the tumor, or into the area around the nipple. That substance travels to the sentinel node, which is then removed to check for cancer.

be done as a separate operation. ALND was the standard operation to remove underarm lymph nodes for many years, and it is still used often. For example, an ALND may be done if a previous biopsy has shown one or more underarm lymph nodes contain cancer cells.

Sentinel Lymph Node Biopsy

In a sentinel lymph node biopsy (SLNB), the surgeon finds and removes the first lymph node(s) into which a tumor drains. This lymph node, known as the sentinel node, is the one most likely to contain cancer cells if they have spread. An SLNB can show whether cancer has spread to lymph nodes without removing all of them.

To perform this type of biopsy, the surgeon first injects a radioactive substance and/or blue dye into the tumor, the area around it, or the area around the nipple. Lymphatic vessels carry the substances to the sentinel node(s). The doctor then uses a special device to detect radioactivity in the sentinel nodes or to look for lymph nodes that have turned blue. These are separate ways to find the sentinel node but are often done together as a safeguard. The doctor then cuts the skin over the area and removes the node(s) containing the dye (or radiation). These nodes (often two or three) are then examined by the pathologist. Because fewer nodes are removed in an SLNB than in an ALND, each one is studied more closely for cancer.

The sentinel lymph nodes can sometimes be checked for cancer during the biopsy by quickly freezing a section of the node(s) and sending it to the pathologist for examination. Until recently, if the sentinel node(s) examined during biopsy contained cancer cells, the surgeon would then go on to do a full axillary lymph node dissection (ALND). If no cancer cells were seen in the sentinel lymph nodes at the time of surgery, the pathologist would examine them more closely over the next several days. If cancer was found in the sentinel node(s) at that point, the surgeon might recommend full ALND at a later time.

Recent research, however, has shown that full ALND may not be needed in all cases. In some cases, it may be just as safe to leave the remaining lymph nodes behind. This determination is based on such factors as the type of surgery used to remove the tumor, the size of the tumor, and what treatment is planned after surgery. Right now, skipping the ALND may be an option only if the main tumor is fairly small (5 cm across or smaller), the lymph nodes are not enlarged, no more than two sentinel nodes show the presence of cancer, and the woman is having breast-conserving surgery followed by radiation. For women who meet these criteria, doing an ALND after the sentinel node biopsy does not seem to help them live longer, but it does increase the risk of side effects from surgery. This information is still new, however, so if your cancer fits this description, you should talk to your doctor before your surgery.

If there is no cancer in the sentinel node(s), it is very unlikely that the cancer has spread to other lymph nodes, and so no further lymph node surgery is needed. The woman can avoid the potential side effects of a full ALND (see the next page).

Not all women are good candidates for sentinel lymph node biopsy. For example, women who have inflammatory breast cancer should not have a sentinel node biopsy. In addition, doing a sentinel lymph node biopsy requires a great deal of skill. It should be done only by a surgical team that has experience with this technique. If you are thinking about having this type of biopsy, ask your medical team how often they do this procedure.

Possible Side Effects of Lymph Node Surgery

As with other operations, possible side effects of lymph node surgery can include pain, swelling, bleeding, and infection. The main possible long-term effect of removing axillary lymph nodes is lymphedema of the arm. The main symptom of lymphedema is persistent swelling. Excess fluid in the arms normally travels back into the bloodstream through the lymphatic system. Removing the lymph nodes can block the drainage from the arm, causing this fluid to remain and build up.

Up to 30 percent of women who have ALND develop lymphedema. It also occurs in up to 3 percent of women who have SLNB. It can be more common if radiation therapy is given after surgery. Sometimes the swelling lasts for only a few weeks and then goes away. In other cases, the swelling might last a long time. There is no cure for lymphedema. With care, lymphedema can often be avoided or kept under control. More information on lymphedema, including ways to help prevent and manage it, can be found in chapter 13.

You might also have short- or long-term limitations in moving your arm and shoulder after surgery. Your doctor will show you exercises to help ensure that you do not have permanent problems with movement, known as a frozen shoulder. Numbness of the skin of the upper inner arm is another common side effect because the nerve that controls sensation in that area travels through the lymph node area.

After lymph node surgery, some women notice a rope-like structure that begins under the arm and can extend down toward the elbow. Sometimes called axillary web syndrome or lymphatic cording, this problem is more common after an ALND than after SLNB. Symptoms may not appear for weeks or even months after surgery. It can cause pain and limit movement of the arm and shoulder. These symptoms often go away without treatment, though some women find physical therapy helpful.

What to Expect with Surgery

For many, the thought of surgery can be frightening. But with a better understanding of what to expect before, during, and after an operation, many fears can be relieved.

Before Surgery

You will usually meet with your surgeon a few days before the operation to discuss the procedure. This is a good time to ask specific questions about the surgery and review potential risks. Be sure you understand how extensive the surgery is likely to be and what you should expect afterward. If you are thinking about breast reconstruction (covered in detail in chapter 15), this is the best time to begin discussing this, too.

You will be asked to sign a consent form giving the doctor permission to perform the surgery. Take your time and review the form carefully to be certain that you understand what you are signing. Sometimes, doctors send material for you to review before your appointment, so you will have plenty of time to read it and will not feel rushed.

You might be asked to donate blood before surgery if the doctors think you could need a transfusion afterward. This is more likely with certain operations, such as mastectomy combined with natural tissue reconstruction. You might feel more secure knowing that you will receive your own blood if a transfusion is needed. If you do not receive your own blood, it is important to know that in the United States, blood transfusion from another person is nearly as safe as receiving your own blood.

Your doctor will review your medical records and ask you about any medicines you are taking to be sure that you are not taking any medications that could interfere with the surgery. For example, if you are taking aspirin, arthritis medicine, or a blood-thinning drug such as warfarin (Coumadin), you will need to stop taking the drug about a week or two before surgery. Tell your doctor everything you take, including vitamins and herbal supplements; some of these substances—such as vitamin E in high doses—can increase the risk for bleeding. Usually, you will be told not to eat or drink anything for eight to twelve hours before surgery.

You will also meet with the anesthesiologist or nurse anesthetist, the health professional who will be giving you anesthesia during your surgery. The type of anesthesia used depends largely on the kind of surgery being done and your medical history.

Surgery

Depending on the likely extent of your surgery, you could be offered the choice of an outpatient procedure (where you go home the same day) or you might be admitted to the hospital. General anesthesia (where you are asleep) is used for most breast surgery. You will have an intravenous (IV) line put in (usually in a vein in your arm), which the medical team will use to give medicines that might be needed during surgery. Usually, you will be hooked up to an electrocardiogram (EKG) machine and have a blood pressure cuff on your arm, so that your heart rhythm and blood pressure can be monitored during surgery.

The length of the operation depends on the type of surgery. For example, a mastectomy with axillary lymph node dissection will usually take from two to three hours.

Questions to Ask Your Medical Team About Side Effects of Surgery

- **What are the risks** of anesthesia?
- **What are the risks of excessive bleeding** or developing an infection?
- **What are the signs** of an infection after surgery?
- **What is my risk of lymphedema, and what** can I do to lessen my risk?
- **Are there any other serious complications** that can come up during or after this surgery?
- **If I already have an implant, am I at higher** risk for side effects from surgery?

If you choose to have breast reconstruction at the same time as the mastectomy, your surgery will take longer. The chart on pages 314–315 gives more information about reconstructive surgery.

After Surgery

After your surgery, you will be taken to the recovery room, where you will stay until you are awake and your condition and vital signs (blood pressure, pulse, and breathing) are stable. The length of your hospital stay depends on the type of surgery being done, your overall state of health and whether you have other medical problems, how well you do in surgery, and how you feel after surgery. Decisions about the length of your stay should be made by you and your doctor and not dictated by what your insurance company will pay. However, it is important to check your insurance coverage before surgery so that you know what to expect.

In general, women having a mastectomy and/or ALND stay in the hospital for one or two nights and then go home. However, some women are placed in a twenty-three-hour, short-stay observation unit before going home. Less involved operations, such as lumpectomy and sentinel lymph node biopsy, are usually done in an outpatient surgery center, and an overnight stay in the hospital is usually not needed.

How long it takes to recover from surgery varies from person to person and depends on what procedures were done. Most women can return to their regular activities within two weeks after a lumpectomy with ALND, whereas it can take as long as four weeks after a mastectomy. Recovery time is longer if breast reconstruction was done as well, and it can take months to return to full activity after some procedures. Talk to your doctor about what to expect after surgery.

Even after the doctor clears you to return to your regular activities, you may still feel some effects of surgery. You may feel stiff or sore for some time, and the skin on your chest or in the underarm area may feel tight. These feelings tend to improve over time. Most doctors will want you to start moving your arm soon after surgery so that it will not get stiff.

You might have a dressing wrapped snugly around your chest over the surgery site. You also may have one or more drains (plastic or rubber tubes) coming out of the breast or underarm area to remove any blood or lymph fluid that collects during the healing process. Your medical team will teach you how to care for the drains, which may include emptying and measuring the fluid and identifying problems that should be reported to your medical team. Most drains stay in place for one or two weeks. They are typically removed when the drainage has decreased to about 20 to 30 cc (one fluid ounce) a day.

You and your caregivers will probably be given written instructions about care after surgery. These instructions should include the following information:

- how to care for the surgical wound and dressing
- how to monitor drainage and take care of the drains
- how to recognize signs of infection
- when to call the doctor or nurse
- when to begin using your arm and how to do arm exercises to prevent stiffness
- when to resume wearing a bra
- when to begin using a prosthesis and what type to use (after mastectomy)
- what to eat and not eat
- when and how to take any necessary medications, including pain medicines and/or antibiotics
- any restrictions on activity
- what to expect regarding sensations or numbness in the breast and arm
- what to expect regarding your feelings about body image
- when to see your doctor for a follow-up appointment
- how to be referred to a Reach To Recovery volunteer

Make sure that your questions are answered before you are discharged.

Most patients see their surgeon seven to fourteen days after the surgery. Your doctor should explain the results of your pathology report and talk to you about the need for further treatment. If you will need more treatment, you will be referred to a radiation oncologist and/or a medical oncologist. If you are thinking about breast reconstruction, you may be referred to a plastic surgeon as well.

Chronic Pain After Breast Surgery

Some women have problems with nerve pain in the chest wall, armpit, and/or arm after surgery that does not go away over time. This problem is called postmastectomy pain syndrome (PMPS) because it was first described in women who had mastectomies. However, it also occurs after breast-conserving surgery. Studies have shown that between 20 and 30 percent of women develop symptoms of PMPS after surgery. The classic symptoms of PMPS are pain and tingling in the chest wall, armpit, and/or arm. Pain might also be felt in the shoulder or surgical scar. Other common complaints include numbness, shooting or pricking pain, and unbearable itching. Most women with PMPS say their symptoms are not severe.

Postmastectomy pain syndrome is thought to be linked to damage done to the nerves in the armpit and chest during surgery, but the causes are not known definitively. Younger women, those who had a full ALND, and women treated with radiation after surgery are more likely to have problems with PMPS. Because ALND is used less often to treat breast cancer today, PMPS is becoming less of a problem.

Talk to your doctor or nurse about any pain or discomfort you are having. This syndrome can cause you not to use your arm the way you should and, over time, you could lose the ability to use it normally. PMPS can be treated. Whereas opioids and narcotics (medicines commonly used to treat pain) may not work well for nerve pain, other types of medicines and treatments do work for this kind of pain. Talk to your doctor to get the pain control you need. For more information on pain management, please see chapter 13.

Follow-Up After Surgery

Most women see the doctor for a follow-up appointment about seven to fourteen days after surgery. Your doctor should explain the results of your pathology report and talk to you about the need for any further treatment. If you do need more treatment, you might be referred to a radiation oncologist and/or a medical oncologist. If you are

Tips for Wearing a Bra After Surgery

Sometimes women have chest tenderness and swelling after surgery, and wearing a bra might be uncomfortable. It may help to attach an extender to your bra. The extender will make the bra bigger to allow a more comfortable fit. Alternately, you might wear one of your older bras that has stretched a little. Leisure and sleep bras are softer and have less support than regular bras. While you are healing, this might be a good choice for you. They are available in department stores, mastectomy boutiques, and maternity shops.

thinking about breast reconstruction and have not already spoken to a plastic surgeon, you might also be referred to one. For more on breast reconstruction, see chapter 15.

The Surgery Pathology Report

As we discussed in chapter 4, your pathology report contains important information that will help your doctor determine your prognosis and how your treatment should proceed. Your doctor will have received a pathology report from your biopsy. If you also have surgery, however, you will have a pathology report from your operation.

The pathology report from surgery usually contains more information than the biopsy pathology report. This information, such as the size of the tumor and the whether cancer is present in the lymph nodes, can be very useful to your doctors in determining next steps in your treatment. This more detailed level of information helps the pathologist determine the cancer's stage, which is often included in the report. Your cancer's stage is important in predicting prognosis and in determining the need for future treatment. Tests that were performed on the biopsy sample, such as tests for hormone receptor and HER2 status, are also done on the surgical specimen. Sometimes the results are not the same, which can change your treatment plan. For example, sometimes a needle biopsy will not show the presence of hormone receptors (receptors for estrogen or progesterone), but the surgical sample will. This can happen because the needle sampled only one small area of the tumor that did not have hormone receptors. Because the receptors were found in the main tumor removed during surgery, the doctor would then prescribe hormone therapy for the patient after surgery.

If you received treatment (such as chemotherapy, hormone therapy, and/or radiation therapy) before your surgery, the findings from surgery (the size of the tumor and the cancer's final stage) will show how well the cancer responded to that treatment. Cancers that respond well to neoadjuvant treatment (treatment before surgery) are less likely to come back later.

See the sample pathology report from a partial mastectomy with lymph node removal on pages 148–159.

Sample Pathology Report from a Partial Mastectomy
with Lymph Node Removal (with Explanatory Comments)

SURGICAL PATHOLOGY REPORT

Patient: Jane Doe   Specimen # XXXXXX
Hospital #YYYYYY   Obtained on: (date)
Birth date: NN/NN/NNNN (Age: #)   Received on: (date)
Sex: F   Reported on: (date)
Submitted by: Doctor X   Department: Surgery

DIAGNOSIS:
1. LYMPH NODE, RIGHT AXILLARY SENTINEL #1, EXCISION, FS1A:
   - ONE LYMPH NODE NEGATIVE FOR MALIGNANCY (0/1)

2. LYMPH NODE, RIGHT AXILLARY SENTINEL #2, EXCISION, FS2A
   - ONE LYMPH NODE NEGATIVE FOR MALIGNANCY (0/1)

3. LYMPH NODE, RIGHT AXILLARY PALPABLE, EXCISION, FS3A:
   - ONE LYMPH NODE NEGATIVE FOR MALIGNANCY (0/1)

4. LYMPH NODE, RIGHT AXILLARY PALPABLE, EXCISION, FS4A
   - ONE LYMPH NODE NEGATIVE FOR MALIGNANCY (0/1)

5. BREAST, RIGHT, PARTIAL MASTECTOMY:
   - INFILTRATING DUCTAL CARCINOMA, NOTTINGHAM GRADE I, 1.5 CM IN MAXIMUM GROSS DIMENSION
   - DUCTAL CARCINOMA IN SITU, INTERMEDIATE NUCLEAR GRADE, SOLID AND CRIBRIFORM TYPES, COMPRISES APPROXIMATELY 5% OF TUMOR MASS.
   - SURGICAL MARGINS FREE OF MALIGNANCY (CLOSEST MARGIN: 0.8 CM FROM THE LATERAL MARGIN).
   - DEFINITIVE ANGIOLYMPHATIC INVASION IS NOT IDENTIFIED.
   - ADJACENT BREAST TISSUE WITH BIOPSY SITE CHANGES AND FIBROCYSTIC CHANGES.
   - MICROCALCIFICATIONS PRESENT IN BENIGN LOBULES.

6. BREAST, RIGHT INFERIOR MARGIN, EXCISION:
   - BENIGN BREAST TISSUE.
   - NEGATIVE FOR MALIGNANCY.

7. BREAST, RIGHT MEDIAL MARGIN, EXCISION:
   - BENIGN BREAST TISSUE WITH FIBROCYSTIC CHANGES.
   - NEGATIVE FOR MALIGNANCY.

8. BREAST, RIGHT LATERAL MARGIN, EXCISION:
   - BENIGN BREAST TISSUE.
   - NEGATIVE FOR MALIGNANCY.

9. BREAST, RIGHT SUPERIOR MARGIN, EXCISION:
   - BENIGN FIBROADIPOSE TISSUE.
   - NEGATIVE FOR MALIGNANCY.

10. BREAST, RIGHT ANTERIOR MARGIN, EXCISION
   - BENIGN BREAST TISSUE.
   - NEGATIVE FOR MALIGNANCY.
   - MICROCALCIFICATIONS ASSOCIATED WITH BENIGN DUCTS AND LOBULES.

This information is essential in assuring that your report doesn't get confused with that of another patient with a similar or identical name and that it gets delivered to your doctor. Every specimen is given a pathology number, which is often based on the year and the number of the specimen in that year.

This is the most important section of the report—the "bottom line."
#1–4: A total of four lymph nodes were removed: Two sentinel nodes and two lymph nodes that were palpable (enlarged enough that they could be felt). None contained cancer.

#5: This indicates the type of procedure/specimen ("breast, right, partial mastectomy"), the type of cancer ("infiltrating ductal carcinoma"), its grade (I), its size (1.5 cm), and states that the edges of the tissue that was removed are free of cancer ("surgical margins free of malignancy"). Ductal carcinoma in situ (DCIS) was also found, but it took up only a small amount of the tumor (5 percent). Benign breast disease ("fibrocystic changes") was also present

#6–10: These detail the examination of each margin (edge of the specimen), none of which contained cancer.

Sample Pathology Report from a Partial Mastectomy with Lymph Node Removal (with Explanatory Comments) (continued)

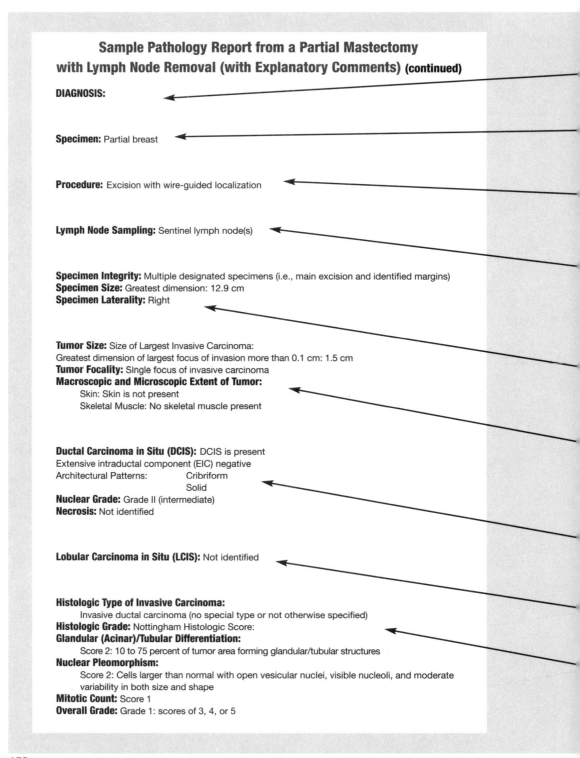

DIAGNOSIS:

Specimen: Partial breast

Procedure: Excision with wire-guided localization

Lymph Node Sampling: Sentinel lymph node(s)

Specimen Integrity: Multiple designated specimens (i.e., main excision and identified margins)
Specimen Size: Greatest dimension: 12.9 cm
Specimen Laterality: Right

Tumor Size: Size of Largest Invasive Carcinoma:
Greatest dimension of largest focus of invasion more than 0.1 cm: 1.5 cm
Tumor Focality: SIngle focus of invasive carcinoma
Macroscopic and Microscopic Extent of Tumor:
    Skin: Skin is not present
    Skeletal Muscle: No skeletal muscle present

Ductal Carcinoma in Situ (DCIS): DCIS is present
Extensive intraductal component (EIC) negative
Architectural Patterns: Cribriform
                               Solid
Nuclear Grade: Grade II (intermediate)
Necrosis: Not identified

Lobular Carcinoma in Situ (LCIS): Not identified

Histologic Type of Invasive Carcinoma:
    Invasive ductal carcinoma (no special type or not otherwise specified)
Histologic Grade: Nottingham Histologic Score:
Glandular (Acinar)/Tubular Differentiation:
    Score 2: 10 to 75 percent of tumor area forming glandular/tubular structures
Nuclear Pleomorphism:
    Score 2: Cells larger than normal with open vesicular nuclei, visible nucleoli, and moderate
    variability in both size and shape
Mitotic Count: Score 1
Overall Grade: Grade 1: scores of 3, 4, or 5

Some pathology laboratories add a summary containing key features of the cancer. Many doctors—and patients—find this useful.

This identifies what type of specimen was obtained and examined.

This explains what procedure was used. In this case, the correct area to remove was determined by a wire that had been placed in the tumor before surgery ("excision with wire-guided localization").

This indicates that some lymph nodes were removed by a sentinel lymph node biopsy, as opposed to removing all of the underarm lymph nodes (a full axillary dissection).

This gives details about the breast tissue submitted to pathology, including how large the tissue specimen is and that it came from the right breast.

This gives details about the cancer/tumor, including the size of the invasive part (1.5 cm), that only one cancer was present, and that the cancer was not growing into skin or muscle.

This gives details about the DCIS that was present.

This indicates that Lobular Carcinoma in Situ (LCIS) was not present.

More details are given about the type of invasive cancer found ["Invasive ductal carcinoma (no special type or not otherwise specified)"] and its grade.

Sample Pathology Report from a Partial Mastectomy
with Lymph Node Removal (with Explanatory Comments) (continued)

SURGICAL PATHOLOGY REPORT

Margins:
Margins uninvolved by invasive carcinoma
Distance from closest margin: Greater than 8.0 mm
Margins uninvolved by DCIS (if present)
Distance from closest margin: Greater than 8.0 mm

Treatment Effect: Response to Presurgical (Neoadjuvant) Therapy: In the breast:
No known presurgical therapy

Lymph-Vascular Invasion
Not identified
Dermal Lymph-Vascular Invasion: No skin present

Lymph Nodes: Number of sentinel lymph nodes examined: 2
Total number of lymph nodes examined (sentinel and nonsentinel): 4
   • Number of lymph nodes with macrometastases (> 0.2 cm): 0
   • Number of lymph nodes with micrometastases (>0.2 mm to 0.2 cm and/or > 200 cells): 0
   • Number of lymph nodes with isolated tumor cells (≤ 0.2 mm and ≤ 200 cells): 0

Pathologic Staging:
   Primary Tumor: pT1c: Tumor > 10 mm but ≤ 20 mm in greatest dimension
   Regional Lymph Nodes: pN0: No regional lymph node metastasis identified histologically
   Distant Metastasis: Not applicable

SPECIMEN:
1. Sentinel lymph node #1, right axilla.
2. Sentinel lymph node #2, right axilla.
3. Palpable lymph node, right axilla.
4. Palpable lymph node, right axilla.
5. Right breast partial mastectomy; one short suture, superior;
   one long suture, lateral.
6. Inferior margin, right breast.
7. Medial margin, right breast.
8. Lateral margin, right breast.
9. Superior margin, right breast.
10. Anterior margin, right breast.

CLINICAL HISTORY/OPERATIVE FINDINGS:
Right wire-directed partial mastectomy, right axillary sentinel lymph node biopsy, right breast cancer.

This comment indicates how close the cancer cells are to the various margins (edges of the tissue removed). If cancer cells are present at the margin, the surgeon will often remove additional tissue. Knowing which margins were positive or how close the cancer cells are to the margins helps the surgeon plan this reexcision. In some cases, the pathologist will add other information in this section. In this case, the margins did not contain cancer cells, and the distance from the cancer/tumor to the edges was at least 8 mm. This is good news—it appears that all of the cancer was removed, so no further surgery would be needed.

The patient didn't receive treatment to try to shrink the cancer before surgery (neoadjuvant therapy).

The cancer is not growing into blood or lymph vessels or the skin.

A total of four lymph nodes were removed and examined; none contained deposits of cancer cells.

This gives details of the pathological stage. The tumor is 1.5 cm (or 15 mm), making it a T1c. The lymph nodes did not contain cancer cells, making them N0. "Distant Metastasis: Not applicable" means that no areas of possible cancer spread were biopsied.

Each specimen (piece of tissue removed) is described and given a number.

This information helps the pathologist and surgeon consider the microscopic findings in the context of your medical situation.

Sample Pathology Report from a Partial Mastectomy
with Lymph Node Removal (with Explanatory Comments) (continued)

GROSS DESCRIPTION:

Ten specimens are received, each labeled with the patient's name and medical record number.

Specimen #1 is received fresh for intraoperative consultation and is labeled "sentinel lymph node #1, right axilla." It consists of a single lymph node measuring 2.5 × 1.5 × 1.0 cm. The lymph node is submitted entirely for frozen section diagnosis in cassette "FS1A."

Specimen #2 is received fresh for intraoperative consultation and is labeled "sentinel lymph node #2, right axilla" and consists of a single portion of soft tissue measuring 2.0 × 1.5 × 1.0 cm. A single lymph node is grossly identified and submitted entirely for frozen section diagnosis in cassette "FS2A."

Specimen #3 is received fresh for intraoperative consultation and is labeled "palpable lymph node, right axilla #1" and consists of a single lymph node measuring 2.5 × 0.8 × 0.6 cm. The lymph node is submitted entirely for frozen section diagnosis in cassette "FS3A."

Specimen #4 is received fresh for intraoperative consultation and is labeled "palpable lymph node, right axilla #2," and consists of a single portion of soft tissue measuring 3.0 × 1.0 × 0.5 cm. A lymph node is identified and submitted entirely for frozen section diagnosis in cassette "FS4A."

Specimen #5 is received fresh in a radiograph container and is labeled with the patient's name and medical record number as "right breast, partial mastectomy; one short suture, superior; one long suture, lateral." The specimen consists of a portion of fibroadipose breast tissue measuring 12.9 × 11.1 × 2.6 cm and weighing 170.1 grams. Two sutures and a radiograph guidewire are present in the specimen for orientation. Within the center of the specimen, near the area delineated by the guidewire, there is a firm fibrotic mass with ill-defined margins measuring 1.5 × 1.3 × 0.9 cm. This mass extends to within 1.0 cm of the anterior edge, 1.2 cm of the superior edge, 1.5 cm of the lateral edge, and 1.9 cm of the inferior edge. At least 2.0 cm of uninvolved tissue exists between the mass and all other edges. The specimen is inked as follows: superior edge, orange; inferior, yellow; anterior, red; medial, green; lateral, blue; deep margin, black. Representative sections are submitted as stated below.

Specimen #6 is received in formalin in a container labeled with the patient's name and medical record number and as "inferior margin, right breast." The specimen consists of a portion of fibroadipose breast tissue measuring 3.1 × 2.4 × 1.0 cm. A suture is present for orientation of the specimen. No lesions are identified in the specimen. The surgical resection margin is inked blue. The specimen is serially sectioned and entirely submitted in cassettes "7A" through "7C."

Specimen #7 is received in formalin in a container labeled with the patient's name and medical record number and as "medial margin, right breast." The specimen consists of a portion of fibroadipose breast tissue measuring 4.4 × 4.1 × 1.6 cm. A suture is present for orientation of the specimen. There is a multiloculated cystic structure filled with inspissated clear fluid measuring 2.1 × 1.0 × 1.0 cm. This structure extends to the surgical resection margin. The surgical resection margin is inked blue. The specimen is serially sectioned and entirely submitted in cassettes "8A" through "8G."

Specimen #8 is received in formalin in a container labeled with the patient's name and medical record number and as "lateral margin, right breast." The specimen consists of a portion of fibroadipose breast tissue measuring 2.6 × 2.0 × 1.6 cm. A suture is present for orientation of the specimen. No discrete masses are present within the specimen. The surgical resection margin is inked blue. The specimen is serially sectioned and entirely submitted in cassettes "9A" through "9C."

Specimen #9 is received in formalin in a container labeled with the patient's name and medical record number and as "superior margin, right breast." The specimen consists of a portion of fibroadipose breast tissue measuring 4.1 × 2.9 × 1.5 cm. No discrete masses are identified in the specimen. The surgical resection margin is inked blue. The specimen is serially sectioned and entirely submitted in cassettes "10A" through "10D."

Specimen #10 is received in formalin in a container labeled with the patient's name and medical record number and as "anterior margin, right breast." The specimen consists of a portion of fibroadipose breast tissue measuring 3.6 × 3.0 × 1.3 cm. A suture is present in the specimen for orientation. No discrete masses are identified in the specimen. The surgical resection margin is inked blue. The specimen is serially sectioned and entirely submitted in cassettes "11A" through "11D."

This gives more detail about the specimens that were submitted, how they looked to the naked eye, and how they were processed for examination under the microscope. The first four were lymph nodes.

The fifth specimen is the breast tissue removed (from the partial mastectomy). The dimensions of the specimen are given using the metric system (one inch is about 2.5 cm). The weight is also given. This specimen contains a guidewire with the end near the tumor. This was placed before surgery to help the doctor know the correct area to remove. The size of the tumor is given. The surgeon placed stitches (sutures) on the tissue so that the pathologist would know which are the superior (top) and lateral (toward the side) margins (edges) of the specimen. The pathologist marked the edges with different colors of ink that can be seen under the microscope to determine how close the cancer cells are to each edge of the sample. Each edge corresponds to a different color marking. This specimen (#5) was sectioned (pieces were removed) so that each margin could be examined under the microscope. These sections were numbered 6 through 10.

Sample Pathology Report from a Partial Mastectomy with Lymph Node Removal (with Explanatory Comments) (continued)

CODE OF MICROSCOPIC SECTIONS:
FS1A: One lymph node, bisected
FS2A: One lymph node, whole
FS3A: One lymph node, bisected
FS4A: One lymph node, bisected
6A: Representative superior deep margin
6B–D: Representative specimen superior and deep
6E: Area immediately superior to mass
6F: Mass and superoanterior edge
6G: Mass and lateral edge
6H: Representative mass
6I: Area immediately inferior to mass
6J: Area immediately anterior to mass
6K: Representative anteroinferior specimen

INTRAOPERATIVE CONSULTATION:
FS1A: SENTINEL LYMPH NODE #1, RIGHT AXILLA (FROZEN SECTION): NEGATIVE. Frozen section results were communicated to the surgical team and were repeated back by Dr. X on DATE at 2:55 p.m.

FS2A: SENTINEL LYMPH NODE #2, RIGHT AXILLA (FROZEN SECTION): NEGATIVE. Frozen section results were communicated to the surgical team and were repeated back by Dr. X on DATE at 2:55 p.m.

FS3A: PALPABLE LYMPH NODE, RIGHT AXILLA (FROZEN SECTION): NEGATIVE. Frozen section results were communicated to the surgical team and were repeated back by Dr. X on DATE at 2:55 p.m.

FS4A: PALPABLE LYMPH NODE, RIGHT AXILLA (FROZEN SECTION): NEGATIVE. Frozen section results were communicated to the surgical team and were repeated back by Dr. X on DATE at 2:55 p.m.

MICROSCOPIC DESCRIPTION:
Microscopic examination performed.

SPECIAL STAINS:
ERQ (88360)	DONE
PRQ (88360)	DONE
HERCEPQ (88360)	DONE
MIB1Q (88360)	DONE

SPECIAL PROCEDURES

BLOCK:
6H
SPECIMEN TYPE:
Fixed paraffin sections.

ESTROGEN RECEPTOR / PROGESTERONE RECEPTOR
Cancer Prognostic Panel
Immunohistochemistry with ChromaVision ACIS
Quantitation Image Analysis

Test Name Assay Type	Staining Intensity Average	Percent Positive (%)	Result
Estrogen Receptor	3+	97	Positive
Progesterone Receptor	3+	93	Positive
HER2	1.9		Equivocal/2+ (FISH ordered)
Ki-67 (MIB-1)	3+	7	Low

Each piece of tissue that was examined was given a code (consisting of numbers and letters) that will be used to refer to that piece of tissue later in the report.

The lymph nodes were examined by the pathologist while the surgery was still going on ('intraoperative consultation"). All were negative.

If the appearance of this cancer under the microscope was in any way unusual, the pathologist would have added a description of its appearance here. Some pathologists briefly describe all cancers. Others describe only the unusual ones. If the pathologist does not add a description, the laboratory computer system automatically adds, "Microscopic examination performed" to confirm that the pathologist checked the sample under the microscope.

This lists the special stains used to examine the tissue. The results are listed separately.

This section lists the results of the special stains. The tumor is positive for estrogen and progesterone receptors. The immunohistochemistry (IHC) test for HER2 showed 2+, which is "equivocal" (not definite either way). As a result, a FISH test for HER2 will be done. A Ki-67 test also was done, which estimates how fast the cancer cells are dividing. If it is high (> 20 percent), it means that the cancer cells are dividing more rapidly, a sign of a more aggressive cancer.

Sample Pathology Report from a Partial Mastectomy
with Lymph Node Removal (with Explanatory Comments) (continued)

REFERENCE RANGES

Test Name	NEGATIVE/ LOW	EQUIVOCAL/ INTERMEDIATE	POSITIVE/HIGH
Estrogen Receptor	< 1%		≥ 1%
Progesterone Receptor	< 1%		≥ 1%
HER2	< 1.8 (1+)	1.8 – 2.1 (2+)	> 2.2 (3+)
Ki-67	< 10%	10% – 20%	> 20%
p53	< 10%		≥ 10%

ER: DAKO ID5, ENVISION +, ANTIGEN RETRIEVAL
PR: DAKO PgR 636, ENVISION +, ANTIGEN RETRIEVAL
HER2: HERCEPTEST, DAKO CYTOMATION, FDA APPROVED
Ki-67: DAKO, MIB-1, ENVISION +, ANTIGEN RETRIEVAL
P53: DAKO, DO-7, ENVISION +, ANTIGEN RETRIEVAL

COMMENT:

Formalin-fixed, deparaffinized sections were incubated with the above panel of monoclonal and/or polyclonal antibodies. Localization is via an avidin biotin, streptavidin biotin, or peroxidase labeled polymer immunoperoxidase method, with or without the use of heat-induced epitope-retrieval techniques. Positive and negative control slides were reviewed and showed appropriate results.

The results of these tests should not be used alone as the sole basis for diagnosis and/or treatment. The results may prove useful when used in conjunction with other diagnostic procedures and clinical evaluations. Use of these results, in this manner, can be considered to fall within the scope of the practice of medicine.

A list of reference ranges for the special stains is given below the results. This lets you see the criteria for what is considered "positive" or high for each test.

The names of each specific assay are listed, often including the name of the company making the test. This is followed by a description of the specific procedures followed to do the special stains.

CHAPTER 9

Other Treatments for Breast Cancer

Surgery is part of the treatment for most women with breast cancer, but it is usually not the only treatment needed—many other types of treatment might be used, too. Depending on the stage of the cancer and other factors, these other treatments might be used along with or instead of surgery. They might also be used alone or in different combinations.

For example, women who have no detectable cancer after surgery are often given adjuvant therapy to try to kill any breast cancer cells that might have been left behind. Adjuvant refers to any treatment given after surgery. This might be in the form of radiation therapy, chemotherapy, hormone therapy, targeted therapy, or some combination of these. Not every patient needs adjuvant therapy, but if the cancer is large or has spread to nearby lymph nodes, adjuvant therapy is more likely to be helpful.

Some patients receive treatment (such as chemotherapy or hormone therapy) before surgery to try to shrink the tumor. This type of treatment is called neoadjuvant therapy. This approach might allow some women with more advanced tumors to become candidates for surgery or allow women who would otherwise need a mastectomy to have breast-conserving surgery instead.

This chapter gives an overview of the types of treatment that may be used for your cancer: radiation therapy, chemotherapy, hormone therapy, targeted therapy, and drugs to protect the bones. This chapter also briefly lists the side effects associated with each type of treatment. Side effects and how to manage them are discussed in more detail in chapter 13. Recommendations about treatment based on the stage and type of cancer (as well as for women who are pregnant) are discussed in the next chapter, "Treatment Options Based on Your Situation."

Radiation Therapy

Radiation therapy uses special equipment to deliver high doses of radiation to cancerous cells, killing or damaging them so they cannot grow, multiply, or spread. Radiation is usually used to destroy cancer cells left behind in the breast, chest wall, or lymph nodes after surgery. It can also be used to help relieve pain or other symptoms if the cancer has spread to other parts of the body. Unlike chemotherapy, which exposes the entire body to cancer-fighting chemicals, radiation therapy targets only the tumor and the surrounding area, so it is sometimes called a local treatment.

External Beam Radiation Therapy

External beam radiation is the most widely used type of radiation therapy. The radiation is focused from a source outside the body onto the area affected by the cancer. The extent of radiation depends on whether lumpectomy or mastectomy was done and whether lymph nodes are involved. If lumpectomy was done, most often the entire breast gets radiation, and an extra boost of radiation is often given to the area in the breast where the cancer was removed to help prevent it from coming back in that area. Depending on the size and extent of the cancer, radiation also might include the chest wall and the lymph nodes under the arm.

When given after surgery, external radiation therapy is usually not started until the tissues have had a chance to heal, often a month or longer. If chemotherapy will also be given, radiation therapy is usually delayed until chemotherapy is complete. External beam radiation therapy is much like getting an x-ray, but the radiation is more intense. The procedure itself is painless. Each treatment lasts only a few minutes, but the setup time—getting you into place for treatment—usually takes longer.

Before your treatments start, the radiation team will take careful measurements to determine the correct angles for aiming the radiation beams and the proper dose of radiation. They will make some ink marks or small tattoos on your skin that they will use later as a guide to focus the radiation on the right area. You might want to talk to your medical team to find out how long these marks will last. Lotions, powders, deodorants, and antiperspirants can interfere with external beam radiation therapy, so you may be told not to use them until treatments are complete.

Radiation treatments are usually given five days a week (Monday through Friday) for about five to six weeks. But this might not be convenient or even possible for some women. Some doctors now give slightly larger daily doses over only three weeks. This approach, which is known as accelerated breast irradiation (because it is given over a shorter period of time), seems to be just as effective.

Newer Approaches to External Beam Radiation Therapy

Newer approaches being studied give radiation over even shorter periods, but it is not yet clear whether these are as good as longer courses of treatment. In one approach, larger doses of radiation are given each day (or even twice a day), and the course of radiation is shortened to only five days. The radiation may be given to the whole breast, or it may be directed only at the site of the tumor (known as accelerated partial breast irradiation).

> ### Questions to Ask Your Medical Team About Radiation Therapy
>
> - **What are the chances** that radiation therapy will achieve the result we want?
> - **If I chose radiation therapy,** how long would it last? Could I travel during the treatment period?
> - **Can the radiation therapy** be given over a shorter period of time and still be as effective?
> - **What side effects should I expect?** When should I expect them? Is there anything that can help reduce side effects?
> - **Am I at risk for lymphedema?** Can I do anything to lessen my risk?
> - **Will any of the side effects** temporarily or permanently change my appearance?
> - **Does radiation therapy increase my chances** of another cancer developing?
> - **Will the rest of my body be protected** while I'm receiving radiation?

Intraoperative radiation therapy (IORT) is another form of accelerated partial breast irradiation under investigation. In this approach, a single large dose of radiation is given in the operating room right after lumpectomy before the breast incision is closed.

Brachytherapy (Internal Radiation Therapy)

Brachytherapy is another way to deliver radiation therapy. Instead of aiming radiation beams from outside the body, radioactive "seeds," or pellets, are placed directly into the breast tissue for a short time near where the cancer was located. It is often used as a way to boost the radiation delivered to the tumor site (along with external radiation to the whole breast). It can be used by itself, too, in which case it is considered a form of accelerated partial breast irradiation. Tumor size, location, and other factors might limit who can get brachytherapy. For example, it may not be a good option for some women whose tumors are close to the skin or to the chest wall.

Intracavitary Brachytherapy

Intracavitary brachytherapy is the most common way to give brachytherapy in women with breast cancer. A source of radiation is put into the space left by lumpectomy for a short time and then removed. There are several different devices that can be used to administer intracavitary brachytherapy: MammoSite, SAVI, Axxent, and Contura. These devices all go into the breast as a small catheter (tube). The end of the device inside the breast is then expanded so that it stays securely in place for the entire treatment. The other end of the catheter sticks out of the breast. For each treatment, a source of radiation (often pellets) is placed down through the tube and into the device for a short time and then removed. Treatment is given twice a day for five days as an outpatient procedure. After the last treatment, the device is collapsed and removed from the breast.

Interstitial Brachytherapy

In interstitial brachytherapy, several small, hollow catheters are inserted into the breast around the area of the lumpectomy and are left in place for several days. Radioactive pellets are inserted into the catheters for short periods each day and then removed. This method of brachytherapy has been around longer (and has more evidence to support it) than intracavitary brachytherapy, but it is not used as much anymore.

Possible Side Effects of Radiation Therapy

The ability to target radiation therapy accurately has increased dramatically over past decades, which has greatly reduced the resulting side effects. Radiation therapy is a painless procedure, but it can cause side effects. You should know about these potential side effects when choosing your treatment. See chapter 13 for more information about managing these side effects.

Fatigue

Fatigue is more than just tiredness. It is a bone-weary exhaustion that does not get better with rest. You might begin to feel tired during or after radiation therapy, and your fatigue might increase as treatment progresses. This tiredness and weakness will go away gradually after your treatment is finished.

Changes in the Skin and Breast

Radiation therapy after lumpectomy can cause swelling and redness in the treated breast. The redness will fade, leaving your skin slightly darker, just as a sunburn fades to a suntan. These changes to the breast tissue and skin usually go away in six to twelve months.

Accelerated Partial Breast Irradiation—Is It Better?

Studies have clearly shown that adding radiation therapy after breast-conserving surgery reduces the risk that the cancer will come back in the breast and helps women live longer. These studies were done with standard courses of external radiation therapy given to the whole breast over several weeks. But standard external radiation therapy can have drawbacks. It can cause side effects, including changes in the way the breast looks and feels. It can also be time-consuming and inconvenient for many women.

Newer types of accelerated partial breast irradiation, such as intraoperative radiation therapy (IORT) and intracavitary brachytherapy (MammoSite, SAVI, Axxent, and Contura), might help overcome some of these problems. First, they are given over shorter periods: IORT is given as a one-time treatment at the time of lumpectomy, whereas intracavitary brachytherapy is given in treatments over five days. In addition, the radiation is focused on the site of the lumpectomy and nearby tissues, as opposed to irradiating the whole breast, which might cut down on side effects.

Some doctors are offering these newer approaches to treatment (currently intracavitary brachytherapy is used more than IORT), but it is not yet clear whether they are as effective as standard external radiation therapy to the whole breast, especially over the long term. Early results suggest they seem to be about as good as standard radiation at keeping the cancer from recurring at the site of lumpectomy for the first few years after treatment. But long-term results are not yet available, and it is not yet clear whether irradiating only the area around the cancer will reduce the chances of recurrence as much as radiation to the whole breast. The results of studies being done now will probably be needed before more doctors recommend accelerated partial breast irradiation as a standard treatment option.

A large study comparing accelerated partial breast irradiation to standard external radiation therapy is under way, but the results may not be available for several years. In the meantime, women considering these options should have open, honest discussions with their doctors about what is known and not known about these treatments right now.

The pores in the skin of your breast might be enlarged and more noticeable after radiation therapy. Some women report increased sensitivity of the skin on the breast, and others report decreased feeling. The skin and the fatty tissue of the breast might feel thicker and firmer than before radiation treatment.

Sometimes the size of your breast changes—it might become larger because of fluid buildup or smaller because of the development of scar tissue. Many women have little or no change in breast size.

Most changes to the breast resulting from radiation therapy happen within ten to twelve months of completing therapy. If you see changes in breast size, shape, appearance, or texture after this time, tell your doctor right away.

Numbness or Weakness in the Shoulder or Arm

Radiation to the breast can sometimes damage some of the nerves to the arm. This condition is called brachial plexopathy, and it can lead to numbness, pain, and weakness in the shoulder, arm, and hand.

Lymphedema

Lymphedema is a buildup of lymph fluid. Generally, the fluid buildup occurs in the arm and is caused by damage to the underarm lymph nodes. It typically affects women who have had their lymph nodes removed, but it can also affect women whose lymph nodes have received radiation therapy. The fluid buildup can also occur in the breast area. It occurs more in women who have breast-conserving surgery and chest wall radiation. See pages 276–285 for more information on preventing and controlling lymphedema.

Low White Blood Cell and Platelet Counts

Radiation therapy can sometimes cause low levels of white blood cells and platelets (the blood cells that normally help your body fight infection and prevent bleeding). However, this is more likely with radiation to areas such as the pelvis. This side effect is unlikely with breast radiation.

Loss of Appetite

Although not common, breast radiation can cause problems with eating and digestion. You might lose interest in food during your treatment. Some people report feeling nauseated.

Questions to Ask Your Medical Team About Side Effects of Radiation Therapy

- How long will I be at risk for side effects from radiation therapy?
- How do I deal with the immediate side effects of radiation?
- What can be done to lessen the side effects?
- What kinds of side effects can radiation have internally?
- Do I increase my risk for other cancers by undergoing radiation?
- How will I know if I'm having a harmful reaction to radiation?
- Will I lose my appetite while I'm undergoing radiation?
- Will my breasts change size? Is there any way of predicting how radiation will affect my breast size?
- Is there anything I can do to reduce pain and swelling from treatment?
- How should I care for my skin during and after radiation therapy?
- How painful will the skin irritation be?

Effects on Sexual Relations

Although most women receiving breast radiation do not report changes in their sexual relations, you might notice a decrease in your level of desire while you are undergoing treatment. Radiation to the breast does not physically decrease a woman's sexual desire, nor does this treatment reduce her ability to produce vaginal lubrication, have normal genital sensitivity, or reach orgasm. However, many women undergoing breast cancer treatment have a loss of sexual desire because of worry, depression, fatigue, nausea, or pain. Emotions or distracting thoughts might keep you from feeling excited and can interfere with your desire for sex.

Effects on Fertility

Technicians will shield your pelvic region during radiation treatments to prevent harm to your ovaries, so treatments should not affect fertility. Radiation therapy is usually not given to pregnant women because it can harm the fetus.

Damage to Nearby Ribs or Other Organs

In rare cases, radiation therapy can weaken the ribs, which could lead to a fracture. In the past, parts of the lungs and heart were more likely to receive some radiation in the course of treatment, which could lead to long-term damage of these organs. However, modern radiation equipment allows doctors to better focus the radiation beams, so these problems are rare today.

Second Cancers

In some very rare instances, radiation therapy can cause a second cancer to occur years later. Rare cancers called angiosarcomas can develop eight to ten years after radiation treatment for breast cancer. These cancers appear as bluish or reddish nodules on the treated breast, usually within the area treated by radiation therapy.

Chemotherapy

Chemotherapy is treatment that uses cytotoxic (cell-killing) drugs to destroy cancer cells. These drugs are usually given intravenously, as an injection, or in pill form (though this is less common). The drugs then travel through the bloodstream and move throughout the entire body.

The Purpose of Chemotherapy

Chemotherapy can be used in different ways according to your situation. For example, if you have a lumpectomy or mastectomy to remove cancer in your breast, your doctor might recommend adjuvant chemotherapy after surgery. As a tumor grows, it can release cancer cells into your bloodstream or lymphatic system. These cells then travel throughout your body. Adjuvant chemotherapy is used to try to kill any cells that have broken away from the original tumor, in order to reduce the chance that the cancer will return.

If you have a large breast tumor, your doctor might recommend trying neoadjuvant chemotherapy before surgery to shrink the tumor. This might make surgery easier or allow for a less extensive operation (such as a lumpectomy instead of a mastectomy). It may also help the doctors determine whether the tumor is likely to respond to the recommended treatment later on.

For women whose breast cancer has already spread outside the breast and underarm area at the time of diagnosis, or if it has spread after initial treatments, chemotherapy might be the main type of treatment. The length of treatment will depend on whether the cancer shrinks, how much it shrinks, and how well the woman tolerates treatment.

Preconceived Notions About Chemotherapy

Chemotherapy is one of the most powerful weapons the medical community has to fight cancer. Many people associate cancer treatment with chemotherapy and have preconceived ideas and fears about this therapy. It is true that chemotherapy, like most other cancer treatments, can cause side effects. But each person's response to chemotherapy is different. Try to keep an open mind. Chemotherapy is typically given in a doctor's office, a clinic, or in the outpatient section of a hospital. Some people might be surprised to find that upon walking into a chemotherapy clinic, they would most likely see people sitting in lounge chairs reading books or watching TV. Aside from the IV lines in patients' arms, there might be few signs they are getting treatment.

This is not to say that everyone has an easy time with chemotherapy—these are powerful medicines that can cause problems for some people. But there are medicines to lessen some of their side effects, such as nausea and vomiting, and these medicines have improved greatly over the years. This has helped make treatment more tolerable than it was in the past.

How Chemotherapy Works

Chemotherapy drugs work by interfering with a cell's process of growth and division. Normal cells tend to grow slowly, and when they have outlived their usefulness, they die. The problem with cancer cells is that they grow and divide very rapidly, and they do not die when they're supposed to. Chemotherapy drugs attack cells that are dividing rapidly. As with radiation therapy, chemotherapy affects both normal and cancerous cells. However, cancer cells are not as good as normal cells at repairing themselves, so they are more likely to be affected by chemotherapy drugs.

Chemotherapy Options

Chemotherapy is given in cycles in order to give the body a chance to recover from some of the effects of treatment. Each cycle consists of one or more days of treatment, followed by a number of days without treatment. The chemotherapy drugs are then started again to begin the next cycle.

The length of the chemotherapy cycle varies according to the specific drug or combination of drugs but is generally two or three weeks. Some cycles are given closer together. Chemotherapy generally continues for a total of three to six months when given as adjuvant therapy, depending on the drugs used. Treatment might last longer for advanced breast cancer, based on how well the treatment is working and what side effects the patient has.

In most cases, chemotherapy is given in combinations of two or three drugs. Many combinations may be used, based on the woman's situation and the preferences of the doctor, but it is not clear that any single combination is clearly the best. Clinical studies continue to compare today's most effective treatments against new combinations that might be better.

Chemotherapy Drugs

These are the chemotherapy drugs most commonly used to treat breast cancer:
- albumin-bound paclitaxel (Abraxane)
- capecitabine (Xeloda)
- cisplatin (Platinol)
- cyclophosphamide (Cytoxan)
- docetaxel (Taxotere)
- doxorubicin (Adriamycin)
- epirubicin (Ellence)
- eribulin (Halaven)
- 5-fluorouracil (5-FU, Fluorouracil, Adrucil)
- ixabepilone (Ixempra)
- liposomal doxorubicin (Doxil)
- methotrexate (Amethopterin, Mexate, Folex)
- mitoxantrone (Novantrone)
- paclitaxel (Taxol)
- vinorelbine (Navelbine)

Many combinations of drugs may be used for adjuvant chemotherapy. These are some of the most common chemotherapy drug combinations*:
- CMF: cyclophosphamide, methotrexate, and 5-fluorouracil
- CAF (or FAC): cyclophosphamide, doxorubicin, and 5-fluorouracil
- EC: epirubicin and cyclophosphamide
- TAC: docetaxel, doxorubicin, and cyclophosphamide
- AC → T: doxorubicin and cyclophosphamide followed by paclitaxel or docetaxel

*Abbreviations of chemotherapy regimens are based on combinations of brand and generic drug names.

- CEF (FEC): cyclophosphamide, epirubicin, and 5-fluorouracil (this may be followed by docetaxel)
- TC: docetaxel and cyclophosphamide
- TCH: docetaxel, carboplatin, and trastuzumab (Herceptin) for HER2/neu positive tumors

Often single drugs are used to treat metastatic breast cancer, such as vinorelbine, paclitaxel (and albumin bound paclitaxel), capecitabine, eribulin, and ixabepilone. Some combinations are also used, such as these:

- gemcitabine plus either cisplatin or carboplatin
- docetaxel with capecitabine
- gemcitabine with paclitaxel
- capecitabine with ixabepilone

Targeted therapy drugs, such as trastuzumab (Herceptin) or lapatinib (Tykerb), might be used with some of these chemotherapy drug combinations for tumors that are HER2-positive. All of these drugs are given intravenously, with the exception of capecitabine, which is given as a pill. Targeted therapy drugs are discussed later on pages 188–192.

How Chemotherapy Is Given

In treating breast cancer, some chemotherapy drugs are given by mouth, but most are given into a catheter that is placed in a vein (intravenously or IV). IV chemotherapy can be given in one of three ways:

> ### "Dose-Dense" Chemotherapy
>
> For adjuvant chemotherapy, doctors have found that giving the cycles closer together might lower the chance that the cancer will come back and improve survival in some women. This approach is known as "dose-dense" chemotherapy. For example, chemotherapy that would normally be given every three weeks is given every two weeks instead. The main problem with this approach is that it can lead to more side effects, such as low white blood cell counts. Doctors give a type of drug known as a growth factor after chemotherapy to bring the white blood cell count back to normal in time for the next cycle. Because this approach can lead to more side effects and can be harder to take, it is usually reserved for treating women with a higher chance of cancer recurrence.

- IV push: The drugs are injected into the catheter quickly from a syringe over the course of a few minutes.
- IV infusion: A mixed drug solution flows from a plastic bag through tubing that is attached to the catheter over a longer period of time—from ten minutes to a few hours. The flow is often controlled by a machine called an IV pump.

- Continuous infusion: The drug solution is given over a day or more, allowing small amounts of medicine to be given over a prolonged period. Continuous infusions are rare in the treatment of breast cancer. They are always controlled by electronic IV pumps. Continuous infusions can be given in the hospital, but there may also be the option of giving the chemotherapy with the use of an ambulatory infusion pump. This is a small pump that you carry (on a strap over your shoulder or hooked to your belt) as you go about your regular activities.

Intravenous drugs are given through either a regular IV catheter or an indwelling vascular access device. A regular IV catheter is a tiny plastic tube about an inch long with a plastic hub. A needle is used to put the catheter into a vein in your forearm or hand, and then the needle is removed, leaving the catheter in the vein with the hub outside of the skin. The catheter can stay in place for a few days at most, so if you need to be treated over the course of weeks or months, you would need to have many IVs placed.

Repeated use of needles and catheters over the course of treatment can scar and damage veins. Another option is an indwelling vascular (or venous) access device (VAD). These are catheters that are placed in large veins and left in for a long time (some can stay in place for years). A VAD allows nurses and doctors to draw blood and give medications. They can be helpful for anyone who is receiving chemotherapy often or over a long period, as they can reduce the need for repeated needle sticks. Most VADs are either put right into large veins in the neck or chest or are placed into a smaller vein (such as in the arm) and then threaded up into a larger vein. When the catheter empties into a large vein in the chest, it is also known as a central venous catheter (CVC). A CVC may be needed to give certain drugs, called vesicants, that can cause serious damage to skin and muscle tissue if they leak outside of a vein. Doxorubicin and epirubicin are vesicants commonly used to treat early-stage breast cancer.

There are different types of vascular access devices with different types of catheters and ports. The type of VAD a woman gets will depend on the specific treatment (such as what drugs are used and how many are given at one time), the length of treatment, the patient's and doctor's preferences, the amount of care required to maintain the VAD, and any problems you have had with previous devices. Cost can also be an issue. Before you agree to have a VAD put in, find out more from the doctor about the type he or she is recommending and why. Also find out whether your insurance will cover it and whether you will have to do anything to take care of it.

The types of VAD used most often in breast cancer patients are the peripherally inserted central catheter and the implantable venous access port.

Peripherally Inserted Central Catheter

A peripherally inserted central catheter, or PICC (pronounced "pick") line, is like a very long IV catheter that is put into a vein in the arm and threaded up to a large vein in the chest near the heart. The hub where the medicines go in stays outside the skin like a regular IV. A PICC can be inserted at the patient's bedside without surgery and can stay in place for weeks or months. The catheter site in the arm needs to be cared for with dressing changes, and care must be taken during bathing so that it does not get wet. The catheter itself must be flushed at least once a day. If it needs to be removed, it can just be pulled out.

The advantages of a PICC include the ease of placement and removal and its relatively low cost. The drawbacks are the care the catheter needs, including dressings and flushes, and the fact that you will have a small tube sticking out of your arm until the device is removed.

Implantable Venous Access Port

An implantable venous access port, with brand names like Port-A-Cath, BardPort, Pass-Port, Medi-Port, and Infusaport, is often just called a "port." It consists of a large catheter with one end that is put either into a large vein in the chest or into a vein in the arm and threaded up into a large chest vein. The other end is attached to a shallow drum-shaped device (the "port"), which is placed under the skin of the arm or chest. The port is made of plastic or metal and is covered with a silicone diaphragm. To access the port to give medicines, a special needle is inserted in the skin and into the diaphragm of the port. This needle is taken out when the medicine has been given, and no special dressing is needed over the site. No special care is needed for bathing or showering when there is no needle in the port—you can even go swimming. If it is not being used, this type of VAD should be flushed about once a month.

Putting in a port is more involved than with a PICC: placement requires a small incision and is usually done as an outpatient surgery. The area is numbed, and the patient is awake but often sedated. Removal also involves sedation and a small procedure. The advantages of a port are that it is easy to care for and can stay in for a long time, even years. The disadvantages are that placement and removal are more involved than with a PICC, it is more expensive than a PICC, and accessing it means piercing the skin.

PICC line

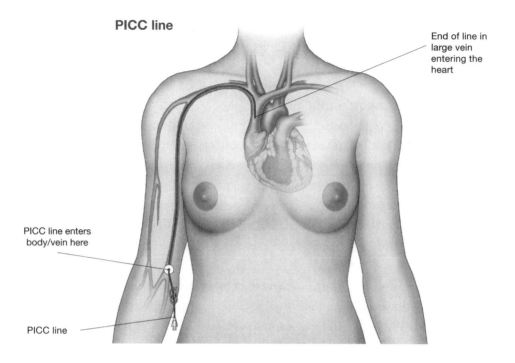

End of line in large vein entering the heart

PICC line enters body/vein here

PICC line

© Sam and Amy Collins

Port

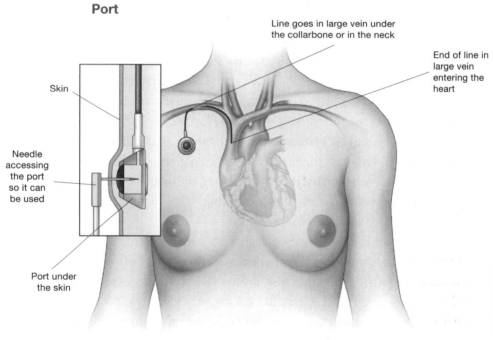

Line goes in large vein under the collarbone or in the neck

End of line in large vein entering the heart

Skin

Needle accessing the port so it can be used

Port under the skin

© Sam and Amy Collins

Other devices are used less often in breast cancer treatment but may be useful for some patients. Some of these are listed below.

- Midline catheter (Per-Q-Cath Midline, Groshong Midline): A midline catheter is placed in a vein in the arm, but the catheter is not threaded as far as a PICC. This catheter is used for intermediate-length therapy when a regular short-term IV is not advisable or available. No surgery is needed to install the device. Care of the external catheter and regular flushing are needed.
- Tunneled central venous catheter (Hickman, Broviac, Groshong, Neostar): This catheter can have multiple separate lumens (channels or tubes) and is surgically placed in a large central vein in the chest. The catheter is tunneled under the skin, but the openings to the lumens remain outside the body. This is a long-term catheter that is good for months to years. Care of the external catheter and regular flushing are needed.

Potential Problems with Central Venous Catheters and Vascular Access Devices

Some problems can occur when the device is put in or shortly after:

- *Bleeding:* Any time you puncture the skin and/or a blood vessel, there is a risk of bleeding. Before the catheter is put in, the doctor will do blood tests to be sure that your blood clots normally. Serious bleeding is rare, but even with normal clotting, blood can leak out of the vein and cause bruising or press on other blood vessels or organs, which can cause pain or cut off circulation and may need to be treated.
- *Infection at incision site:* Any time you puncture the skin, there is a risk of infection. Infection can develop at the site of the incision or where the catheter enters the skin. This risk is minimized by cleaning the skin well beforehand and by using a sterile technique when placing the catheter. You can help lower your risk by following any instructions about caring for the incisions as they heal and by changing the catheter dressing as instructed.
- *Pneumothorax:* Sometimes when a central venous catheter is placed in the chest or neck, the lung is nicked by the needle. Air leaks out and collects in the chest between the lung and the chest wall—this is called pneumothorax. If severe, it can cause the lung to collapse. Pneumothorax is treated by putting a tube or catheter in the space between the chest wall and the lungs to suck out the air. If the doctor uses ultrasound or fluoroscopy (an imaging technique using x-rays)

to guide the placement of the device, the risk of pneumothorax is greatly decreased.

- *Arrhythmia:* If the catheter is inserted too far, it can touch the heart, causing changes in the normal heart rhythm. This is usually temporary and stops when the position of the catheter is changed. It rarely causes serious problems.

- *Error in placement:* In rare cases, the catheter is put in the wrong place, like into an artery instead of a vein or into the space around the lung. If this happens, the catheter will have to be taken out. If there are no other complications, the puncture usually heals by itself. This is rare today because ultrasound or other imaging tests are used to look at the vein before the catheter is put in and to be sure the catheter is in the right place.

The following problems can occur after the VAD is in place, over the course of the time the device is in the body:

- *Infection:* Infection can develop at the insertion site, and sometimes the catheter inside the body can become infected, leading to more serious bloodstream infections. When this happens, the catheter often needs to be removed. The chance of infection can be minimized by washing hands carefully before handling the catheter, changing the dressing carefully, checking the skin each time the dressing is changed, and following a sterile technique when using the catheter.

- *Fluid leak:* A hole or break in the catheter can lead to a fluid leak. It is important not to clamp the catheter in the same spot each time, which can weaken that area. Never use too much force when flushing the catheter.

- *Catheter blockages:* Any type of catheter can become blocked by clotted blood. You can minimize this risk by carefully flushing the catheter as instructed. Once a catheter becomes blocked off (occluded), it can sometimes be opened by injecting certain medicines, but in some cases the catheter may need to be removed or replaced.

- *Dislocation:* Some catheters may move or be pulled out accidentally. This is not an issue with an implantable venous access port but can be for a PICC.

- *Air in catheter:* If the catheter is not managed properly, air can get into it, which can then get into the bloodstream. A large amount of air can create an emergency that causes chest pain or shortness of breath. This complication is very rare.

- *Blood clot:* A blood clot can develop in the vein the catheter is in, which can cause swelling in the arm, shoulder, neck, or head. A blood clot is treated with blood thinners, but the catheter also may have to be removed.
- *Damage to the vein:* The catheter can irritate the vein, leading to the formation of scar tissue. This can lead to stenosis—abnormal narrowing of the vein that can slow the blood flow and cause swelling.

Be sure you understand the benefits and risks of having a vascular access device. Know what problems to watch for, what to do about them, and when to call your doctor.

Side Effects of Chemotherapy

The side effects of chemotherapy depend on the drugs used, the amount given, the length of treatment, and other factors. As mentioned before, chemotherapy drugs act on cells that divide rapidly, especially cancer cells. But some normal cells in your body divide rapidly, too—those in the bone marrow, digestive tract, reproductive system, and hair follicles, for example—and they can be affected by chemotherapy.

Many side effects are short-term and go away after treatment is finished. And in many cases, medicines can help you manage these side effects. For example, drugs can be given to help prevent or reduce nausea and vomiting. For many women, these medicines have helped to make chemotherapy more tolerable than it was in the past. It is important to let your medical team know if you have any side effects.

Nausea, fatigue, hair loss, and lowered blood cell counts are among the most common side effects of chemotherapy, but even the same chemotherapy drugs can affect people differently. Some people go through chemotherapy without experiencing significant side effects, so it is important not to assume the worst before treatment begins.

The more common side effects of chemotherapy are described briefly in the following paragraphs. For information on managing these side effects, see chapter 13.

Fatigue

Fatigue is an unusual and constant feeling of tiredness that can occur with cancer or cancer treatment. It is one of the most common side effects of cancer and its treatments, including chemotherapy. Fatigue tends to become more pronounced as more chemotherapy is given. You might feel a lack of energy and less able to do physical and mental work, and you might have difficulty thinking, forgetfulness, and trouble concentrating. Fatigue related to cancer is different from normal tiredness; getting more rest often does not make this fatigue go away.

Hair Loss

Some chemotherapy drugs are more likely to cause hair loss than others. When it does occur, hair loss is almost always temporary, and usually begins two to three weeks after chemotherapy has started. The extent of hair loss depends on which drugs you are taking, their doses, and the length of your treatment. Usually, less hair is lost from the eyebrows, eyelashes, pubic region, and other body areas than from the scalp.

Hair loss can be one of the most distressing side effects of chemotherapy for many women, because it is an outward sign you are being treated for cancer. It can in turn cause depression, loss of self-confidence, and grief. Once chemotherapy treatment ends, your hair will grow back, but its color or texture might be different at first.

Nausea and Vomiting

Many chemotherapy drugs can cause nausea and vomiting, which can begin minutes, hours, or even days after your treatment. The severity and length of time these symptoms last can also vary greatly. Nausea can be accompanied by sweating, lightheadedness, dizziness, and weakness. Medicines to help prevent or reduce the severity of nausea and vomiting are commonly given with certain chemotherapy drugs; ask your doctor or nurse for more information. Some complementary methods may also be effective against nausea.

Low Blood Cell Counts

Many chemotherapy drugs can damage the bone marrow, which makes the main cells of the bloodstream: red blood cells, white blood cells, and platelets (which are technically fragments of cells). If the bone marrow is damaged, you might have fewer blood cells than normal during chemotherapy. A low red blood cell count, called anemia, can lead to fatigue. If your white blood cell count is low, you might be more prone to serious infections. Having a low platelet count can increase your risk of bleeding or bruising after minor cuts or injuries.

Constipation or Diarrhea

Constipation and diarrhea can occur because of certain chemotherapy drugs. Women with constipation might also have excessive bloating, increased gas, cramping, or pain.

The amount and duration of these symptoms depends on which drugs are being taken, their doses, and the length of treatment.

Mouth and Throat Sores

Some chemotherapy drugs can cause mouth or throat sores within a week or two of starting treatment. The first sign of mouth sores is a pale, dry lining of the mouth. Later, your mouth, gums, and throat might feel sore and become red and inflamed. Your tongue might feel coated and swollen, which can cause problems with swallowing, eating, and talking. These sores can lead to bleeding, painful ulcers, and infection.

Appetite and Weight Changes

Some chemotherapy medicines can cause appetite changes—either increased or decreased appetite. Any appetite change you notice will generally be temporary, and your regular appetite will probably return a few weeks after chemotherapy is finished.

Cancer treatments can also alter your sense of taste, which can reduce your appetite and lead to undernourishment. Changes in taste and smell might continue as long as your chemotherapy treatments continue, but they should return to normal several weeks after treatment has ended.

Some women gain weight during chemotherapy. Although the reasons are unclear, weight gain might be related to intense food cravings that develop despite the nausea.

Nail Changes

During chemotherapy with certain drugs, your nails might become brittle or cracked, and they might develop vertical bands or darken in color.

Hand-Foot Syndrome

Certain chemotherapy drugs, such as capecitabine and liposomal doxorubicin, can irritate the skin covering the palms of the hands and the soles of the feet. This is called hand-foot syndrome. Early symptoms include numbness, tingling, and redness. If it gets worse, the hands and feet can become swollen and uncomfortable or painful. The skin might blister, leading to peeling of the skin. There is no specific treatment, but these symptoms gradually get better when the drug is stopped or the dose is decreased. The best way to prevent severe hand-foot syndrome is to tell your doctor when early symptoms come up, so that the drug dosage can be changed.

Nerve Damage

Several drugs used to treat breast cancer, including the taxanes (docetaxel and pacli-taxel), platinum agents (carboplatin, cisplatin), vinorelbine, ixabepilone, and eribulin, can damage nerves outside of the brain and spinal cord. This condition is called periph-eral neuropathy. It can sometimes lead to symptoms such as numbness, pain, burning or tingling, sensitivity to cold or heat, or weakness. These symptoms occur mainly in the hands and feet. In most cases, this side effect goes away once treatment is stopped, but it can be long-lasting in some women.

Heart Damage

Doxorubicin, epirubicin, and some other drugs can cause permanent heart damage if used for a long time or in high doses, so doctors often check the heart's function before the patient starts taking one of these drugs. They also carefully control the doses and use echocardiograms or other tests to monitor heart function. If the heart function begins to decline, treatment with these drugs will be stopped. In some patients, heart damage can take a long time to develop. They might not show signs of poor heart func-tion until months or years after treatment stops. Heart damage from these drugs happens more often if the targeted therapy drug trastuzumab is used at the same time, so doctors are more cautious when trastuzumab is part of the regimen.

"Chemo Brain"

Many women who get chemotherapy for breast cancer report changes in mental functioning. Some problems with concentration and memory can last a long time. Still, most women do function well after chemotherapy. In studies that have found "chemo brain" to be a side effect of treatment, the symptoms usually go away, though it may take some time to resolve.

Effects on the Sexual Organs

Reproductive and sexual problems can occur after chemotherapy. These problems include temporary or permanent infertility, irregular menstrual periods or lack of menstruation, premature menopause, lessened sexual desire, and discomfort during intercourse because of vaginal dryness or irritation. Whether you have any reproductive problems as a result of treatment (and if so, which ones) will depend on your age when treated, the dose and duration of your chemotherapy, and the chemotherapy drug(s) given to you.

Lack of sexual desire: Women often have reduced desire for sex during the time they are undergoing chemotherapy. The physical effects of treatment, including upset stomach and weakness, might leave women with little energy to put into a sexual relationship. Women receiving chemotherapy might feel unattractive—hair loss, weight loss, other changes in appearance, and changes from other treatments such as breast surgery can affect a woman's sexual self-image. Sexual desire usually returns when a woman feels better. For a while, this might mean only the few days before the next treatment. After chemotherapy ends, side effects slowly fade and sexual desire often returns to normal.

Premature menopause: Younger women getting chemotherapy might show symptoms of early menopause. These symptoms can include hot flashes, vaginal dryness, tightness during intercourse, and irregular or absent menstrual periods. The older a woman is when she receives chemotherapy, the more likely it is that she will become infertile or menopausal as a result. Symptoms of premature menopause are often more severe than the slow changes that happen during natural menopause. Women who have premature menopause sometimes have decreased sexual desire and pleasure.

Menstruation and infertility: Chemotherapy can significantly alter the menstrual cycle. Your period might stop or become irregular. This might be temporary or permanent. It might still be possible for you to get pregnant, even if your menstrual cycle is interrupted. Although it is possible to conceive a child during chemotherapy, the toxicity of some drugs may cause birth defects. For this reason, it is important that premenopausal women who are sexually active talk with their doctors about birth control options.

Spotting: As the lining of the vagina thins, light spotting of blood after intercourse is common. Light spotting should not be a cause for worry. If spotting gets heavier or does not stop, talk to your doctor or nurse right away.

Vaginal dryness: Some chemotherapy drugs irritate all mucous membranes in the body, including the lining of the vagina, which can become dry and inflamed. Using a vaginal lubricant can help make intercourse more comfortable.

Yeast infections: Another possible side effect of chemotherapy is yeast infections, particularly in women taking steroids and in those taking antibiotics to prevent bacterial infections. Yeast cells are a natural part of the vagina's cleansing system, but if too many grow, a woman can experience itching or burning in the vagina, sometimes accompanied by a whitish discharge that looks like cottage cheese. Yeast infections inflame the lining of the vagina, which can cause a burning sensation during intercourse.

Side effects for women with sexually transmitted diseases: Women who have had genital herpes or genital wart infections in the past might have flare-ups during chemotherapy. It is especially important for women undergoing chemotherapy to have any vaginal infections treated.

Other Side Effects

Outlined next are some possible but uncommon side effects that occur in some patients receiving chemotherapy. Ask your doctor if these are likely to occur with your treatment and, if so, find out more information about them.

Questions to Ask Your Medical Team About Chemotherapy

- **Why are you recommending chemotherapy** for me? What are the possible benefits?
- **What are the chances that the tumor** will respond to chemotherapy?
- **How is the chemotherapy given?** Would I receive it orally, intravenously, or by injection? Will I have a "port" for my chemotherapy?
- **What are the names of the drugs** I will be taking? What are their possible side effects?
- **Am I likely to lose my hair?** How soon might this happen?
- **Will I have nausea** during or after my first treatment?
- **Are there any foods or beverages** I should avoid during treatment?
- **Is there anything I can do** during treatment to decrease my risk for side effects?
- **How should I expect fatigue** to affect my daily routine?
- **What are my chances of premature menopause** due to chemotherapy?
- **How will my fertility and menstrual cycle** be affected?
- **How can I reduce my risk** for getting yeast infections?
- **Can chemotherapy damage my organs** or nervous system?
- **Are there any other side effects** I should know about?
- **Will chemotherapy increase my risk** for other cancers?
- **What local resources can help me** deal with side effects such as hair loss?

Liver damage: Some chemotherapy drugs can damage the liver. Signs of this damage can include yellowing of the skin and the whites of the eyes, fatigue, and pain under the lower right ribs or right upper abdomen. Older women and those who have had hepatitis are at increased risk for liver damage while undergoing chemotherapy. Most often, the damage is temporary and resolves a few weeks after treatment is stopped.

Kidney and urinary system damage: Certain chemotherapy drugs can cause kidney or bladder damage. Signs and symptoms of damage include headache, pain in your lower back, fatigue, weakness, nausea, vomiting, increased blood pressure, faster breathing, a change in the pattern of urination, a change in the color of your urine, an urgent need to urinate, and swelling or puffiness of the body.

Hearing loss or tinnitus (ringing in the ears): Both hearing loss and ringing in the ears can be long-term side effects of some drugs.

Cancer: Development of a second cancer, although very rare, is a great concern for women who have had breast cancer. Certain chemotherapy drugs can slightly raise the risk of leukemia, a cancer of white blood cells. When a second cancer does develop, it usually occurs within ten years of treatment.

Hormone Therapy

Hormones are natural chemicals produced by the body that control processes such as metabolism and reproduction. A woman's ovaries are the main source of the hormone estrogen until menopause. After menopause, smaller amounts of estrogen are still made in the body's fat tissue, where a hormone made by the adrenal glands is converted into estrogen.

Estrogen promotes the growth of breast cancers that contain receptors for the hormones estrogen (ER–positive cancers) and/or progesterone (PR–positive cancers). Such tumors represent about two out of three breast cancers overall. Using hormone therapy, doctors can reduce the level or effects of estrogen in order to treat hormone receptor–positive breast cancers. Hormone therapy will not help treat a cancer that is both ER– and PR–negative.

Hormone therapy is used most often after surgery to help reduce the risk of cancer returning, but it can also be used as neoadjuvant treatment (before surgery) and to treat cancer that has spread or has come back after treatment.

Options for Hormone Therapy

Doctors can use several approaches to block the effects of estrogen or to lower estrogen levels, including drugs such as anti-estrogens, aromatase inhibitors (blockers), and luteinizing hormone-releasing hormone (LHRH) analogs (mimicking drugs). In the past, removing the ovaries (in premenopausal women) or the adrenal glands (in post-menopausal women) were often effective treatments. Today, drugs such as tamoxifen (Nolvadex) and aromatase inhibitors are more commonly used.

Anti-estrogens

Tamoxifen and toremifene are drugs that work by temporarily attaching to the estrogen receptors on breast cancer cells, preventing estrogen from binding to them. The anti-estrogen tamoxifen has been around for decades and is still among the most widely used hormone drugs, especially in premenopausal women. It is taken daily as a pill.

For women with hormone receptor–positive cancers, taking tamoxifen after surgery for at least five years reduces the chances of the cancer coming back by about half and helps patients live longer. Recent studies have shown that taking it for ten years can be even more helpful. Tamoxifen can also be used to treat metastatic breast cancer and to reduce the risk of breast cancer in women at high risk. Toremifene works like tamoxifen, but it is not used as often and is only approved for patients with metastatic breast cancer.

The most common side effects of these drugs include fatigue, hot flashes, vaginal dryness or discharge, and mood swings. Some patients whose cancer has spread to their bones may have a "tumor flare" and experience pain and swelling in the muscles and bones. This usually subsides quickly, but, rarely, the patient can also develop a high blood calcium level, a condition called hypercalcemia. If this occurs, treatment may need to be stopped for a time.

Rare but more serious side effects are also possible. These drugs can increase the risk for cancers of the uterus (endometrial cancer and uterine sarcoma) in post-menopausal women. Report any unusual vaginal bleeding (a common symptom of both of these cancers) to your doctor right away. Most uterine bleeding is not caused by cancer, but this symptom always needs prompt attention.

Another possible serious side effect of hormone therapy is blood clots, usually in the legs. In some cases, these blood clots can lead to a heart attack, stroke, or blockage in the lungs (called a pulmonary embolism). Call your doctor or nurse right away if you develop pain, redness, or swelling in your calf; shortness of breath; chest pain; sudden, severe headache; confusion; or trouble speaking or moving.

Depending on a woman's menopausal status, tamoxifen can have different effects on the bones. In premenopausal women, tamoxifen can cause some bone thinning, but in postmenopausal women, it is often good for bone strength. The effects of toremifene on bones are less clear.

A newer anti-estrogen, fulvestrant (Faslodex), is sometimes used for women whose breast cancer has spread and is no longer responding to tamoxifen. Unlike tamoxifen, which has both estrogen-like (estrogenic) and anti-estrogenic properties, fulvestrant is a pure anti-estrogen. It is given by injection once a month. Hot flashes, mild nausea, fatigue, and pain at the injection site are the major side effects.

Aromatase Inhibitors

Aromatase inhibitors work by blocking aromatase, an enzyme responsible for making small amounts of estrogen after a woman goes through menopause. They cannot stop premenopausal women's ovaries from making estrogen, so the drugs work only in post-menopausal women. Aromatase inhibitors include anastrozole (Arimidex), exemestane (Aromasin), and letrozole (Femara). They are taken daily as pills.

Using these drugs after surgery, either alone or after tamoxifen, has been shown to reduce the risk of cancer recurrence more than using tamoxifen alone for five years. The following schedules are known to be helpful:

- tamoxifen for two to three years, followed by an aromatase inhibitor to complete five years of treatment
- tamoxifen for five years, followed by an aromatase inhibitor for five years
- an aromatase inhibitor for five years

For postmenopausal women whose cancers are hormone receptor–positive, most doctors now recommend using an aromatase inhibitor at some point during adjuvant therapy. But it is not yet clear whether starting adjuvant therapy with one of these drugs is better than giving tamoxifen and then switching to an aromatase inhibitor. It is also not known whether any one of these drugs is better than the others. Studies are being done now that should help answer these questions.

Aromatase inhibitors tend to have fewer serious side effects than tamoxifen—they do not cause uterine cancers and very rarely cause blood clots. They can, however, cause muscle and joint pain and stiffness. This side effect might improve by switching to a different aromatase inhibitor, but it has led some women to stop drug treatment. If this occurs, most doctors recommend using tamoxifen to complete five years of hormone treatment.

Because aromatase inhibitors remove all estrogens from women after menopause, they also cause bone thinning, sometimes leading to osteoporosis and even fractures. Many women treated with an aromatase inhibitor are also given medicines to strengthen their bones, such as bisphosphonates or denosumab (described on pages 192–193).

Ovarian Ablation

In premenopausal women, removing or shutting down the ovaries (which are the main source of estrogen) effectively makes the women postmenopausal. This process is called ovarian ablation, and it may allow some other hormone therapies to work better.

Permanent ovarian ablation can be done by surgically removing the ovaries. This operation is called an oophorectomy. More often, ovarian ablation is done with drugs that mimic luteinizing hormone-releasing hormone (LHRH), such as goserelin (Zoladex) and leuprolide (Lupron). These drugs stop the signal that the brain sends to the ovaries to make estrogens. They can be used alone or with tamoxifen as hormone therapy in premenopausal women with metastatic breast cancer. They are also being studied as adjuvant therapies with tamoxifen or aromatase inhibitors in premenopausal women.

Chemotherapy drugs might also damage the ovaries of premenopausal women and cause them to stop producing estrogen. In some women, ovarian function returns

Hormone Therapies Commonly Used to Treat Breast Cancer		
Anti-estrogens	Aromatase Inhibitors	Luteinizing Hormone-Releasing Hormone (LHRH) Analogs
fulvestrant (Faslodex) tamoxifen (Nolvadex) toremifene (Fareston)	anastrozole (Arimidex) exemestane (Aromasin) letrozole (Femara)	goserelin (Zoladex) leuprolide (Lupron)

months or years later, but in others, the damage to the ovaries is permanent and leads to menopause. This can sometimes be a helpful (if unintended) consequence of chemotherapy with regard to breast cancer treatment, although it has other negative effects, such as leaving the woman infertile.

All of these methods of ovarian ablation can cause a woman to have symptoms of menopause, including hot flashes, night sweats, vaginal dryness, and mood swings.

Other Drugs

Other hormone therapies include progesterone-like drugs such as megestrol acetate (Megace), testosterone-like drugs such as fluoxymesterone (Android-F), and estrogens such as ethinyl estradiol (Estinyl), which is sometimes effective if given in high doses. These drugs were used more in the past. Today, they are usually reserved for women whose cancers do not respond to the hormone therapies described previously.

All of these drugs can have significant side effects. Megestrol acetate can cause weight gain. Testosterone-like drugs can cause masculine characteristics, such as an increase in body hair and a deeper voice. High doses of estrogens can cause nausea and increase the risk of blood clots.

Questions to Ask Your Medical Team About Hormone Therapy

- **Is my particular cancer** estrogen receptor–positive and/or progesterone–receptor positive? How does this affect my treatment options?
- **How will my status** as someone who has or has not reached menopause affect my treatment?
- **How does my family history** of breast, ovarian, or endometrial cancer affect my hormone therapy options?
- **How long will I need to** take hormone therapy?
- **Which type of hormone therapy** do you think would be best for me? Why?
- **What are the possible side effects** of different types of hormone therapy?
- **Is there anything I can do** to lower my risk of side effects?
- **Are phytoestrogens** (the estrogen-like substances from certain plant sources, such as soy products) an option for me?
- **Am I eligible for clinical trials** testing hormone therapy?

Who Should Get Hormone Therapy

Not all types of breast cancer can be treated with hormone therapy. Women whose biopsies show that their tumors are estrogen receptor–positive (ER+) or progesterone receptor–positive (PR+) are likely to benefit from hormone therapy, but women whose tumors are negative for these receptors are not. Hormone therapy is typically part of the treatment for nearly all women with breast cancers that are ER+ or PR+, regardless of whether the cancer is at an early or advanced stage.

Targeted Therapy

As researchers have learned more about the gene changes in cells that cause cancer, they have been able to develop newer drugs that specifically target these changes. These targeted drugs work differently from standard chemotherapy drugs. They often have different (and less severe) side effects. For breast cancer, these drugs are used most often with chemotherapy.

Drugs that Target the HER2/neu Protein

About 20 to 25 percent of breast cancers have too much of a growth-promoting protein known as HER2/neu (or just HER2) on the surface of the cancer cells. Breast cancers with too much of this protein tend to grow and spread more quickly, but some newer drugs that target this protein can help treat these cancers.

All of these drugs can harm and even cause death to a fetus if taken by someone who is pregnant. Women who could become pregnant need to use effective birth control during treatment.

Trastuzumab (Herceptin)

Trastuzumab is a type of drug known as a monoclonal antibody—an artificial version of a very specific immune system protein. It attaches to the growth-promoting HER2 protein on breast cancer cells and blocks its effects. Trastuzumab can help slow the growth of cancer cells and might also stimulate the immune system to attack the cancer more effectively.

Trastuzumab is given as a slow injection intravenously (by IV), usually once a week or as a larger dose every three weeks. When chemotherapy is given for early HER2-positive breast cancer, trastuzumab is started with the chemotherapy and then continued by itself to complete one year of treatment. This treatment reduces the risk of recurrence compared with giving chemotherapy alone and can be started before or after surgery. Starting this treatment before surgery also helps shrink the tumor.

Trastuzumab can also shrink some HER2-positive advanced breast cancers that return after chemotherapy or continue to grow during chemotherapy. Treatment with trastuzumab and chemotherapy has been shown to work better than chemotherapy alone in many patients. If a cancer progresses while a woman is taking trastuzumab and receiving chemotherapy, often the trastuzumab is continued and the type of chemotherapy is changed.

Compared with chemotherapy drugs, the side effects of trastuzumab are relatively mild. They can include fever and chills, weakness, nausea, vomiting, cough, diarrhea, and headache. These side effects occur less often after the first dose. A more serious possible side effect is congestive heart failure, in which damage to the muscle of the heart affects its ability to pump blood properly. Symptoms of congestive heart failure can include shortness of breath, leg swelling, and severe fatigue. For most (but not all) women who have this side effect, it is temporary and improves when the drug is stopped. The risk is higher when this drug is given with certain chemotherapy drugs, such as doxorubicin (Adriamycin) or epirubicin (Ellence). For this reason, heart function is checked regularly during treatment with trastuzumab.

Pertuzumab (Perjeta)

Like trastuzumab, pertuzumab is a monoclonal antibody that attaches to the HER2 protein. This is a newer drug that seems to target a different part of the protein than trastuzumab. Pertuzumab is used to treat advanced breast cancer. In one study, when pertuzumab was given along with docetaxel and trastuzumab to patients with advanced breast cancer who had not yet received chemotherapy, tumors got smaller or stopped growing for about six months longer than in patients treated with docetaxel and trastuzumab alone.

Pertuzumab is given as an infusion into a vein every three weeks. When given with trastuzumab and docetaxel, common side effects include diarrhea, hair loss, nausea, fatigue, rash, and low white blood cell counts (sometimes with fever). Many side effects, such as hair loss, nausea, and fatigue, occur at about the same rate as in patients taking just docetaxel and trastuzumab.

Although pertuzumab has not yet been shown to affect heart function, there is concern that it can, so it cannot be given to patients with poor heart function. As with trastuzumab, your doctor will check tests of heart function every few months while you are treated with this drug.

Pertuzumab is also being studied for use earlier in the treatment of advanced cancer, as well as for treatment of earlier-stage disease.

Ado-trastuzumab Emtansine (Kadcyla)

Ado-trastuzumab emtansine is a newer kind of targeted therapy drug known as a chemo-labeled antibody or antibody-drug conjugate. It is made up of the trastuzumab antibody attached to the chemotherapy drug DM-1. In this kind of drug, the antibody acts as a homing device, taking the chemotherapy drug directly to the cancer cells.

Targeted Therapies Commonly Used to Treat Breast Cancer

lapatinib (Tykerb)

trastuzumab (Herceptin)

pertuzumab (Perjeta)

ado-trastuzumab emtansine (Kadcyla)

everolimus (Affinitor)

Ado-trastuzumab emtansine is used to treat advanced breast cancer. A study of women with advanced breast cancer who had previously been treated with trastuzumab and a taxane (either paclitaxel or docetaxel) compared giving ado-trastuzumab emtansine with lapatinib combined with capecitabine. The women who got ado-trastuzumab emtansine were more likely to have their tumors shrink. They also lived an average of five months longer.

This drug is given as an injection into a vein (by IV) every three weeks. Common side effects include fatigue, nausea, muscle and bone pain, low platelet counts, headache, and constipation. This drug can also cause more serious side effects, such as severe allergic reactions, liver damage, heart damage, and lung problems. In studies, the liver damage was severe in some cases and even led to death, although this was rare.

Ado-trastuzumab emtansine is also being studied for use earlier in the treatment of advanced cancer, as well as for treatment of earlier-stage disease.

Lapatinib (Tykerb)

Lapatinib is another drug that targets the HER2 protein. This drug is taken daily as a pill. It is used most often in women who have advanced breast cancer that is no longer responding to chemotherapy and trastuzumab. It can also be used with hormone therapy for patients with metastatic breast cancer that is estrogen receptor–positive and HER2-positive. It is being studied for use as an adjuvant therapy in women with HER2-positive cancers, as well as for use with trastuzumab for advanced breast cancer.

The most common side effects of this drug include diarrhea, nausea, vomiting, rash, and hand-foot syndrome. Diarrhea is a common side effect and can be severe, so it is very important to let your medical team know about any changes in bowel habits as soon as

Bevacizumab (Avastin) and Breast Cancer

Bevacizumab (Avastin) is a monoclonal antibody that targets vascular endothelial growth factor (VEGF), a protein that helps tumors create new blood vessels. By blocking VEGF, bevacizumab is thought to limit the growth of new blood vessels, which in turn should limit how large a tumor can grow. When used with chemotherapy, this drug has been shown to be helpful for several types of cancer, including colorectal and lung cancers. Doctors have been hopeful that bevacizumab might also help against breast cancer.

In early 2008, the US Food and Drug Administration (FDA) granted accelerated approval for bevacizumab to be used along with chemotherapy in women with metastatic breast cancer. This was based on a study that found that adding bevacizumab to the chemotherapy drug paclitaxel increased the time until the cancer began growing again (known as progression-free survival) by a few months, although it did not help the women live longer. As a condition of the accelerated approval, the drug's manufacturer had to conduct more studies to determine just how effective bevacizumab was.

Unfortunately, later studies (reported in 2010) confirmed that bevacizumab does not help women live longer. In addition, the benefit seen with progression-free survival was less in these studies than in the original study. In late 2011, the FDA withdrew its approval of bevacizumab for breast cancer, stating that, in its opinion, the risks of bevacizumab outweighed the possible benefits. The drug is still available to treat other types of cancer (where the evidence of its usefulness is more convincing), and some doctors may still prescribe it "off-label" for patients with breast cancer. However, its benefits in treating breast cancer remain unclear. The drug is expensive, and some insurance companies will no longer cover its costs for the treatment of breast cancer. If you are considering taking bevacizumab, check with your insurance company beforehand.

Bevacizumab can cause rare but potentially serious side effects, including bleeding, holes forming in the colon (which require surgery to correct), and slow wound healing. More common side effects include high blood pressure, fatigue, blood clots, low white blood cell counts, headaches, mouth sores, loss of appetite, and diarrhea.

they happen. In rare cases, lapatinib can cause liver problems or a decrease in heart function, although these side effects seem to go away once treatment with lapatinib is finished.

Everolimus (Affinitor)

Everolimus is a type of targeted therapy that blocks mTOR, a protein in cells that normally promotes their growth and division. By blocking this protein, everolimus can help stop cancer cells from growing. Everolimus may also stop tumors from developing new blood vessels, which can help limit their growth. In the treatment of breast cancer, this drug seems to help hormone therapy drugs work better.

Everolimus is approved to treat advanced hormone receptor–positive, HER2-negative breast cancer in women who have gone through menopause. It is meant to be used with the drug exemestane in these women if their cancers grew while they were being treated with either letrozole or anastrozole. In a study, giving everolimus with exemestane was better than exemestane alone in shrinking tumors and stopping their growth in postmenopausal women with hormone receptor–positive, HER2-negative breast cancer that had stopped responding to letrozole or anastrozole. Everolimus is also being studied for use with other hormone therapy drugs and for earlier-stage breast cancer.

Everolimus is a pill taken once a day. Common side effects include mouth sores, diarrhea, nausea, fatigue, feeling weak or tired, low blood cell counts, shortness of breath, and cough. Everolimus can also increase blood lipids (cholesterol and triglycerides) and blood sugars, so your doctor will check your blood work periodically while you are on this drug. It can also increase your risk of serious infections, so your doctor will watch you closely for infection while you are undergoing treatment.

Drugs to Protect the Bones

The spread of breast cancer to the bones is a serious concern for many women and their doctors. Some drugs can slow the growth of cancer in the bones or may even help prevent breast cancer from spreading there in the first place. These drugs are often used in addition to chemotherapy or targeted therapy drugs.

Bisphosphonates

Bisphosphonates are drugs that help strengthen bones. They can reduce the risk of fractures in bones weakened by metastatic breast cancer. Examples include pamidronate (Aredia) and zoledronic acid (Zometa). These drugs are given intravenously (IV). Bisphosphonates may also help counteract weak bones (osteoporosis), which can be caused by treatment with aromatase inhibitors or by early menopause as a side effect of chemotherapy.

Bisphosphonates can have side effects, including flu-like symptoms and bone pain. They can also lead to kidney problems, so women with poor kidney function may not be able to take these drugs. A rare but serious side effect of intravenous bisphosphonates is osteonecrosis of the jaw (ONJ), or destruction of bone in the jaw. ONJ often appears as an open sore in the jaw that will not heal. It can be triggered by having a tooth removed while being treated with bisphosphonates, and it can lead to loss of teeth or infections of the jawbone. Most

---

Drugs that Block Bone Destruction

pamidronate (Aredia)

zoledronic acid (Zometa)

denosumab (Xgeva)

---

doctors recommend that women have a dental checkup and have any tooth or jaw problems treated before they start taking bisphosphonates. Maintaining good oral hygiene by flossing, brushing, and making sure that dentures fit properly can also help prevent this side effect.

RANKL Inhibitors

When cancer spreads to the bone, it causes increased levels of a substance called receptor activator of nuclear factor kappa-B ligand (RANKL), which is important in bone metabolism. Higher levels of RANKL stimulate cells called osteoclasts to destroy bone. A newer drug called denosumab (Xgeva) works against RANKL and can help protect bones. When given to patients with breast cancer that has spread to the bones, it can help prevent such problems as fractures, possibly working better than bisphosphonates. For some women, denosumab also seems to help after bisphosphonates stop working. Studies are now looking at whether giving denosumab to patients with early-stage breast cancer can help prevent metastasis. Denosumab can also be used to strengthen bones in breast cancer patients who have weak bones as a result of treatment with aromatase inhibitors.

Denosumab is given as an injection under the skin (subcutaneously). In women whose cancer has spread to the bones, the drug is given every four weeks. When it is used to increase bone strength in women taking aromatase inhibitors, it is given less often (usually every six months). Side effects can include low blood levels of calcium and phosphate and osteonecrosis of the jaw. Unlike bisphosphonates, this drug does not seem to affect the kidneys, so it is safe to give to women with kidney problems.

CHAPTER 10

Treatment Options Based on Your Situation

This chapter explores some of the standard treatment options for breast cancer, based on the stage of the cancer and other factors. In addition, it includes a discussion of advanced cancer and some of the issues it can bring about, as well as information about breast cancer during pregnancy.

Each woman's situation is unique, and your doctor might have reasons to suggest a treatment plan that differs from the general treatment options discussed here. Treatment options are also constantly changing as doctors look for newer and better ways to treat breast cancer. Be sure to ask your doctor if you have any questions about your proposed treatment plan.

Treatment of Stage 0 (Noninvasive) Breast Cancer

The two types of noninvasive breast cancer, lobular carcinoma in situ (LCIS) and ductal carcinoma in situ (DCIS), are treated very differently.

Lobular Carcinoma in Situ

Because lobular carcinoma in situ (LCIS) is not a true cancer, no immediate treatment is recommended for most women with LCIS. But if LCIS is found based on a needle biopsy (as opposed to a surgical biopsy), the doctor may recommend surgery to remove it so that a wider area (or larger specimen) can be examined more closely.

Because having LCIS increases your risk of an invasive breast cancer later on, close follow-up is very important. This usually includes a yearly mammogram and a clinical breast examination. Close monitoring of both breasts is important because women with

Questions to Ask Your Medical Team About Your Personal Treatment Plan

When deciding upon a course of treatment, you will want to set up an appointment to ask your doctor questions about your treatment plan, including how it will affect your body, your life, and your family.

PREPARING FOR TREATMENT

- Are there things I should or should not do to get ready for treatment?
- Should I follow a special diet before, during, or after treatment?
- What medicines or vitamins should I avoid during treatment?
- How long will this treatment last? How is the treatment given?
- Will I be hospitalized during any of the treatment? If so, for how long?
- Will the treatment affect my ability to have children later?
- What is the average recovery time for people receiving this treatment?
- How soon can I resume my normal activities?

MY TREATMENT TEAM

- How much experience do you have with this type of cancer and with the treatment plan you are recommending?
- Who will coordinate and monitor my treatment? What other specialists will take part in my care? Will they all be involved throughout my treatment?
- Whom should I call with questions? When is the best time to call? Will this person communicate with the rest of my treatment team?
- Who will be in charge of monitoring my health after I have finished treatment?
- Can I speak to someone who has undergone this treatment under your care?

EVALUATING MY TREATMENT

- How will you know if my treatment is working?
- What will my checkup schedule be after treatment?
- What tests will I undergo at my checkups?
- What are the chances that my cancer might come back after the treatment options we have discussed? What would my options be at that point?

PAYING FOR TREATMENT

- How much does this treatment cost?
- Is this treatment covered by most insurance or health care plans? Is it covered by my plan?
- How will I be billed? For example, will I receive separate bills for the hospital, surgeon, anesthesiologist, pathologist, and radiologist?

LCIS in one breast have an increased risk of cancer developing in either breast. Although there is not enough evidence to recommend routine use of magnetic resonance imaging (MRI) in addition to mammography for women with LCIS, it is reasonable for women to talk with their doctors about the benefits and limits of being screened yearly with MRI.

Women with LCIS might also consider taking tamoxifen or raloxifene, which could reduce their risk of breast cancer. They might also wish to discuss other possible prevention strategies (such as losing weight or starting an exercise program) with their doctor. Some women with LCIS choose to have a bilateral mastectomy (removal of both breasts) to reduce their risk, especially if they have other risk factors, such as a strong family history of breast cancer. Mastectomy can be followed by immediate or delayed breast reconstruction.

Ductal Carcinoma in Situ

Unlike LCIS, ductal carcinoma in situ (DCIS) can become an invasive breast cancer in some cases if it is not treated, so treatment is recommended. In most cases, a woman with DCIS can choose between breast-conserving surgery (lumpectomy, usually followed by radiation therapy) and simple mastectomy. Lymph node removal (axillary lymph node dissection) is usually not needed, but sentinel lymph node biopsy is sometimes recommended. Many doctors will do a sentinel lymph node biopsy if a mastectomy is done.

Lumpectomy without radiation therapy may be an option for women who had small areas of low-grade DCIS that were removed with large enough surrounding margins of normal tissue. But most women who have a lumpectomy will need radiation therapy.

Mastectomy might be needed if any of the following conditions exist:

- the area of DCIS is very large
- the breast has several areas of DCIS
- cancer cells are found at or near the edge of the surgical specimen (called positive or close margins) after lumpectomy and repeat excision

Mastectomy for DCIS can typically be followed by immediate or delayed reconstruction.

If the DCIS contains receptors for estrogen (ER–positive) and/or progesterone (PR–positive), treatment with tamoxifen (Nolvadex) for five years after surgery can lower the risk of another DCIS or invasive cancer developing in either breast. Women with

DCIS might want to talk with their doctors about the pros and cons of tamoxifen and other ways to reduce risk.

Treatment of Invasive Breast Cancer by Stage

For most invasive breast cancers, surgery to remove the cancer is a major part of treatment. In many cases, other treatments are also recommended to offer you the best chance of getting rid of the cancer completely.

Breast-conserving surgery (such as lumpectomy) is often appropriate for earlier-stage invasive breast cancers if the cancer is small enough, although mastectomy is also an option. If the cancer is larger, mastectomy might be necessary, unless preoperative chemotherapy can shrink the tumor enough to allow breast-conserving surgery. In either case, the lymph nodes will need to be checked and, if they contain cancer, removed. Radiation therapy will be needed afterward for almost all patients who have breast-conserving surgery and for some who have mastectomy.

Chemotherapy, trastuzumab (Herceptin), and/or hormone therapy are typically recommended after surgery for all but the smallest cancers. The types of treatments recommended depend to some extent on the hormone receptor status and HER2/neu status of the tumor.

Stage I Breast Cancer

These cancers are still relatively small and have not spread to the lymph nodes (or there is a tiny area of metastasis in the sentinel lymph node).

Stage I cancers can be treated with either breast-conserving surgery (lumpectomy or partial mastectomy) or simple mastectomy. Nearby lymph nodes also should be examined. This is most often done by sentinel lymph node biopsy but, in some cases, it may be done by axillary lymph node dissection. Breast reconstruction can be done at the same time as the main surgery or later.

Radiation therapy is almost always given after breast-conserving surgery. Some women might be able to have breast-conserving surgery without radiation therapy, if all of the following are true:

- They are age seventy years or older.
- The tumor is small (T1, which is 2 cm or less across) and has been removed completely.
- None of the nearby lymph nodes contain cancer.
- The tumor is ER– and/or PR–positive and adjuvant hormone therapy is given.

Some women who do not meet these criteria might be tempted to avoid radiation therapy, but studies have shown that not having radiation increases the chances of the cancer coming back in the breast.

Most doctors will discuss the pros and cons of using hormone therapy after surgery (either tamoxifen or an aromatase inhibitor) with all women who have an ER– or PR–positive breast cancer, no matter how small the tumor is. Women with tumors larger than 0.5 cm (about a quarter of an inch) across might be more likely to benefit from hormone therapy than those with smaller tumors.

Chemotherapy is usually recommended after surgery for women with tumors larger than 1 cm (about half an inch) across. It might also be offered for some women with smaller tumors, especially if the cancer has any worrisome features (such as being high-grade, ER– and PR–negative, or HER2/neu-positive). If your tumor is ER– or PR–positive and HER2/neu-negative, a gene panel such as Oncotype DX (described on pages 51–52) can help determine whether you are likely to benefit from chemotherapy along with hormone therapy. For HER2/neu-positive cancers, adjuvant trastuzumab is usually recommended with chemotherapy.

Stage II Breast Cancer

These cancers are larger and/or have spread to a few nearby lymph nodes. Surgery and radiation therapy options for stage II breast cancers are similar to those for stage I cancers. Because these cancers are more advanced, breast-conserving surgery might be harder to do in some cases.

Some women might want to have breast-conserving surgery instead of a mastectomy, but the tumor may be too large for this to be an option. One option for some of these women is to have chemotherapy, hormone therapy (if the tumor is ER– or PR–positive), and/or trastuzumab (if the tumor is HER2/neu-positive) before surgery to try to shrink the tumor. If treatment shrinks the tumor enough, the woman may be able to have breast-conserving surgery and radiation therapy. This would be followed by more hormone therapy and/or trastuzumab, if appropriate. Further chemotherapy might also be considered.

If therapy before surgery does not shrink the tumor enough for breast-conserving surgery, mastectomy may be required. Mastectomy might be followed by chemotherapy (if chemotherapy was given before surgery, different drugs would be used after surgery). Radiation to the chest wall may be considered if the tumor is large—more than 5 cm (about two inches) across—or if the cancer cells are found in several lymph nodes.

Hormone therapy is recommended if the tumor is ER– or PR–positive. Hormone therapy can be given both before and after surgery.

After surgery, hormone therapy, chemotherapy, trastuzumab, or some combination of these therapies is typically recommended for all women with stage II breast cancer. The type of treatment(s) recommended will depend on the woman's age, ER/PR status, and HER2/neu status.

Stage III Breast Cancer

Stage III breast cancers include tumors that are large (more than 5 cm or about 2 inches across) or growing into nearby tissues (the skin over the breast or the muscle underneath the breast), as well as cancers that have spread to many nearby lymph nodes. Some inflammatory breast cancers are considered stage III. Treatment of inflammatory breast cancer is discussed on pages 204–205.

Before surgery, most women with stage III breast cancers are first treated with chemotherapy to try to shrink the tumor and to determine its response to a particular therapy regimen. Trastuzumab is added to chemotherapy if the tumor is HER2/neu-positive. Some women with smaller stage IIIA cancers that have not spread far into the lymph nodes may not need this treatment.

Regardless of whether the woman underwent chemotherapy before surgery, most stage III cancers are removed by simple mastectomy. Breast-conserving surgery (such as lumpectomy) might be an option if the tumor is smaller or if it shrinks enough after chemotherapy. Sentinel lymph node biopsy is an option for some patients, but most will need an axillary lymph node dissection.

For women who received chemotherapy before surgery, it might be continued after surgery if the full course has not been completed. Radiation therapy is given to the breast and nearby lymph node areas but, in most cases, radiation is delayed until chemotherapy is completed. If the woman wants breast reconstruction, that procedure may be delayed until after radiation therapy. Trastuzumab will also be part of this treatment if the tumor is HER2-positive, and it is usually continued for up to a year. Hormone therapy will be recommended if the tumor is ER–positive or PR–positive, and it is usually started once chemotherapy treatments are completed.

Adjuvant Therapy for Stages I to III Breast Cancer

For cancers that have not spread to distant parts of the body, adjuvant therapy might be recommended after surgery, based on the tumor's size, spread to lymph nodes, and other features. If your doctor recommends adjuvant therapy, you might get chemotherapy, trastuzumab, hormone therapy, or some combination of these treatments.

Hormone Therapy

Hormone therapy is typically recommended for all women with ER–positive or PR–positive invasive breast cancers, regardless of the size of the tumor or the number of lymph nodes involved. Hormone therapy is not helpful for women with ER– and PR–negative tumors.

Women who have stopped having periods or are known to be in menopause at any age and who have ER– and PR–positive tumors generally receive adjuvant therapy either with an aromatase inhibitor (typically for five years) or with tamoxifen for a few years followed by an aromatase inhibitor for a few more. For women who cannot take aromatase inhibitors because of their side effects, an alternative is to take tamoxifen for five years.

Women who are still having periods and who have ER– and/or PR–positive tumors can be treated with tamoxifen, which blocks the effects of estrogen. Some doctors also prescribe a luteinizing hormone-releasing hormone (LHRH) analog, which temporarily shuts down the ovaries. Another option, though permanent, is surgical removal of the ovaries (called an oophorectomy). If the woman becomes postmenopausal within five years of starting tamoxifen (either naturally or because her ovaries are removed), she might be switched from tamoxifen to an aromatase inhibitor.

Sometimes a woman will stop having periods after chemotherapy or while taking tamoxifen, but this does not necessarily mean she is truly postmenopausal. The woman's doctor can do blood tests for certain hormones to determine her menopausal status. The menopausal status is important because aromatase inhibitors are beneficial only to postmenopausal women.

Many questions are still unanswered about the best way to use tamoxifen and aromatase inhibitors. For example, it is not clear whether starting adjuvant therapy with one of the aromatase inhibitors is better than giving tamoxifen for some length of time and then switching to an aromatase inhibitor. The best duration of treatment with aromatase inhibitors has not been determined, either. Studies now under way should help answer these questions. You might want to talk about these issues with your doctor.

If chemotherapy is also to be given, hormone therapy is given after chemotherapy is completed.

(continued, next page)

Chemotherapy

Chemotherapy is usually recommended for all women whose invasive breast cancer is ER– and PR–negative (and who therefore will not benefit from hormone therapy). It is also recommended for women with ER– and/or PR–positive tumors who might get additional benefit from having chemotherapy and hormone therapy, based on the stage and characteristics of their tumors.

Adjuvant chemotherapy might lower the risk for the cancer coming back, but it does not remove the risk completely. Before deciding whether it is right for you, it is important to understand the chances of your cancer returning and how much adjuvant chemotherapy might lower that risk. The benefits of chemotherapy need to be weighed against the possible downsides, including side effects.

Your doctor should discuss what specific drug regimens are best for you based on the stage and grade of the cancer, your other health issues, and your preferences. Some of the typical regimens used for adjuvant chemotherapy are listed on page 170. These regimens usually take from four to six months to complete. In some cases, the doctor may recommend dose-dense chemotherapy, in which the same chemotherapy doses are given over a shorter period of time.

Trastuzumab

Trastuzumab is a targeted drug that attaches to the HER2/neu protein on some breast cancer cells. Women who have HER2/neu-positive cancers are usually given trastuzumab with chemotherapy as part of their adjuvant treatment.

A common chemotherapy regimen is doxorubicin (Adriamycin) and cyclophosphamide (Cytoxan) together for about three months, followed by paclitaxel (Taxol) and trastuzumab. The paclitaxel is given for about three months, and the trastuzumab is given for a year. A concern among doctors is that giving the trastuzumab so soon after doxorubicin can cause heart problems, so tests such as echocardiograms are used to watch heart function closely during treatment.

To try to lessen the possible effects on the heart, doctors are also looking for effective chemotherapy combinations that do not contain doxorubicin. One such regimen, called TCH, uses the chemotherapy drugs docetaxel (Taxotere) and carboplatin (Paraplatin) given every three weeks along with trastuzumab for six cycles. This is followed by trastuzumab either given weekly or every three weeks to complete a year of treatment.

Making Decisions About Adjuvant Therapy

It is not always clear which women will benefit from adjuvant therapy and which will do as well without it. This prediction is important because adjuvant therapy can have side effects.

(continued, next page)

Some doctors use new gene-pattern tests to help decide whether women with certain stage I or stage II breast cancers should receive adjuvant chemotherapy. Examples of such tests include Oncotype DX and MammaPrint, which are described in more detail on pages 51–52. These tests, which are done on a sample of the breast cancer tissue, look at the function of several genes in the cancer cells to help predict the risk of the cancer returning after treatment and how much benefit you are likely to get from chemotherapy. The tests do not tell your doctor which is the best hormone therapy or chemotherapy to recommend.

Doctors might also use other tools that rely on data from large numbers of previously treated women to predict whether adjuvant treatment is likely to be helpful. One example is Adjuvant! Online (www.adjuvantonline.com). This program, designed for use by health care professionals, helps doctors determine the risk of the cancer returning within the next ten years and what benefits you might expect from hormone therapy and/or chemotherapy. You might want to ask your doctor if he or she uses this program.

Stage IV Breast Cancer

Stage IV cancers have spread beyond the breast and lymph nodes to other parts of the body, such as the bones, brain, liver, or lungs. Although surgery and/or radiation might be useful in some situations, these treatments cannot reach cancers in all parts of the body, so systemic therapy is the initial main treatment. Depending on many factors, systemic therapy could include hormone therapy, chemotherapy, a targeted therapy such as trastuzumab or lapatinib (Tykerb), or some combination of these. These treatments can help shrink tumors, improve symptoms, and help patients live longer, but they are unlikely to cure these cancers.

If the tumor is ER–positive or PR–positive and the cancer is not in a vital area or causing symptoms, hormone therapy is often the first treatment chosen. For ER– and PR–negative tumors (or ER– and PR–positive tumors for which hormone therapy is no longer working), chemotherapy is typically the main treatment. Trastuzumab is added to the chemotherapy if the tumor is HER2/neu-positive.

If cancer has spread to the bones, your doctor is likely to also recommend a bone-protecting drug such as denosumab (Xgeva), zoledronic acid (Zometa), or pamidronate (Aredia). These drugs strengthen bones and help prevent fractures due to the cancer. Calcium and vitamin D supplements might also be recommended.

All of these treatments have potential side effects. Your doctor should explain the benefits and risks of these treatments to you before prescribing them. Make sure to get clear answers to all of your questions before beginning treatment.

Radiation therapy and/or surgery might also be used in certain situations, such as to treat a small number of metastases in a certain area (such as the brain), to help prevent bone fractures or blockages in the liver, or to ease pain or other symptoms. If the cancer metastasis is limited and responds well to initial systemic therapy, some doctors might recommend breast surgery and possible lymph node removal to help control the cancer, but this is still being studied. If your doctor recommends surgery and/or radiation therapy, it is important that you understand the goal of treatment—whether it is trying to cure the cancer or to prevent or treat symptoms.

In some cases, regional chemotherapy (where drugs are delivered directly into a certain area, such as the fluid around the brain) might also be useful.

Treatment of Inflammatory Breast Cancer

Inflammatory breast cancer (IBC) tends to grow more quickly and aggressively than more common types of breast cancer. It is already considered at least stage IIIB when first diagnosed. Inflammatory breast cancer is classified as stage IV if it has spread to distant parts of the body. It is often harder to treat successfully than other types of breast cancer.

If the cancer has not spread to distant areas, treatment typically starts with chemotherapy. Anthracyclines (doxorubicin or epirubicin) and taxanes (paclitaxel or docetaxel) are among the most effective chemotherapy drugs for IBC, and most women with IBC get a combination that includes one of each of these drugs. If the cancer does not respond (and the breast is still very swollen and red), different chemotherapy drugs may be tried and/or the breast may be treated with radiation therapy. If the cancer is HER2/neu-positive, trastuzumab is given with chemotherapy. If the tumor shrinks with this treatment, surgery may then be an option.

Surgery is typically done next if the cancer has not spread too far to be removed completely. The usual operation for inflammatory breast cancer is a modified radical mastectomy. Because IBC involves so much of the breast and skin, lumpectomy and skin-sparing mastectomy are not treatment options. Sentinel lymph node biopsy—where only one or a few nodes are removed—is not reliable in IBC and so is also not an option.

After surgery, radiation therapy is typically given to the chest and lymph nodes. Radiation is usually given once a day for about six weeks, but in some cases, more intense treatment (twice a day) might be used. Chemotherapy might be given after surgery if the full course of chemotherapy is not completed beforehand. Trastuzumab might also be part of treatment if the tumor is HER2/neu-positive, and it is usually continued for up to a year. Hormone therapy is recommended if the tumor is ER– or PR–positive. It is usually started once chemotherapy is completed, although it might be started with radiation.

If inflammatory breast cancer has already spread to other parts of the body at the time of diagnosis, treatment is similar to that for other stage IV breast cancers. The main treatment is usually chemotherapy. Typically, trastuzumab is also given if the tumor is HER-positive, and hormone therapy is given if the tumor is ER– or PR–positive. The drug pertuzumab may be given along with trastuzumab.

Participation in a clinical trial may also be a good option, as IBC is rare, and these studies can allow access to drugs not available for standard treatment.

Treatment of Advanced Cancer that Progresses After Treatment

Treatment for advanced (metastatic) breast cancer can often shrink or slow the growth of the cancer (often for many years), but it will likely stop working after a time. For ER– and PR–positive cancers that were being treated with hormone therapy, switching to another type of hormone therapy is sometimes helpful. Starting a new hormone drug along with everolimus is also an option. If hormone drugs stop working, chemotherapy is usually the next step.

For cancers that are not responding to one chemotherapy regimen, trying another is often helpful. Many different drugs and combinations can be used to treat breast cancer. However, each time a cancer progresses during chemotherapy, it becomes less likely that further treatment will be as effective.

HER2/neu-positive cancers that are not responding to trastuzumab might respond to lapatinib, another drug that attacks the HER2 protein. Lapatinib is usually given with the chemotherapy drug capecitabine (Xeloda), but it may be used with other chemotherapy drugs, with trastuzumab, or even alone (without chemotherapy). Ado-trastuzumab emtansine (Kadcyla) is also an option.

Although in most cases, breast cancer that has spread beyond the nearby lymph nodes is not curable, treatments can shrink the tumors and help with some of the problems the cancer is causing. Further treatment at this point depends on several factors, including previous treatments, where the cancer is located, and a woman's age, general health, and desire to continue treatment. The main goals of treatment for metastatic disease are helping you feel better and live longer.

Here we will talk about the common sites of breast cancer metastasis, what problems can occur, and some of the possible treatments for those problems. Most often, treatment of metastatic breast cancer includes chemotherapy or hormone therapy. In some women, surgery might be an option to control local disease. For other problems, such as pain and fractures, radiation may also be used.

Because current treatments are unlikely to cure advanced cancer, patients in otherwise good health are encouraged to think about taking part in clinical trials of other promising treatments. Clinical trials are discussed in chapter 11.

If Cancer Has Spread to Bones

One of the most common sites of breast cancer metastasis is bone. Bone metastasis can cause symptoms or it can be found on an x-ray or other imaging study before any symptoms occur. In addition to anticancer treatment, people with bone metastases receive medicine to help strengthen and protect the bones, such as a bisphosphonate or denosumab (Xgeva). This medication is given monthly once bone metastases are diagnosed.

Bone pain: The main symptom from bone metastases is pain. Women often notice pain in the spine or hips, but any bone can be affected. Often, the cancer has spread to many places in the bones but causes pain in only a few. Treatment can include medicines for pain, including nonsteroidal anti-inflammatory drugs (NSAIDs), such as ibuprofen or naproxen. Stronger opioid pain medicines (like morphine) may also be needed to control the pain. Some other treatments include drugs that strengthen bones (bisphosphonates and denosumab) and radiation therapy to painful areas.

Broken bones: When cancer spreads to the bones, it can make them weak and more likely to fracture. The bone can become so weak that a break can occur with little or no injury. When a bone breaks because it is weakened by cancer, it is known as a pathologic fracture. These fractures occur most often in the leg bones near the hips, which support most of your weight. However, other bones can be affected, too. The cancer can cause severe pain for a time before the bone actually breaks. An x-ray can show that the bone is likely to break and, if the weakened bone is found in time, a surgeon can put a metal rod through the weak part of the bone to prevent a fracture. This procedure is done under general anesthesia.

If the bone has already broken, other methods are used to support the bone. Usually, a surgeon will put a steel support over the area of the broken bone. After surgery, treatments such as chemotherapy or radiation therapy are often used to stop the cancer from causing further damage and help with pain.

Radiation therapy can be given to stop the cancer from growing and prevent any more damage. Usually about ten to fifteen treatments are needed, although some doctors give the total dose of radiation in only one or two treatments. This treatment will not make the bone stronger, but it can stop further damage and help with pain. Surgery may still be needed after radiation to prevent a fracture.

If bones of the spine are fractured, vertebroplasty is sometimes used to support them. In this procedure, the surgeon injects acrylic cement into the damaged bones. The area is numbed first and an imaging scan, such as a CT scan, is used to guide the needle to the right place. Vertebroplasty often reduces pain right away and can be done as an outpatient procedure.

High blood calcium levels: When cancer spreads to the bones, it can cause calcium to be released, leading to a high level of calcium in the blood. This is called hypercalcemia. Hypercalcemia may be found on a routine blood test, but it can also cause symptoms. Early symptoms of hypercalcemia include constipation, frequent urination, feeling sluggish or sleepy, extreme thirst, and drinking large amounts of fluid. If the high calcium level is left untreated, problems with muscle weakness, muscle and joint aches, confusion, coma, and kidney failure can occur.

The main treatment of hypercalcemia is intravenous fluids and medicine to lower calcium levels. A bisphosphonate, such as zoledronic acid or pamidronate, is used most often. Denosumab can also lower blood calcium levels, but it is not approved for this use by the FDA. Other medicines can be used if these measures do not work. If the cancer cannot be treated, the calcium level might go up again and require more treatment.

Pressure on the spinal cord: Cancer sometimes spreads to the bones in the spine or the area around the spinal cord. As the tumor grows, it can put pressure on the nerves in the spinal cord. This is called spinal cord compression. Symptoms can range from back pain to weakness or even paralysis. The pressure on the spinal cord can affect the nerves controlling the bladder and bowel, leading to problems passing urine or even trouble passing stool (causing feelings of constipation). If left untreated, early problems with leg weakness can progress into paralysis, which is often not reversible.

Symptoms to watch for include severe back pain (especially pain in the middle of the lower back), leg numbness or weakness, and trouble passing urine. If you have these symptoms, tell your doctor right away. This is considered a medical emergency and needs immediate treatment. An MRI of the spine will be done to see whether the cancer is pressing on your spinal cord. Treatment with steroid drugs, such as prednisone or dexamethasone, will begin right away to reduce spinal cord swelling and preserve nerve function. These will also help with pain, although other drugs for pain will likely be needed. Depending on how much pressure is on the spinal cord, surgery may be done to remove all or part of the tumor in the spine and to make the spine more stable. Surgery is often followed by radiation therapy to help keep the cancer from growing back right away. If surgery is not needed, radiation is started right away to shrink the tumor.

If Cancer Has Spread to the Chest or Lungs

Pleural effusion: Breast cancer can spread to the pleura—the tissue that coats the outside of the lungs. This may cause fluid to build up around the lungs (called pleural effusion). The fluid keeps the lung from being able to expand fully when you take a breath, leading to shortness of breath.

Pleural effusion is often treated by using a needle to remove the fluid that has built up around the lungs. This is called thoracentesis. The cancer must then be treated to keep the fluid from building up again. If the fluid keeps coming back, a chemical or talc can be put into the space to prevent further fluid buildup. This is called pleurodesis. If pleurodesis does not work, a catheter can be inserted into the space around the lungs to allow the fluid to be drained.

Shortness of breath: The cancer can spread to the lung tissue itself, leading to shortness of breath and cough. If the cancer spreads to one of the airways leading to the lungs, it can prevent that lung from expanding all the way when a breath is taken, leading to lung collapse.

Shortness of breath can be treated with oxygen and opioid drugs (such as morphine). If an area of cancer spread is blocking an airway, all or part of the tumor might be able to be removed with laser treatment. Sometimes radiation therapy is used instead.

Pericardial effusion: Breast cancer can also spread to the sac surrounding the heart (the pericardium). This is not common, but it can cause fluid to build up around the heart (called a pericardial effusion). The fluid can press on the heart so that it cannot pump blood well. Symptoms include shortness of breath, low blood pressure, swelling, and feeling tired.

Removing the fluid with a long, hollow needle can relieve a pericardial effusion. This procedure, called pericardiocentesis, is usually done in the hospital so that the heartbeat can be monitored. This procedure is often followed by surgery to put a small hole in the pericardium to prevent further fluid buildup. Sometimes radiation therapy and/or putting a chemical into the pericardium will also be tried to prevent further fluid buildup.

If Cancer Has Spread to the Brain

The most common symptoms of cancer spreading to the brain are headaches and losing movement in part of your body, such as in an arm or leg. Some other common symptoms are nausea and sleepiness. Problems with hearing, eyesight, and even passing urine can also occur. Seizures are another possible symptom of cancer in the brain. They are not common, but they can be very upsetting and scary for you and those around you.

Treatment with steroid drugs, such as dexamethasone, can often help with symptoms. Medicines called anticonvulsants might be given to help prevent seizures. If there are only one or two areas of cancer spread in the brain, they may be removed surgically or treated with a type of radiation therapy known as stereotactic radiosurgery. This may be followed by radiation to the entire brain (whole brain irradiation). If there are many areas of cancer metastasis in the brain, treatment generally consists of whole brain irradiation and steroids.

If Cancer Has Spread to the Meninges

Cancer can also spread to the meninges—the tissues that coat the brain and spinal cord. This is called leptomeningeal spread. This can cause problems with weakness in the arms and legs, slurred speech, trouble swallowing, double vision, and weakness of the facial muscles. To diagnose leptomeningeal spread, the doctor must do a lumbar puncture (also called a spinal tap) to remove some of the fluid that surrounds the brain and spinal cord (called cerebrospinal fluid). The fluid is examined under the microscope to see whether it contains cancer cells.

Treatment for metastasis to the meninges can include injecting chemotherapy into the cerebrospinal fluid (called intrathecal chemotherapy). Radiation to the brain and spinal cord can also be used.

If Cancer Has Spread to the Liver

If cancer spreads to the liver, you may lose your appetite and feel tired. Some people feel pain in the upper right part of the abdomen, where the liver is. The pain is usually not severe and is less of a problem than the tiredness and appetite loss. If there is a lot of cancer in the liver, the eyes and skin might turn yellow. This is called jaundice. Metastasis to the liver is most often treated with chemotherapy or hormone therapy to shrink the tumors, but it can be hard to treat with chemotherapy. This is because many of these drugs are broken down by the liver, and drug levels can get dangerously high if the liver is not working well.

If Cancer Has Spread to the Skin

When cancer spreads to the skin, it can cause lumps on the skin. Sometimes these lumps open up, becoming painful sores. If the sores become infected, they can smell bad, too. Treatment might include radiation therapy to the sores to shrink them and dry them out. This can be done only if the area has not received radiation therapy before. Certain chemotherapy drugs can be put directly on the tumors to help dry them up. If the sores are infected, antibiotic pills or cream can help.

Other Problems

Advanced cancer can also lead to problems that are not caused by a specific area of metastasis. Left untreated, these problems can severely impair your quality of life. These can include constipation and diarrhea, depression, fatigue, nausea and vomiting, and pain. These side effects and ways to cope with them are discussed in chapter 13.

Pregnancy and Breast Cancer Treatment

Breast cancer is not often diagnosed in pregnant women. Because more women are now choosing to have children later in life, however, and because the risk of breast cancer increases as women get older, a breast cancer diagnosis during pregnancy is more common than in the past. Two important and related issues are how the pregnancy will affect the woman's cancer treatment options and how cancer treatment will affect the current or future pregnancies. Fertility after cancer treatment is discussed more in chapter 13.

Treatment During Pregnancy

If you are pregnant at the time of your breast cancer diagnosis, your treatment options will likely be affected by your condition. The type and timing of treatment will depend on many things, including the stage of the cancer, how far along the pregnancy is, and your preferences.

When possible, surgery is the first treatment for any woman with breast cancer who is pregnant. Surgery poses little risk to a fetus and is the safest treatment option for pregnant women. Many doctors, such as a high-risk obstetrician, a surgeon, and an anesthesiologist, will need to work together to decide the best time to perform the surgery. If it is done later in the pregnancy, the obstetrician may be there in case there are problems with the baby during surgery. Together, these doctors will also decide which drugs and techniques are the safest for both mother and baby.

Radiation therapy during pregnancy is known to increase the risk of birth defects, so it is not recommended for pregnant women. For this reason, breast-conserving surgery (lumpectomy with radiation therapy) is an option only when the radiation can wait until after the baby is born. Otherwise, mastectomy should be done instead. If the cancer is found during the third trimester of pregnancy, breast-conserving surgery might be an option, as there would be very little delay in radiation treatments. A woman who would be undergoing chemotherapy before radiation may also have little or no delay in her radiation treatments. But cancers found early in the pregnancy may mean a longer delay in starting radiation. Treatment during pregnancy must always be considered on a case-by-case basis.

Chemotherapy usually is not given during the first trimester of pregnancy. The risk of birth defects or miscarriage is greatest during this time. The safety of chemotherapy during this period has not been studied because of concerns about damage to the fetus. All chemotherapy drugs were once thought to harm the fetus, but some chemotherapy drugs have been shown not to raise the risk for birth defects or stillbirths when used during the second and third trimesters (the fourth through ninth months of pregnancy).

If a woman is already in her third trimester when the cancer is diagnosed, chemotherapy might be delayed until after the birth. Labor might be induced a few weeks early in these cases. Chemotherapy should not be given during the three to four weeks before delivery, as it can lower the mother's blood cell counts, which could cause bleeding and increase the chances of infection during birth. Holding off on chemotherapy for the last few weeks before delivery allows the mother's blood cell counts to return to normal levels before childbirth.

The targeted drugs trastuzumab, pertuzumab, lapatanib, and everolimus (Affinitor) are not recommended during pregnancy. The use of hormone therapy, such as tamoxifen or aromatase inhibitors, after surgery or as treatment for advanced breast cancer has not been studied well in pregnant women, so its effects are not known. Most infants born to women taking tamoxifen have been normal, but there have been reports of miscarriages, fetal deaths, and birth defects of the head and face in a few babies born to women who took tamoxifen early in pregnancy. More study in this area is needed, but it is recommended that hormone therapy for breast cancer not be started until after the woman has given birth.

Breastfeeding During Cancer Treatment

Most doctors recommend that women who are about to be treated for breast cancer stop (or not start) breastfeeding. If surgery is planned, stopping breastfeeding can help reduce blood flow to the breasts and make them smaller, which can help with the operation. It also helps reduce the risk of infection in the breast and can help prevent breast milk from collecting in biopsy or surgical areas. In addition, many chemotherapy and hormone therapy drugs can enter breast milk and be passed on to the baby, so breastfeeding is not recommended during chemotherapy or hormone therapy.

If you have specific questions, such as when it might be safe to start breastfeeding, talk with your medical team. If you wish to resume breastfeeding after stopping for a while, you will need to plan ahead. You might need extra help from breastfeeding experts.

CHAPTER 11

Clinical Trials

Clinical trials are research studies in people to help find ways to improve health and cancer care. These studies are used to learn more about certain diseases and conditions. They are also used to find better ways to prevent, diagnose, or treat diseases such as cancer. Some people just call clinical trials research studies.

Clinical trials can offer benefits for many people during their cancer experience. These can include access to newer or more treatment options, getting more involved medical care, and having a greater sense of control over the situation. But by their nature, clinical trials involve some possible risks and disadvantages, and they may not be right for everyone. Your decision about whether to consider a clinical trial should be based on a realistic understanding of the possible risks and benefits.

What Are Clinical Trials?

When most people think of clinical trials, they think of studies of new drugs and treatments. But clinical trials are done to study many different areas of a disease, including the following:

- who gets it
- how to prevent it
- how to find it early (screening)
- diagnosis
- treatment options
- supportive care (including control of pain and other symptoms and methods to help people recover after treatment)

- patient quality of life
- psychological impact of the disease

Not every type of research study directly affects your medical care. Some simply gather information through medical records and questionnaires or ask that your blood or tumor tissue be used to learn more about your cancer. These types of studies are very important in terms of advancing knowledge about cancer.

Who Can Take Part in a Clinical Trial

All clinical trials have guidelines about who can and cannot take part. These are called eligibility criteria. Each person has to match these criteria to be eligible for the study. For instance, some studies look for volunteers with a certain type of illness or a certain stage of disease, whereas others look for healthy volunteers. Some studies look for people who have been treated for their illness, and others look for people who have not.

The factors that allow a person to sign up for a study are called inclusion criteria, whereas some factors can exclude a person from a study—these are called exclusion criteria. For example, if a study is looking for people of a certain age, then older and younger people cannot take part. Having certain medical conditions might mean that you can't take part in a study, as can taking certain drugs. These criteria are often used to be sure that the people in the study can take part safely. They also help make sure that the researchers will be able to answer their questions.

For cancer treatment clinical trials, eligibility criteria often include the following:
- the type of cancer a person has
- the stage of the cancer
- what previous treatments the person has had
- the length of time since the last treatment
- results of certain laboratory tests
- what medicines the person is taking
- other medical conditions the person has
- any history of another type of cancer
- a person's activity level (also known as performance status)

Other factors, such as a person's age or sex, might also be part of the criteria. There are usually other criteria for each study, too.

Things to Think About When Deciding to Take Part in a Clinical Trial

Possible Benefits

If you meet the criteria for a clinical trial, your doctor may recommend that you participate. The decision is up to you—all clinical trials are voluntary. Keep in mind that although there are risks associated with taking part in a clinical trial, there are also many potential benefits:

- You may have access to treatment that is not otherwise available, which might be safer or work better than current treatment options.
- You will probably get more attention from your medical team and more careful monitoring of your condition and the possible side effects of treatment.
- Some study sponsors may pay for part or all of your medical care and other expenses during the study. (This is not true for all clinical trials. Be sure you know who is expected to pay for your care before you enroll in the study.)
- You may feel you have more control over your situation and are taking a more active role in your health care.
- You may help others who have the same condition in the future by helping to advance cancer research.

Some of our most powerful advances in cancer treatment have been made through participation in clinical trials.

Possible Risks

Are there risks associated with taking part in a clinical trial? Yes. But risks are a part of any medical test, drug, or procedure. The risk might be greater in certain clinical trials because some aspects of any new treatment are unknown. This is especially true of early clinical trials of drugs or other treatments: early on, scientists do not know the effects or side effects that the treatment might have in people. For later studies, the biggest risk may be that the new treatment is not as good as the standard one.

A more important question is whether the possible benefits outweigh the risks. People with cancer are often willing to accept a certain amount of risk for a chance to be helped, but it is always important to have a realistic idea about the actual chance of being helped. Some people decide that any chance of benefit is worth the risk, whereas others choose to be more cautious. Weighing all of these factors will help you make a more informed decision—one that's right for you.

Costs and Insurance Coverage

It is important to learn about costs and insurance issues before deciding to take part in a clinical trial. Although the overall costs of taking part in a clinical trial are not much more than the costs of treatment outside of a study, insurance coverage can vary widely. Sometimes all of the care related to a clinical trial is free, but some insurance companies will not cover costs when a new treatment is being tested. Check to see whether your insurance policy has an exclusion for experimental treatment. When insurers do cover costs related to clinical trials, it is usually only for tests, treatments, or doctor visits that would have been part of your treatment plan even if you were not taking part in a study. In other words, they are not likely to pay for special tests or treatments you are getting just because you are in the study.

For new drugs, the study sponsor (whether it is the government or a pharmaceutical or biotechnology company) usually provides the new treatment free and pays for special testing or extra doctor visits. But this is not always the case. For some studies (often those looking for healthy volunteers), the sponsors might pay you a small stipend (meant to compensate you for things such as travel time and mileage). It is important to find out what you can expect before entering the study.

Recognizing the importance of clinical trials, many states have passed laws about insurance coverage for research studies. A few states without such laws have worked out voluntary agreements with insurance companies to cover clinical trials. The federal government has become involved, too. One of the goals of the Patient Protection and Affordable Care Act of 2010 was to make coverage available for cancer treatment given within clinical trials, allowing more people to take part in them. As of January 2014, insurers will not be able to drop or limit existing coverage because a person chooses to take part in a clinical trial. This will apply to clinical trials related to cancer or other life-threatening conditions.

Be sure that the paperwork your doctor submits to your insurance company describes your treatment in terms that will not jeopardize your coverage. It might help if the doctor includes studies supporting the treatment, its benefits, and its acceptance by the medical community. If your claim is turned down, try submitting it again. If turned down again, ask your medical plan about its appeals process. If you still have to pay for some or all of the treatment, you can try to negotiate a lower cost.

For more information on clinical trials and insurance, contact the American Cancer Society at 800-227-2345.

Questions to Ask Your Medical Team About Clinical Trials

- Do members of my medical team participate in clinical trials? If so, what type?

- Am I eligible for a national or local clinical trial?

- What is the study trying to find out? Is it trying to find the safest dosage of a new drug or to see whether one treatment is more effective than another?

- Who is sponsoring the study? Has it been reviewed by a respected national group, such as the NCI? Which institutional review board or ethics committee approved the study?

- What results could I reasonably expect from the trial treatment?

- In early studies, how has the trial treatment compared to current treatments?

- How is my cancer likely to progress or change if I join this study? What treatment plan would I pursue if I didn't join the study?

- How would being in the study affect my daily life? Would I be able to continue work?

- Would I have to be hospitalized? How often and for how long?

- What kinds of additional tests, such as blood tests or biopsies, would I need to have for the study? What are the side effects or risks of these tests?

- How long would my participation in the study last, assuming I complete all of it?

- What short-term and long-term side effects are possible with the treatments being tested? Are any of these likely to be permanent or life-threatening?

- Could I continue taking my other medicines?

- If I am harmed during the study, to what care would I be entitled for problems related to the trial treatment? Would the study sponsor pay to treat these problems?

- Where would I be treated and evaluated? Would I have to travel? How often?

- How would you know if the treatment was working properly or if I was responding to it?

- What type of follow-up care would I receive after I'm done participating?

- How much would my personal doctor be involved in my follow-up care?

- Who would be responsible for my health care while I'm in the clinical trial?

- Would the treatment involve additional expense?

- Would any or all of the costs be covered? Are there other sources I can turn to for help?

- Do you know of any organizations that could help me persuade my insurance company plan to cover the costs?

What Kind of Care Can I Expect?

You might worry that you are being a "guinea pig" if you agree to be in a research study. People who participate in clinical trials will receive excellent care. Instead of being treated by one or two doctors, study participants' health and well-being are monitored by multiple specialists.

In some studies, the health of patients who are given a placebo (an inactive substance) is compared with that of patients who receive an active treatment, so that researchers can gauge the effectiveness of treatment versus no treatment at all. However, clinical trials of anticancer drugs are not usually designed to have participants receive a placebo (even when the current standard is no treatment). Participants in cancer clinical trials generally receive either a standard cancer treatment or a new treatment that is hoped to be better than current treatments. When there is no accepted treatment for a certain cancer, the new treatment is often compared to "best supportive care," which is something that every patient is given.

Clinical Trials of Treatments

Promising new treatments are studied in clinical trials. Clinical trials are designed to help the medical community find out whether a new treatment is "safe and effective"— whether it works without being too toxic. To learn this, the treatment is given under controlled conditions to a certain number of patients. Information is collected to see how well the treatment works and what problems the patients have during and after treatment. Each patient who takes part in a clinical trial provides information on the effectiveness and risks of the new treatment.

Laboratory research allows the development of medical and scientific advances. Before any new treatment is given to people, it is carefully studied in cells and animals in the laboratory. This laboratory research identifies which new methods are most likely to succeed and can help show how to use them safely and effectively. But this early research cannot predict exactly how a new treatment will work in people or identify all the side effects that might occur. After all, people and animals can be very different in the way their bodies absorb, process, and get rid of substances. A treatment that works against cancer in mice may or may not work in people. And people may have side effects or other problems that did not appear when the treatment was studied in mice.

Thousands of clinical trials of cancer treatment are currently under way in the United States. By doing clinical trials, researchers try to answer questions about a new treatment, such as the following:

- Is the treatment safe? What side effects does it cause?
- How does this new type of treatment work?
- Is the treatment helpful? Does it help people live longer?
- Does it work better than current treatments?
- Are the side effects greater or less than with standard treatments?
- Do the benefits outweigh the risks (side effects)?
- Which patients are most likely to be helped by the treatment?

Answering these questions, while exposing as few people as possible to an unknown treatment, often requires several different clinical trials.

Phases of Clinical Trials

Clinical trials are carried out in steps called phases. Each phase is designed to answer certain types of questions, while trying to ensure the people taking part are kept as safe as possible. New treatments are tested in two or more phases of clinical trials before being considered "safe and effective." Researchers analyze the information gathered at each stage to decide whether the treatment is promising enough to continue the study and progress to the next phase.

Phase I

Phase I trials are mainly dose-finding studies. Small numbers of people take part in this type of study, which investigates the best way to give a drug, how often it should be given, and what dose(s) can be used. In general, everyone in the study receives the drug the same way (for example, by IV) and on the same schedule (weekly, for example), but they might not all get the same dose. The first few patients get the lowest dose, and if serious side effects do not occur, the next few patients get a higher dose. This process continues to find the highest dose that can be given that still has acceptable side effects. Often, patients taking part in phase I studies have tests done (usually blood tests) to look at levels of the drug in the blood and to see how the body breaks down the drug. At this stage, scientists are trying to learn what happens to a drug in the human body and what side effects may occur at different dosages. These studies are not designed to find out whether the new treatment works against cancer.

A phase I trial is often the first time a new drug is given to people. Sometimes phase I studies are used to see what doses to use when combining two approved drugs for the first time. For many drugs or treatments, the phase I study will enroll patients with different types of cancer. If a treatment is designed for a certain cancer, though, only people with that type of cancer will be included. When this is the case, the phase I study might be combined with another study to see whether the treatment works for that type of cancer. This combination is known as a phase I/II study.

Phase II

In phase II trials, researchers try to figure out how effective the studied treatment is in people with a specific type of cancer. In a typical phase II trial, all the patients are treated and all get the same dose of the drug. No placebo or inactive treatment is used. In some phase II studies, though, patients are split into two or more treatment groups, much like what is done in phase III trials. These groups may get different doses or get the treatment in different ways to see which provides the best balance of safety and effectiveness. If a treatment shows enough benefit without too many risks and side effects, it often moves to phase III study. Still, about 70 percent of phase II cancer drugs do not advance to phase III studies, usually because they do not work well enough. Some drugs may be approved for use against cancer based on a phase II study, but this really only happens for rare cancers when there is no other approved treatment.

Phase III

A phase III trial is often the final round of study before a new drug is approved for use in people. This type of study involves large numbers of patients. Phase III trials help doctors decide how the new treatment or drug compares to the accepted standard treatment. Some phase III studies are designed to see whether a new drug is better than the standard treatment. Others are designed to see whether the new drug or treatment is as good as standard treatment (called an equivalence study) or is not worse than the standard treatment (called a noninferiority trial).

Because doctors do not know at this stage of the study which treatment is better, patients are often assigned at random to get either the standard treatment or the new treatment (this is called randomization). The group getting the standard treatment may be called the "control group." If possible, the type of treatment the patient is getting will be kept secret from both the patient and the medical team. This type of study is called a double-blind study. This is often impractical in cancer treatment trials.

As with other studies, patients in phase III trials are watched closely for side effects, and treatment is stopped if side effects get too bad. Placebos might be used in some phase III studies, but only if no effective treatment exists.

Based on the possible expected outcome, a phase III trial will enroll a certain number of patients. This is to give the study statistical "power" to find at least a certain difference (or even a lack of difference) between the two treatments. Often, patient outcomes are analyzed at a midpoint, before all the patients are enrolled. This is called an interim analysis and is used to see whether continuing the study is warranted. For example, if one group has much better results than the other, the study may need to be stopped so that everyone can get the better treatment. The study might also be stopped early if the evidence clearly shows that the results at the end of the trial are likely to be negative (if the new drug is not better than the old one, for example). This approach is sometimes called futility analysis.

Phase IV

Even after testing a new medicine on thousands of people, scientists might not know the full effects of the treatment. Some questions often still need to be answered. For example, a drug might be approved by the US Food and Drug Administration (FDA) because it has been shown to reduce the risk for cancer recurrence or cause the cancer to shrink. But does this mean that people who take the drug are more likely to live longer? Are there rare side effects that have not been seen yet, or side effects that show up only after a person takes the drug for a long time? These types of questions can take many years to answer fully, and they might not be critical for getting a medicine to market. Phase IV clinical trials often address such questions.

Phase IV studies look at drugs that have already been approved by the FDA. The drugs are already available for doctors to prescribe for patients, but these studies are still needed to answer important questions.

When thinking about taking part in a phase IV trial, you should know that the drug has already been approved for use. You do not need to enroll in the study to get the medicine. At the same time, the care you would get in these types of studies often is very much like what you could expect if you were to get the treatment outside of a clinical trial. You should be reassured that in taking part, you would be getting a form of treatment that has already been studied a lot and that you would be doing a service to future patients.

FDA Approval

In the United States, when clinical trials show that a new drug treatment is better in some way than the current standard treatment, the drug's manufacturer submits a new drug application (NDA) to the FDA for approval. Most often, the results of phase III studies are needed before the company can submit an NDA, but sometimes phase II results are enough, as in the case of some drug treatments for rare diseases that lack effective standard treatments. The FDA then reviews the results from the clinical trials and other relevant information. In general, the FDA looks to see whether the new drug is more effective and/or safer than current treatments. If the FDA has questions, it may ask the drug company for more information or even require that the company conduct more studies, which can extend the approval process to more than five years.

Based on its review, the FDA decides whether it will approve the treatment for use in patients with the type of illness for which it was tested. This approval might be very specific; for example, a drug might be approved for use only for a certain type and stage of cancer and only after certain other treatments have been used first. This set of requirements is known as an *indication*. The drug company can market the drug only for the indications approved by the FDA. Still, once a drug has been approved, it is available to anyone who might need it. Doctors can legally prescribe it for people and diseases not included in the FDA indication. This is known as off-label prescribing. Off-label use of drugs is very common, but it can be a gray area. Often, but not always, there are good data to support a particular off-label use. Another factor to consider is that your insurance company may not cover off-label treatments.

How Can I Learn More About Clinical Trials?

There are several ways to learn about clinical trials. Most people who enter clinical trials do so after hearing about them from their doctors. Many cancer patients actively look for clinical trials on the Internet or in other places, hoping to find more options for treatment. Some clinical trials are advertised directly to patients. No one source can offer information about all of the cancer clinical trials now enrolling patients. Clinical trial lists and clinical trials matching services are the primary resources for locating trials for your specific situation.

Clinical Trial Lists

Clinical trial lists provide the names and descriptions of clinical trials of new treatments. If you are interested in a particular study, you will probably be able to find it in a list. The list will often include a description of the study, the criteria for eligibility, and a contact person. If you (or your medical team members) are willing and able to read through descriptions of all the studies listed for your cancer type, then a list might be all you need. Some organizations that provide lists can help you narrow the list a little, according to the kind of treatment you're looking for (chemotherapy, radiation therapy, hormone therapy, etc.) and the stage of your cancer.

Clinical Trials Matching Services

Several organizations have developed computer systems that match patients with studies for which they might be eligible, called a clinical trials matching service. This service is often offered online. Each might differ somewhat in how it works. Some services let you search for clinical trials without registering at the website. If you do have to register, the service should assure you that your information will be kept confidential. Either way, you will probably have to enter certain details, such as the type of cancer, the stage of the disease, and any previous treatments you might have had. With this information, these systems can find clinical trials for which you might be eligible and save you the time and effort of reading descriptions of studies that are not relevant. Some groups also allow you to subscribe to mailing lists so that you're informed as new studies open up.

Although they are usually free to users, most clinical trials matching services get paid to list studies or get a finder's fee from those running the studies when someone enrolls. This might affect how and in what order the services rank the studies.

How to Choose a Clinical Trials Matching Service

Because different services work differently, be sure you understand how the service you are looking at operates. Ask the following questions. (Note that the answers do not necessarily mean that the service is not worth using.)

- Is there a fee for using the service?
- Do I have to register to use the service?
- Does the service keep my information confidential?
- How does the service get its list of clinical trials?
- Does the service rank the studies in any particular order? Is this based on fees they get?
- Can I contact the service through the Internet or by telephone?

American Cancer Society Clinical Trials Matching Service: The American Cancer Society works with the Coalition of Cancer Cooperative Groups—a nonprofit service organization dedicated to ensuring access to clinical trials—to provide a free, confidential, and reliable matching and referral service for patients looking for clinical trials. The TrialCheck database, developed and maintained by the Coalition, is a comprehensive database of studies being sponsored by the Coalition groups, the National Cancer Institute, and drug/biotechnology companies. To our knowledge, this is the most complete matching database of cancer clinical trials.

This clinical trials information is not biased in any way. It is updated every day, as is the contact information that allows people to get in touch with the doctors and nurses at cancer centers running each of the studies. You can access the TrialCheck system by visiting www.cancertrialshelp.org/trialcheck or calling 877-227-8451.

Other clinical trials lists and matching services: The National Cancer Institute (NCI) sponsors most government-funded clinical trials for cancer. The NCI has a list of active studies (those currently enrolling patients) and some privately funded studies. You can find the list by visiting www.cancer.gov/clinicaltrials or calling 800-4-CANCER (800-422-6237). You can search the list by the type and stage of cancer, by the type of study (for example, treatment or prevention), or by ZIP code.

The National Institutes of Health (NIH) has an even larger database of clinical trials at www.clinicaltrials.gov, but not all of these are cancer studies.

EmergingMed provides a free and confidential matching and referral service for people looking for cancer clinical trials at www.emergingmed.com, or you can call 877-601-8601.

CenterWatch (www.centerwatch.com) is a publishing and information services company that keeps a list of industry- and government-funded clinical trials for cancer and other diseases.

Private companies, such as drug and biotechnology firms, may list the studies they are sponsoring on their websites or offer toll-free numbers so you can call and ask about them. Some of these companies also offer matching services for the studies they sponsor. This can be helpful if you are interested in research on a particular experimental treatment and know which company is developing it.

Taking Part in a Clinical Trial

Informed Consent

Enrollment in a clinical trial is completely up to you. The people running the study are required to get your written informed consent before you take part in any way (often even before you have any needed tests to see whether you are eligible for the study). During the informed consent process, the researchers (doctors or nurses) will explain the details of the study to you and answer your questions and concerns.

You will then be given a consent form to sign. Consent forms are not all the same, but they should include the following:

- the reason for the study (what the researchers hope to find out)
- who is eligible to take part in the study
- what is known about the treatments being studied
- the possible risks and benefits of the treatments (based on what is known so far)
- other treatments that might be an option for you
- the design of the study (whether it is randomized, double-blinded, uses a placebo, etc.)
- how many and what types of tests and doctor visits are involved
- who must pay for the costs of the trial (tests, doctor visits, etc.) and any other care you might need because you took part in the trial
- a statement about how your identity will be protected
- a statement saying that taking part in the study is voluntary and that you have the right to leave the study at any time without your care being affected
- contact information if you have further questions

Before you sign the consent form, ask questions. Be sure someone from the research team goes over the study and the form with you in detail. Researchers try to make consent forms easy to understand, but some words or ideas can still be confusing. You might want to bring someone with you to the meeting to help make sure all your concerns are addressed.

Be sure you understand what is involved and what is expected of you. Explain what you heard to your doctor or nurse to make sure you've got it right. According to recent surveys, most people are satisfied with the informed consent process, but more than half do not understand some of the main points on the consent form.

Finally, do not feel rushed into making a decision. Take the consent form home with you if you want to. Ask trusted family members and friends what they think. If possible, you might want to get a second opinion from another doctor, too.

Taking Part in the Study

Once you've signed the consent form, you will be ready to take part in the study. You will probably need to have blood tests or imaging tests done before you start treatment (if you have not had them recently). A full medical history and physical examination are also usually done. The results are needed before you start the actual study, to make sure that you meet the eligibility criteria and to help keep you safe.

Some studies might need you to stay in a hospital for a day or two to get treatment. In other studies, the participants are treated much the same way as other patients who are not in a clinical trial.

You may need to have tests done more often to find out how well the treatment is going and to see how you are doing. You will likely get more attention as a study participant than you would otherwise. The doctors and nurses may examine you more often and will ask about any side effects (called adverse events) you are having.

Because the research team might not know all of the possible complications of the study treatment, it is very important to let them know about anything out of the ordinary. They can then decide whether your symptoms are related to the study, whether the symptoms need treatment, and whether your study treatment should be changed.

You might stop taking part in the study for any number of reasons:
• you finish the study treatment
• the treatment does not appear to be working for you
• you have serious side effects while in the study
• the study itself is stopped early because the treatment has been proven to work, has not been proven to work as well as standard treatment, or has been found to be too harmful
• you decide to leave the study for your own reasons

Once you have left the study, the researchers might still watch you for a time, so they can continue to get an idea of how you're doing.

Some studies let you keep taking the new treatment even after the study ends. This is known as open-label treatment, because you and your doctors both know which treatment you are getting. This option varies among trials, so be sure to ask about it before you begin.

What If I Want to Leave the Study Early?

You will be told many times before you enter the study that taking part in the study is always voluntary. This is an important point. You have the right to leave the study at any time, for any reason. Your doctor will still take care of you to the best of his or her ability.

In a study, the researchers might ask whether they can follow up with you from time to time to see how you're doing. This might give them important information and help keep you safe, even though you are no longer taking part in the study.

CHAPTER 12

Complementary and Alternative Therapies

Tens of millions of Americans spend billions of dollars a year on complementary and alternative therapies for a wide variety of diseases, ailments, and medical complaints, including cancer. The growing popularity of complementary and alternative therapies has had an enormous impact on every aspect of health care in the United States, Europe, and elsewhere in the developed world. Based in the 1960s back-to-nature movement, the rise of complementary and alternative medicine has particularly influenced people with cancer. Accurate figures are difficult to obtain, but it's believed that as many as 50 percent of people living with cancer have sought out some type of complementary or alternative therapy.

What Are Complementary and Alternative Therapies?

The terms complementary and alternative can be confusing. Not everyone uses them the same way, and they are used to refer to many different methods. These terms are often used interchangeably, but in this book, we make important distinctions between them.

Complementary therapies are used along with your regular medical care, or standard treatment. Some of these therapies can help relieve symptoms and improve quality of life by reducing the side effects of treatments or by providing psychological or physical benefits. Many women today have a growing interest in the use of complementary therapies to help enhance their quality of life, especially while dealing with breast cancer. Examples of complementary therapies include meditation (to reduce stress), ginger tea (to relieve nausea), and acupuncture (to relieve nausea). Some complementary therapies, such as massage therapy, yoga, and meditation, have also been referred to as supportive care. Some insurance plans offer their members discounts on complementary therapies. Complementary treatments can sometimes be dangerous, though, if they interfere with your cancer treatment, causing it to be less effective or have more side effects.

Alternative therapies, on the other hand, are unproven treatments that are used instead of conventional treatment. They may be used to try to prevent, treat, or cure disease. One of the greatest dangers of alternative medicine is that people with cancer may use alternative therapies instead of the conventional therapy that has been shown to help treat cancer and prolong survival. According to the American Cancer Society, 90 percent of women who receive a diagnosis of breast cancer survive at least five years if they receive standard medical care, which can include surgery, chemotherapy, and radiation therapy. Time spent pursuing alternative therapies is time spent delaying care that has been proven to be effective. Unneeded delays and interruptions in standard therapies are dangerous. Alternative therapies can also be toxic in and of themselves.

Talking to Your Doctor About Complementary and Alternative Therapies

Many cancer patients do not discuss complementary or alternative therapies with their doctors. However, communicating with your doctor is crucial. It's true that many doctors may not know about the uses, risks, and potential benefits of unconventional treatments. But this does not have to stop you. You can help bridge the knowledge gap in a number of ways:

- Gather as much information as you can about the therapy you are considering. Look for information from respected sources regarding the treatment's potential benefits and risks. For example, see the resource guide at the end of this book for information on some reputable organizations from which you can seek information.

- When you share information with your doctor, try to convey that you know your doctor wants what is best for you. Let him or her know that you are thinking about a complementary treatment and that you want to make sure it will not interfere with your regular medical treatment.

- Do not delay or forego conventional therapy. If you are thinking about stopping or not using conventional treatment, discuss this decision with your doctor. Sometimes a treatment delay can make a big difference in your prognosis.

- Let your doctor know which complementary and alternative therapies you are using now and before you begin using any others. This includes vitamins, minerals, supplements, and special diets. Even treatments thought to be safe in most cases can have harmful interactions with some cancer treatments. For example, doses of vitamin E that are normally safe can cause dangerous bleeding if you take them in the weeks immediately before surgery. Many supplements can interact in harmful ways with other medicines, so talk with your doctor and pharmacist, and report any changes in supplement use to your medical team.

- Ask the doctor about any studies on the therapy you are considering and whether you have other options. Ask questions—if it is helpful, make a list and bring it with you to your appointment. Let your doctor know you are an educated consumer and are seeking as much information as you can.

- Work with your doctor. If your doctor has not heard of the particular therapy you are interested in, do not become discouraged. Ask your doctor to help you find out more about it. Listen to what the doctor has to say, and try to understand his or her point of view. If the treatment you are considering will cause problems with your current treatment, discuss safer options together.

- Be sure to ask your doctor whether there are mainstream methods for treating the side effects or symptoms you are having. There are many supportive medical treatments that can help you feel better.

- Ask your doctor to help you identify possibly fraudulent products. See the information about "red flags" to watch for on the next page.

- Follow up after conversations with your medical team. Be sure to continue your conversation about complementary and alternative therapies from appointment to appointment (as appropriate). Your team may or may not agree with your decisions, but it is important that they know which treatments you are taking so they can give you the best possible care.

- Be open to change. New studies can yield new information about complementary and alternative methods of managing cancer, which could change your treatment plan.

- Though this will not apply to most people with breast cancer, be aware that complementary and alternative therapies can be especially risky if you are pregnant or breastfeeding. Never give herbal medicines to children without talking to their doctors first.

Researching Complementary and Alternative Therapies

Find out all you can about any type of treatment before getting your hopes up or taking something that could be harmful. Many alternative treatments have not been proven to be effective, so get all the facts. Keep an eye out for fraud. If something sounds too good to be true, it usually is. This can be hard to think about if you are looking for and hoping for a miracle. If you are not sure, talk to your doctor or nurse before moving ahead. You may want to use the following checklist to help you spot fraudulent treatments:

- Does the treatment promise a cure for all cancers or other serious illnesses? Be suspicious of claims that any unconventional treatment can cure cancer. Claims that a treatment can cure all cancers, or that it can cure cancer and other hard-to-treat diseases (such as chronic fatigue, multiple sclerosis, AIDS, etc.) are certain to be fraudulent.
- Are you told to use the treatment instead of using standard medical treatment?
- Is the treatment or drug a secret that only certain people can give?
- Is the treatment or drug offered by only one person or only one clinic? Keep in mind that once a treatment is found to be helpful, it will be used by other qualified professionals. Beware of treatments only available in one clinic, especially if the clinic is located in a country with less patient protection than the United States or the European Union.
- Do the promoters use terms such as "scientific breakthrough," "miracle cure," "secret ingredient," or "ancient remedy"?
- Are you offered personal stories of amazing results, but no actual scientific evidence?
- Do the promoters attack the medical or scientific community?
- Do the promoters promise no side effects? Many treatments promise to help you without causing any side effects, but even herbs and vitamins have side effects. If the treatment is marketed as having no side effects, it has not likely been studied in rigorous clinical trials, where side effects would be seen.

If you suspect fraud, contact the US Food and Drug Administration (FDA) at www.fda.gov or 888-463-6332.

When looking at information about a substance or treatment, particularly on the Internet, try to determine whether the information is provided by someone selling a product (such as a supplement or book). If a product is being promoted for sale, then information will likely be slanted toward helping to sell the product. The objectivity and accuracy of the information might not be reliable.

The American Cancer Society, the National Cancer Institute, and the National Center for Complementary and Alternative Medicine are reliable sources for information about complementary and alternative therapies. For contact information for these organizations, see the resource guide, starting on page 443.

Questions to Ask About Complementary and Alternative Therapies

- **What is my medical team's experience** with complementary therapies?
- **Does my hospital or medical facility offer these therapies?** If not, where can I go to find out more about them?
- **What claims are made for the treatment?** Does it reportedly cure the cancer, help conventional treatment work better, or relieve symptoms or side effects, for example?
- **What are the credentials of people** supporting the treatment? Are they recognized experts in cancer treatment? Have they published their findings in trustworthy medical journals?
- **How is the therapy promoted?** Is it promoted only in the mass media (the Internet, books, magazines, TV, and radio talk shows) rather than in scientific journals?
- **What are the costs** of therapy?
- **Is the treatment widely available** for use within the health care community, or is it controlled, with limited access to its use?
- **If I use the treatment in place** of conventional therapies or clinical trials, will the ensuing delay in standard treatment affect my chances for cure or advance the cancer stage?
- **Will the treatment help ease my pain** or decrease my anxiety?
- **Are there any books or videos about the treatment** that my medical team can recommend?
- **How do I find a licensed** or trained practitioner for the treatment?
- **Are there any complementary** treatments I should avoid?
- **Which treatment would my health care provider** most highly recommend?
- **Will my insurance cover** complementary treatments?

Complementary Therapies

Complementary therapies can be used along with conventional cancer treatments to decrease side effects and improve quality of life. For example, a special diet prescribed by a dietitian might help a woman with breast cancer stay healthy even though she is vomiting and losing weight because of chemotherapy. Complementary therapies related to the mind, body, and spirit—such as meditation, yoga, and prayer—might help relieve anxiety, nausea, and pain that can occur during cancer treatment. Complementary therapies do not directly alter the growth or spread of cancer.

Because many complementary therapies involve some form of physical or mental relaxation, they may help you better deal with emotional or psychological stress during and after breast cancer treatment. Many complementary therapies are also used during cancer treatment to help ease side effects.

Books, videos, and websites offer information on many different mind and body techniques, such as tai chi and aromatherapy. You can usually find classes on some of these methods at fitness and community centers in your area. Some hospitals and health centers offer training in these techniques.

The following complementary therapies are meant to be used with conventional treatment to help you deal with physical or emotional side effects and to promote well-being. Talk with your doctor before starting any exercise that involves manipulation of your joints or muscles. The complementary therapies used most often by people with cancer are discussed next.

Acupuncture

Acupuncture began two thousand to three thousand years ago as an important component of traditional Chinese medicine. With this technique, very thin needles of varying lengths are inserted at specific locations in the skin, called acupoints, and left in place for about half an hour. There are a number of different acupuncture techniques, including some that use sound waves, tiny electrical charges, and some that use actual needles. Skilled acupuncturists cause little to no pain, and the procedure is generally considered to be safe when performed by a licensed or certified practitioner.

Although no evidence supports the use of acupuncture as an effective treatment for cancer, clinical studies have proven its effectiveness in treating nausea caused by chemotherapy drugs and surgical anesthesia. It can also help with the hot flashes caused by hormone treatments.

Aromatherapy

Aromatherapy is the use of essential oils (fragrant substances distilled from plants) to alter mood or improve health. The use of aromatic, perfumed oils dates back thousands of years to ancient Egypt, China, and India. In Egypt, such oils were used after bathing and for embalming mummies. The Greeks and Romans used fragrant oils for both medicinal and cosmetic purposes. However, it was the medieval physician Avicenna who first extracted these oils from plants.

There are about forty essential oils commonly used in aromatherapy. These highly concentrated aromatic substances are either inhaled or applied as oils during massage. For inhalation, a few drops of the essential oil are placed in steaming water, an atomizer, or a humidifier that is used to spread the water vapor and oil combination throughout the room. Sometimes the oil is placed in a heatproof dish over a candle or other flame to diffuse the scent.

Essential oils also can be applied to the skin during massage or added to bathwater. For application to the skin, the oils are combined with another substance (called a carrier), usually vegetable oil. Some essential oils can be used directly on the skin. Oils may also be used to make salves, creams, and compresses. Some people also apply drops of certain essential oils to their pillows. Essential oils should never be taken internally. People should not directly breathe in the oil or keep it on the skin for long periods, either.

Aromatherapy is promoted as a natural way to help people cope with chronic pain, depression, and stress and to produce a feeling of well-being. Some evidence suggests that these effects might be real. Aromatherapy is self-administered or applied by an aromatherapist. Many aromatherapists in the United States are trained as massage therapists, psychologists, social workers, or chiropractors, and they use the oils as part of their practices.

Art Therapy

Art therapy is a form of treatment that uses creative activities such as painting, drawing, and sculpting to help people with physical and emotional problems express their emotions. Modern-day art therapy is based on the work of artist Hana Kwiatkowska, who introduced ways to evaluate and treat people by means of art therapy at the National Institute of Mental Health in 1958.

Art therapy provides a way for people to come to terms with emotional conflicts, increase self-awareness, and express unspoken and often unconscious concerns about their cancer. This therapy views the creative act as healing, which helps reduce stress, fear, and anxiety. Art therapy also can be used to distract people whose illnesses or treatments cause pain. Many medical centers and hospitals include art therapy as part of inpatient care. Although uncomfortable feelings can be stirred up at times, this is considered part of the healing process. Art therapists work with individuals or groups. The job of the art therapist is to help people express themselves through their creations.

Biofeedback

Biofeedback is a treatment method that uses monitoring devices to help people consciously control physical processes that the body usually controls automatically, such as the heartbeat, blood pressure, temperature, sweating, and muscle tension. For centuries, followers of ancient Eastern practices such as meditation and yoga have claimed they could control physical processes. Biofeedback has been approved by an independent panel convened by the National Institutes of Health as a useful complementary therapy for treating chronic pain and insomnia. It can also regulate or alter other physical functions that might be causing discomfort.

Biofeedback therapists use various monitoring devices to measure information that controls bodily processes. They must be trained and certified to control the monitoring equipment and to interpret changes. The monitoring/control process is repeated as often as needed until a person can reliably use conscious thought to change physical functions.

Hypnosis

Hypnosis can be an effective tool for reducing blood pressure, pain, anxiety, nausea, vomiting, phobias, and aversions to certain cancer treatments. It is a way to put people in a state of restful alertness that helps them focus on a certain problem or symptom. People who are hypnotized have selective attention and can achieve a state of heightened concentration while blocking out distractions. This allows people to be open to images, suggestions, and ideas for resolving issues and improving quality of life.

Most types of hypnotic techniques begin with an induction. While the person is sitting or lying quietly, the hypnotherapist talks in gentle, soothing tones, describes images, and repeats a series of verbal suggestions that allow the person to become relaxed, yet deeply absorbed and focused on his or her awareness. People under hypnosis might appear to be asleep, but they are actually in an altered state of concentration and can focus on a specific goal.

Contrary to what many believe, people under hypnosis are not under the control of the hypnotherapist, nor can they be made to do something they would not ordinarily do. Hypnosis is not brainwashing, and ideas are not "planted" in people's minds to make people do things against their will. Quite the opposite is true. Hypnosis is used to help people gain more control over their actions, emotions, and body. Make sure to use a hypnotherapist that is a trained, licensed professional.

Imagery and Visualization

Imagery involves mental exercises designed to enable the mind to influence the health and well-being of the body. Imagery is believed to have been used as a medical therapy for centuries. Some even say the techniques go back to the ancient Babylonians, Greeks, and Romans. Some people with cancer believe that imagery can ease nausea and vomiting associated with chemotherapy, relieve stress, enhance the immune system, aid in weight gain, combat depression, and lessen pain.

There are many different imagery techniques. One common technique, called guided imagery, involves visualizing a specific image or goal to be achieved and then imagining achieving that goal. One type of guided imagery used for people with cancer, the Simonton method, has the person imagine his or her body fighting the cancer cells and winning the battle.

Imagery techniques can be self-taught with the help of books, audio recordings, or they can be practiced under the guidance of a trained therapist. Imagery sessions with a health care professional might last between twenty to thirty minutes.

Massage

Massage involves the manipulation, rubbing, and kneading of the body's muscles and soft tissues. Massage was first used in many ancient cultures, including those of China, India, Persia, Arabia, Greece, and Egypt. Massage has been shown to decrease stress, anxiety, depression, insomnia, and pain. It is also known to relax muscles. Many people find that massage brings a temporary feeling of well-being and relaxation. Massage is also used to increase mobility, rehabilitate injured muscles, and reduce pain associated with headaches and backaches. There is also some evidence that massage can stimulate nerves, improve concentration, increase blood flow and the supply of oxygen to cells, and help circulation in the lymphatic system. In one study, massage of the feet, known as reflexology, and scalp massage both improved relaxation and quality of life in women after breast surgery.

Massage strokes can vary from light and shallow to firm and deep. The choice will depend on the needs of the person and the style of the massage therapist. If a person has a particular complaint, the therapist might focus on the area of pain or discomfort. Typical massage therapy sessions last from thirty minutes to one hour. Massage therapy appears to have few serious risks if it is used appropriately and provided by a trained massage professional.

Meditation

Meditation is a mind-body process that uses concentration or reflection to relax the body and calm the mind to create a sense of well-being. The ultimate goal of meditation is to separate oneself mentally from the outside world. Meditation is an important part of ancient Eastern religious practices, particularly in India, China, and Japan, but it can be found in all cultures of the world.

Meditation is a useful complementary therapy for treating chronic pain and insomnia. Meditation might also increase longevity and quality of life and reduce anxiety, high blood pressure, and blood cortisol levels initially brought on by stress.

Meditation can be self-directed or guided by doctors, psychiatrists, other mental health professionals, or yoga teachers. Some practitioners recommend two fifteen- to twenty-minute sessions a day.

Music Therapy

Music therapy consists of the active or passive use of music to promote healing and enhance quality of life. Music has been used in medicine for thousands of years. Ancient Greek philosophers believed that music could heal both the body and the soul. Native Americans have included singing as part of their healing rituals for centuries.

When used along with standard treatment, music therapy can help reduce pain and anxiety and relieve chemotherapy-induced nausea and vomiting. It might also relieve stress and provide an overall sense of well-being. In some studies, music therapy has lowered the heart rate, blood pressure, and breathing rate and has eased depression and sleeplessness. Some medical experts believe it can aid healing, improve physical movement, and enrich a person's quality of life.

Music therapists design sessions for individuals and groups based on their needs and tastes. Music therapy can include improvisation, receptive listening, songwriting, lyric discussion, imagery, performance, and learning through music. People can also perform their own music therapy at home by listening to music or sounds that help relieve their symptoms. Music therapy can be conducted in hospitals, cancer centers, hospice centers, at home, or anywhere people can benefit from its calming or stimulating effects.

Prayer and Other Spiritual Practices

Spirituality is generally described as an awareness of something greater than the individual self and is usually expressed through religion and/or prayer. Since the beginning of recorded history, cultures throughout the world have developed systems of religion and spirituality. Earlier religions of ancient Egypt and Greece have given way to more modern religions such as Christianity, Judaism, Hinduism, Buddhism, Islam, and others. Spirituality, especially in the form of prayer, is practiced by billions of people throughout the world.

Spirituality and religion can be very important to the quality of life for some people with cancer. The benefits of prayer can include reduction of stress and anxiety, promotion of a more positive outlook, and the strengthening of the will to live. Proponents of spirituality claim that prayer can decrease the negative effects of disease, speed recovery, and increase the effectiveness of medical treatments. Religious attendance has been associated with the improvement of various health conditions, such as cancer, and of overall health status.

Prayer can be silent or spoken out loud and can be done alone or in groups, as in a church or temple. One form of spirituality, regular attendance at a church, temple, mosque, or other house of worship, can involve supplication (prayer that focuses on one's self) or intercessory prayer (praying for others). Prayers often ask a higher being for help, understanding, wisdom, or strength in dealing with life's problems.

Many medical institutions and practitioners include spirituality and prayer as important components of healing. In addition, hospitals have chapels and contracts with ministers, rabbis, and voluntary organizations to serve the spiritual needs of people with cancer.

Relaxation

Relaxation can relieve pain or keep it from getting worse by reducing tension in the muscles. It can help you fall asleep, give you more energy, make you feel less tired, reduce your anxiety, and make other methods of relieving pain work better.

Relaxation cannot be forced. It might take up to two weeks of practice to feel the first results of relaxation. Use it regularly for at least five to ten minutes twice a day. Check for tension throughout the day by noticing tightness in each part of your body from head to foot. Relax any muscles that feel tense.

There are different relaxation methods. Visual concentration involves opening your eyes and staring at an object, or closing your eyes and thinking of a peaceful, calm scene. Rhythmic massage is done by firmly massaging an area of pain with the palm of your hand in a circular pattern. Inhaling and exhaling involves breathing deeply while tensing your muscles or a group of muscles, holding your breath and keeping your muscles tense for a second or two more, and then letting go and breathing out while letting your body go limp. You can practice slow, rhythmic breathing while staring at an object or while closing your eyes and concentrating on your breathing or on a peaceful scene. You can also use relaxation CDs or downloads. These recordings give step-by-step instructions in relaxation techniques. Other methods include using imagery (imagining yourself in a comfortable, peaceful place), listening to slow, familiar music through earphones or a headset, and progressive relaxation of body parts.

Special Diets

Staying well nourished during cancer treatment can be especially challenging. Some people are tempted to go to extremes, restricting their diets to only a few types of foods. Although certain foods, such as fruits, vegetables, and whole grains, can provide general health benefits, no diet can cure cancer.

A vegetarian diet consists mainly or entirely of food that comes from plant sources such as fruits and vegetables. Some vegetarians (the lacto-ovo type) also consume milk products and eggs, but vegans do not. Some studies have linked vegetarian diets to lower risk for heart disease, diabetes, high blood pressure, obesity, and colon cancer. Although a diet emphasizing plant-based foods is naturally high in fiber and can help people maintain a healthy weight, vegetarian diets can still contain sugar, refined grains, processed foods, and fried foods. These foods are not a part of a macrobiotic diet. A macrobiotic diet consists largely of whole grains, cereals, and vegetables and is based on simplicity and avoidance of "toxins" that come from eating dairy products, meats, and processed or oily foods. A macrobiotic diet can provide general health benefits associated with low-fat, high-fiber diets. However, there is no scientific evidence that either a vegetarian or macrobiotic diet is an effective cancer treatment, and both diets can lead to poor nutrition if overly restrictive or not properly planned.

There is no proof that any other special diet (such as the China, Gerson, Hallelujah, Livingston-Wheeler, and "detoxification" diets) has any anticancer effects. In fact, some can be harmful. Fasting, or not taking in any food and drinking only water or certain liquids, also can harm your health and should be avoided. Even a short fast can have harmful effects.

If you want to follow a particular diet during cancer treatment, discuss your plans with your medical team. Cancer treatment can cause such side effects as nausea, diarrhea, altered taste, and reduced appetite. These can make it especially difficult to maintain good nutrition, especially if your diet limits your intake of certain foods. Referral to a dietitian can be helpful.

Tai Chi

Tai chi is an ancient Chinese form of martial arts. It is a mind-body, self-healing system that uses movement, meditation, and breathing to improve health and well-being. Tai chi is based on the philosophy of Taoism, a Chinese belief system first developed in the sixth century B.C. Tai chi originated as a martial art and has been practiced as an exercise in China for many centuries. Its slow, graceful movements, accompanied by rhythmic breathing, relax the body and the mind. Tai chi relies entirely on technique rather than strength or power. It requires learning a number of different forms or movement groups.

Research has shown that tai chi used as a form of exercise can improve posture, balance, muscle mass and tone, flexibility, stamina, and strength in older adults. Tai chi is also recognized as a method to reduce stress and lower heart rate and blood pressure. People who practice the deep breathing and physical movements of tai chi claim that it makes them feel more relaxed, younger, and more agile. This general sense of well-being is said to reduce stress and lower blood pressure. Practitioners claim it is particularly suited for older adults or for others who are not physically strong or healthy.

Tai chi is taught in many health clubs, schools, and recreational facilities. Practitioners believe that daily practice is needed to get the most benefit from tai chi. Once an individual has mastered a form, it can be practiced at home.

Yoga

Yoga is a form of exercise that involves a program of precise posture and breathing activities. Yoga was first practiced in India more than five thousand years ago.

Yoga can be a useful tool to help relieve some of the symptoms associated with chronic diseases, such as cancer, arthritis, and heart disease, and to increase relaxation and physical fitness. Yoga might enhance quality of life. People who practice yoga claim that it leads to a state of physical health, relaxation, happiness, peace, and tranquility. There is some evidence showing that yoga can lower stress, increase strength, and provide a good form of exercise. Proponents also claim that yoga can be used to eliminate insomnia and increase stamina. Studies of yoga in breast cancer patients have found that women practicing yoga experienced improved mood and had less anxiety.

There are different variations and aspects of yoga. The most common form of yoga in the United States, Hatha yoga, involves the use of movement, breathing exercises, and meditation to achieve a connection with the mind, body, and spirit.

Practitioners say yoga should be done at either the beginning or the end of the day. A typical session can last between twenty minutes and an hour. A session might include guided relaxation, meditation, and sometimes visualization. It often ends with the chanting of a mantra (a meaningful word or phrase) to achieve a deeper state of relaxation. Becoming proficient in yoga requires several sessions a week. Yoga can be practiced at home without an instructor, in adult education classes, or in classes offered at health clubs and community centers. Many books and videos on yoga are available, too.

Herbs, Vitamins, Minerals, and Other Supplements

These therapies include a wide range of natural and biology-based products. Some people with cancer use supplements as an alternative to cancer treatment, but more often they are used along with standard therapies to relieve the mental stress and physical side effects associated with both cancer and its treatment.

It is important to remember that because many supplements are natural products, they do not have to be tested for safety before they come on the market. These products may not come in standard potencies or doses. Some can have very dangerous side effects, especially for patients undergoing cancer treatment. None of these therapies have been proven to halt or reverse the progression of cancer in people, and they should not be considered a substitute for conventional treatment. Consult your doctor before you start taking any herbs, vitamins, minerals, or other supplements—especially if you are pregnant or breastfeeding.

For more information about supplements, please visit the American Cancer Society at www.cancer.org or see our book, the *American Cancer Society Complete Guide to Complementary and Alternative Cancer Therapies, Second Edition*. The Memorial Sloan-Kettering Cancer Center website is also a good source of information about complementary and alternative therapies (www.mskcc.org/aboutherbs).

Regulation of dietary supplements: Dietary supplements are regulated differently than prescription medicines and drug products by the FDA. Drugs must be proven safe and effective by the manufacturer before being allowed on the market. Dietary supplements, however, are officially classified as "foods." Because of this classification, dietary supplements do not need FDA approval before they can be marketed to the public.

The manufacturers of dietary supplements are responsible for labeling their products accurately and making them safe for consumption. However, some dietary supplements have been found to contain contaminants or not to include ingredients listed on the product label. Current regulation of these products cannot ensure that these products are safe and effective before they become available to consumers. Manufacturers of dietary supplements are required to report adverse events to the FDA's Center for Food Safety and Applied Nutrition, but risks and side effects are not always reported. Ultimately, the FDA has to show that a specific product is unsafe before it can take action to remove a dietary supplement from the marketplace.

Possible dangers of herbal therapies for cancer patients: For people with cancer, herbal therapies can cause severe side effects, such as allergic reactions and excessive bleeding, and they can interact in dangerous ways with prescribed therapies. For example, some doctors have expressed concern that antioxidants may cause radiation and chemotherapy to be less effective.

There is also evidence that some commonly used herbal therapies might be harmful to people having surgery. It is best to tell your doctors about everything that you are taking, including vitamins, minerals, herbal medicines, and other supplements.

Alternative Therapies

Unlike conventional medicine, which uses therapies that have been proven to be effective using scientific evidence, there is little or no evidence supporting the use of alternative treatments. If alternative methods are used instead of evidence-based treatment, people can suffer, either from the lack of helpful treatment or because the alternative treatment itself is harmful.

Some alternative therapies are based on remedies thousands of years old, whereas others are newly formulated. None of these therapies have been proven to halt or reverse the progression of cancer. They should never be considered a substitute for conventional treatment.

The Appeal of Alternative Therapies

Many alternative therapies have gained widespread attention lately, often on the basis of anecdotal reports and testimonial stories. Television news shows, magazines, and even product advertisements often carry compelling stories about children and adults with cancer who turned to an alternative treatment instead of receiving conventional treatment or after conventional treatment did not work. Hearing stories from people who claim that an alternative treatment cured their disease can be quite powerful, especially for people with cancer. Because the person is alive to tell his or her story and appears to be restored to health, there is a strong implication that the alternative treatment is safe and effective, even if there is no scientific evidence to support the claim.

When it comes to anecdotal reports or personal testimonials about the effectiveness of alternative treatments, it is important to remember that if something sounds too good to be true, it usually is. Read the fine print describing how a product works rather than relying on one person's experience with it. Claims about alternative treatments that promise to instantly cure cancer, make tumors disappear, or prevent the disease from ever occurring are not based on scientific evidence and can be dangerous and misleading. Keep in mind that cancer can go into remission by chance, and one person's experience does not necessarily represent other people's experiences.

The promise of a cure: The most outlandish claim is that the alternative therapy can cure any and all cancer. Even conventional cancer therapies such as surgery, chemotherapy, and radiation therapy cannot guarantee a cure. However, if certain cancers are diagnosed early enough in their development, conventional therapies can remove the cancer or prolong survival. Many cancer specialists do not use the term "cure" at all, preferring to say that a cancer is in remission. Alternative therapies cannot cure cancer, and any claims for a cure should be treated with skepticism.

No side effects: Another appeal of alternative cancer therapies is the claim that they have no harmful side effects. Often, this claim is backed up by the statement that because the treatment is "natural," it is safe. You should be skeptical of these claims. Just because something is natural does not mean it is safe—a great many poisons are natural. Also, for most of these treatments, side effects have not really been studied well. Promoters of certain treatments often simply refer to testimonials from some people who have used the therapies. Consumers, including some people with cancer, may accept word-of-mouth claims made by friends, reports found in magazines, or even assertions made over the Internet by advocates of alternative medicine.

The reality is that some alternative therapies can cause serious side effects, including infections, heart problems, nutritional deficiencies, and harmful interactions with conventional cancer drugs and therapies. Some have even resulted in death.

Buyer Beware

Consumers should know the ingredients in herbal medicines and other dietary supplements they take. The FDA recommends that you consider these suggestions if you are considering using dietary supplements:

- **Look for products with the USP notation,** indicating that the maker of the product followed standards set by the US Pharmacopeia during manufacturing.
- **Realize that the use of the term "natural"** on an herbal product is no guarantee that the product is safe. Poisonous mushrooms, for example, are natural but not safe.
- **Take into account the name and reputation** of the manufacturer or distributor. Herbal products or other dietary supplements made by nationally known food or drug manufacturers are more likely to have been made under tight quality controls because these companies have reputations to uphold.
- **Write to the manufacturer or visit their website** for more information about the supplement. Ask about the company's manufacturing practices and the quality-control conditions under which the product was made.

Immune-boosting effects: Laws forbid companies that make or sell dietary supplements, such as vitamins, minerals, and herbal treatments, from claiming that their products can cure or prevent disease, so many of them claim that their products "boost the immune system" to help the body fight disease naturally. This commonly used phrase leads the customer to believe that the product will increase the function of their immune system. Yet these claims are often made with no evidence to back them up. All claims should be evaluated on the basis of scientific evidence. The same standard of proof should apply to claims that an herbal product or other alternative cancer therapy can prevent the growth or spread of tumors or destroy cancer cells. In some cases, these claims might be based on solid evidence; in most instances, however, they are not.

The Placebo Effect

If a positive effect resulting from a treatment remained and brought about long-lasting health, it would be considered a new effective treatment. But the effectiveness of many alternative therapies might simply be a placebo effect: the person believed in the treatment and wanted it to work, and so it did—or he or she believed that it did.

A placebo is a substance or other kind of treatment that seems therapeutic but is actually inactive. Because people do not know when they are taking a placebo, and because they believe in the treatment and in their doctor, some people will react to the placebo as though it were the active treatment. Their pain will lessen, or they will feel generally better. This change in signs or symptoms as a result of receiving a placebo is called a placebo effect. Placebos can be so effective that they can actually produce the same unwanted side effects as an actual treatment, including headaches, nervousness, nausea, and constipation.

The placebo effect is real. It has been the subject of many careful scientific tests and gives solid evidence that the mind can directly affect the physical sensations people feel in their bodies. Some scientific evidence suggests that the placebo effect might be due to the release of endorphins (the body's own morphine-like painkillers) in the brain. A recent study showed that when people were told that the inactive treatment could help through a mind-body effect, they experienced the placebo effect even when they knew that they were not getting an "active" treatment. Science is just beginning to learn exactly how the placebo effect works.

PART FOUR

Living with the Effects of Treatment

For many women, one of the biggest concerns is what to expect from treatment. Treatment for cancer can cause many side effects and changes in your life, both physical and emotional. Most women with breast cancer have some type of surgery, such as lumpectomy or mastectomy. This may be followed by chemotherapy, radiation therapy, and/or hormone therapy. Treatment can leave you fatigued and dealing with such side effects as nausea and vomiting, pain, and skin irritation. In the long term, there can be problems with concentration and sexual side effects. You may be worried about the risk of lymphedema. If you are having a mastectomy, you will decide whether to have breast reconstruction.

The effects of treatment will be different for each person. Talk with your doctor about what to expect, and be aware of your risk for such side effects as lymphedema. For many problems, the sooner you notice symptoms, the more easily the problem can be managed. Awareness of your emotional well-being is key as well: coping with the stresses of cancer and treatment can be difficult.

In the next few chapters, we discuss side effects of treatment and how to manage them, ways to keep yourself emotionally healthy, and breast reconstruction.

CHAPTER 13

Coping with Symptoms and Side Effects

In chapter 9, we discussed which side effects are associated with the most common treatments for breast cancer. In this chapter, we will discuss ways to manage symptoms and side effects.

Sometimes cancer and its treatments cause other short- or long-term health problems. Usually the trade-offs for women with breast cancer are clear: To save your life, you might need to give up part or all of your breast, or you might have to experience side effects such as nausea or hair loss while treatment kills the cancer in your body and extends your life.

Most side effects will go away once treatment is finished. Others, however, may persist for some time after treatment, and some will change your life forever, such as changes in fertility. For women who have had surgery and/or radiation, lymphedema, or the risk of it developing, will be

> ## Questions to Ask Your Medical Team About Each Treatment's Side Effects
>
> You'll probably want answers to the following questions no matter what type of treatment you're getting. Make notes of your doctor's answers and ask for more information when you need it.
>
> - **What are the possible side effects** for this treatment?
> - **How long** will these side effects last?
> - **Is there anything I can do** to lower my risk of side effects?
> - **What services or programs can help** me cope with side effects?

something you live with for the rest of your life. It is important to be aware of your risk for side effects. In many cases, the sooner a problem is dealt with, the easier it will be to manage.

Side Effects Log

Date and Time	Side Effect/ symptom	Did anything trigger the problem?	What I did about it (What helped, what didn't?)	Name and amount of any medicine taken	Was the doctor notified? (What I was told to do.)

Some women may become depressed after a diagnosis of breast cancer. For information on depression and ways to stay emotionally healthy during and after treatment, see chapters 14 and 20.

As you go through treatment, it might be helpful to write down any side effects you experience. This will help you and your doctors track your reactions to treatments and prevent or lessen side effects. See the Side Effects Log on the previous page.

Short-Term Side Effects of Cancer and Treatment

Among the most common short-term side effects of cancer and cancer treatments are fatigue, pain, and problems sleeping. In addition to these more common problems, this section discusses how to manage these possible side effects: appetite and weight changes, constipation and diarrhea, hair loss, mouth sores and sore throat, nail changes, nausea and vomiting, and skin changes. Your doctor should tell you what to do if you notice these or other symptoms or side effects, and he or she might tell you how to prevent or ease them.

Appetite and Weight Changes

Some chemotherapy drugs can cause a decrease in or loss of appetite. Appetite changes are usually short-term and will get better a few weeks after the chemotherapy is finished.

Chemotherapy can also affect your eating habits in other ways. Some chemotherapy drugs can cause mouth and throat sores, which can make it hard to eat. Cancer treatments can also alter how things taste and smell, which can in turn affect your appetite. Changes in taste and smell might continue throughout your chemotherapy treatments but should return to normal within several weeks of your treatment ending.

Radiation therapy can also cause problems with eating and digestion, although that is relatively uncommon in women with breast cancer. You might lose interest in food during your treatment. Some people report feeling nauseated. These effects can occur if the esophagus and part of the stomach receive some radiation.

Even if you are not hungry, it is important to keep up your protein and calorie intake. Your body needs calories and nutrients to heal. Maintaining good nutrition can also help you deal with other possible side effects of cancer treatment. A registered dietitian may have suggestions to help you maintain your weight. If needed, ask your medical team about medicines that could help improve your appetite.

Managing Weight Loss and Poor Appetite

Consider the following ways to help you manage weight loss and poor appetite:

- Talk with your doctor about what might be causing your poor appetite.
- Eat as much as you want, but do not force yourself to eat.
- Try to think of food as a necessary part of treatment.
- Start the day with breakfast.
- Eat small, frequent meals of favorite foods.
- Try to eat foods high in calories that are easy to eat, such as pudding, gelatin, ice cream, sherbet, yogurt, and milk shakes.
- Add sauces and gravies to meats, and cut meats into small pieces to make them easy to swallow.
- Use butter, oils, syrups, and milk in foods to increase calories. Avoid low-fat foods unless fats cause heartburn or other problems.
- Try adding strong flavorings or spices.
- Create pleasant settings for meals. Soft music, conversation, and other distractions might make eating more enjoyable.
- Eat with other family members or friends.
- Drink beverages between meals instead of with meals—drinking liquids at mealtime can lead to early fullness.
- Try light exercise one hour before meals.
- If it is okay with your doctor, try a glass of beer or wine before eating (alcohol can help stimulate the appetite).
- Eat a snack at bedtime.
- When you do not feel like eating, try liquid meals, such as flavored supplements (Ensure, Sustacal, Boost, Carnation Instant Breakfast, and others). Using a straw might help, too.

Managing Weight Gain

Some women gain weight during cancer treatment. Although the reasons are unclear, weight gain could be related to intense food cravings. Other factors, such as physical inactivity and retaining water (a common side effect of certain medicines), might contribute to weight gain, too.

Consider the following suggestions if you gain weight during cancer treatment:

- Talk to your doctor or nurse about limiting fluid or salt intake if your ankles are swollen. In some cases, medicines might be needed to help rid the body of excess fluid.
- Limit your intake of high-calorie foods.
- Talk to your doctor or nurse about when you can safely engage in light exercise or activity.
- Ask your doctor or nurse to refer you to a registered dietitian.

Constipation and Diarrhea

Constipation is the infrequent, difficult, or incomplete passage of hardened feces from the bowels. Diarrhea is excessive and frequent passage of watery feces.

Constipation and diarrhea can occur with certain chemotherapy and other drugs. Opioid medicines prescribed for pain control often cause constipation. The amount and duration of these problems depends on which medicines are taken and the dose and length of treatment.

Managing Constipation

Consider the following ways to help relieve constipation:

- Drink more fluids. Pasteurized fruit juices and warm or hot fluids in the morning can be especially helpful.
- Increase your intake of high-fiber foods, such as whole grain breads and cereals; fresh raw fruits with skins and/or seeds; fresh raw vegetables; fruit juices; dried fruits such as prunes, dates, and dried apricots; and nuts.
- Avoid gas-producing foods and beverages, such as cabbage, broccoli, and carbonated drinks.
- Avoid or cut back on any foods that make you constipated, such as cheese and eggs.
- Get as much light exercise as you can.
- Use stool softeners or laxatives as instructed by your doctor or nurse.
- Go to the bathroom as soon as you have the urge to have a bowel movement.
- Keep a record of your bowel movements so that problems can be noticed quickly.

Call your doctor or nurse if you have not had a bowel movement in three days, if there is blood in your stool, or if you have abdominal cramps or vomiting that won't stop.

Managing Diarrhea

Consider the following ways to help relieve diarrhea:

- Eat small meals or snacks every few hours.
- Eat foods that are easy to digest, such as rice, bananas, applesauce, yogurt, mashed potatoes, low-fat cottage cheese, and dry toast. If the diarrhea improves after a day or two, start eating small regular meals.
- Avoid high-fiber foods, which can make diarrhea worse and cause cramping.
- Drink plenty of liquids, such as water, weak tea, sports drinks, peach nectar, clear broth, ice pops, and plain gelatin.
- Avoid acidic drinks, such as tomato juice, citrus juices, and fizzy soft drinks.
- Avoid foods that are very hot or spicy, greasy foods, bran, raw fruits and vegetables, and caffeine.
- Avoid pastries, candies, rich desserts, jellies, preserves, and nuts.
- Do not drink alcohol or use tobacco.
- Avoid milk or milk products if they seem to make diarrhea worse.
- Be sure your diet includes foods that are high in potassium (such as bananas, potatoes, apricots, and sports drinks, such as Gatorade or Powerade). Potassium is an important mineral that can be lost when you have diarrhea.
- Monitor the amount and frequency of bowel movements.
- Clean your anal area with a mild soap after each bowel movement, rinse well with warm water, and pat dry. You can also use baby wipes to clean yourself after each bowel movement.
- Apply a water-repellent ointment, such as A&D Ointment or petroleum jelly, to the anal area after each bowel movement to protect the skin.
- Sitting in a tub of warm water or a sitz bath can help reduce discomfort.
- Take medicine for diarrhea as prescribed by your doctor.

Call your doctor or nurse if you have watery diarrhea or loose bowel movements for more than two days without improvement, you have blood in your stool, or you develop a fever with diarrhea.

Fatigue

Fatigue is one of the most common side effects of cancer and its treatments. It is the feeling of being tired physically, mentally, and emotionally. Cancer-related fatigue is defined as an unusual and persistent sense of tiredness that can occur with cancer or its treatment. It can develop over time or appear suddenly, and it can be overwhelming. It is not always relieved by rest, and it can last for several months after treatment ends.

Fatigue can show itself in many ways. You might feel like you have no energy and lack the desire to take part in normal activities. You might want to sleep all day, and when you wake up, you may still be tired. Fatigue can also make it hard for you to focus your thoughts.

The exact cause of cancer-related fatigue is still unknown. Cancer itself can cause fatigue by forming toxic substances in the body that interfere with normal cell functions. Cancer can also spread to the bone marrow, causing anemia (low red blood cell count). Some factors that can add to fatigue are pain, emotional distress, medication side effects, poor nutrition or hydration, sleep problems, and decreased physical activity.

Most people begin to feel tired after a few weeks of radiation therapy, and you may feel tired as soon as the next day after chemotherapy. Fatigue usually gets worse as treatment progresses.

Managing Fatigue

Consider the following suggestions to help you manage fatigue:
- Do not push yourself to do more than you can manage.
- Talk to your medical team about possible causes of your fatigue. Ask whether there are medicines or other treatments that can help ease your fatigue.
- Save your energy. You may need to accept the fact that you cannot do everything you want to do. Identify your priorities and plan rest periods to save energy for the most important things.
- Schedule necessary activities throughout the day rather than all at once.
- Try to follow a structured daily routine, keeping as normal a level of activity as possible.
- Engage in light exercise—studies have shown that exercising during treatment can help reduce fatigue. Always talk with your doctor before you start an exercise program.
- Balance rest and activities. Get enough rest and sleep, but avoid excessive bed rest. Try not to nap too much during the day, as it can interfere with nighttime sleep.
- Try not to spend too much time in bed, which can make you feel weak. Most people find that a few short rest periods are better than one long one.

- Unless you are given other instructions, eat a healthy diet that includes protein (meat, milk, eggs, and beans), and drink plenty of water each day.
- Let others help you with meals, housework, and errands. Ask for help and delegate when you can.
- Learn ways to deal with stress. Try different methods to reduce stress, such as deep breathing, visual imagery, meditation, prayer, talking with others, reading, listening to music, painting, writing in a journal, or any other activity that gives you pleasure.

Call your doctor or nurse if you have trouble getting out of bed for more than twenty-four hours, if you start to feel short of breath, or if your fatigue gets worse.

Hair Loss

If hair loss or thinning occurs with chemotherapy, it is almost always temporary and usually starts a few weeks after treatment has started. How much hair is lost depends on which chemotherapy drugs you are using, their doses, and the length of your treatment. It is understandable that many women find this side effect traumatic, and it is normal to feel upset about it. Aside from being a visible reminder of your treatment, losing your hair can cause a loss of self-confidence. Your hair will grow back once chemotherapy treatment ends, but its color or texture might be different.

Coping with Hair Loss

Consider the following ways of coping with hair loss:
- Be gentle when brushing and shampooing your own hair. Hair loss can be somewhat reduced by avoiding too much brushing or pulling of hair and by avoiding heat (such as from electric rollers, hair dryers, and curling irons). Avoid styles that pull on the hair, such as braids or ponytails.
- If you are bothered by hair falling out, think about cutting your hair very short or even shaving your head.
- To deal with hair that's coming out in clumps, wear a hair net at night or sleep on a satin pillowcase.
- If you think you might want a wig, buy it before treatment begins or at the very start of treatment. Ask whether the wig can be adjusted—your wig size can shrink as you lose hair. If you buy a wig before hair loss begins, the wig shop can

Look Good. . . Feel Better®

Appearance-related side effects such as hair loss and skin and nail changes can be especially upsetting for many women. The American Cancer Society's Look Good. . . Feel Better program teaches beauty techniques to women to help manage the side effects of cancer treatment. This free, nonmedical national public service program is designed to help you look good, improve your self-esteem, and manage your cancer treatment and recovery with confidence.

Look Good. . . Feel Better group programs include step-by-step makeover sessions led by cosmetology professionals using products donated by the cosmetic industry. Groups are open to all women getting chemotherapy, radiation therapy, or other forms of cancer treatment. In each two-hour, hands-on workshop, professionals teach women about skin care, nail care, and how to apply makeup; provide information about types of wigs and how to care for them; and demonstrate the use of other types of head coverings, including turbans, scarves, and hats. This program is offered jointly by the American Cancer Society, the Personal Care Products Council Foundation, and the Professional Beauty Association.

Look Good. . . Feel Better programs are offered in treatment centers, hospitals, and community centers nationwide. To find a program near you, call 800-395-5665 or visit www.lookgoodfeelbetter.org.

better match your hair color and texture. Or you can cut a swatch of hair from the top front of your head, where hair is lightest, to use for matching.

- Get a prescription for the wig from your doctor, because the cost might be covered by insurance.
- Get a list of wig shops in your area from your doctor, nurse, other cancer patients, the phone book, or online. You can also order wigs, hats, and other accessories from the American Cancer Society's "*tlc*"™ catalog (for women with hair loss due to cancer treatment) by calling 800-850-9445 or by visiting www.tlcdirect.org.
- Try on different wigs until you find one that you really like. Consider buying two wigs: one for everyday wear and one for special occasions.
- Synthetic wigs need less styling than human hair wigs. They might be easier to care for if you have low energy during cancer treatment.
- Turbans or scarves can be used instead of wigs. Cotton items tend to stay on a smooth scalp better than nylon or polyester.

- If you choose not to wear a wig, wear a hat or scarf outdoors in cold weather to prevent loss of body heat. In warmer weather, use sunscreen or a hat to protect your scalp from the sun.
- Be gentle with eyelashes and eyebrows, which are sometimes affected, too. All body hair can be affected by chemotherapy.

When new hair starts to grow, it might break easily at first. Avoid perms and hair color for the first few months. Keep hair short and easy to style.

Mouth Sores and Sore Throat

Sometimes chemotherapy will cause sores to develop in the mouth, throat, or esophagus within a week or two of treatment. The first sign of mouth sores is often a white or yellow film in the mouth or on the tongue. Later, your mouth, gums, and throat might feel sore and become red and inflamed. Your tongue may feel coated and swollen, leading to trouble swallowing, eating, and talking. Sores in the mouth can lead to painful, bleeding ulcers and infection.

If it hurts when you chew and swallow, ask your medical team about using powdered or liquid diet supplements, available at drugstores and supermarkets. You can use these alone or combined with other foods such as puréed fruit or milk shakes.

Soothing Mouth Sores and Sore Throat

Consider the following suggestions for coping with mouth sores and sore throat:
- Thirty minutes after eating and every four hours while awake, unless your doctor or nurse gives you other instructions, follow these steps:
  - Brush your teeth with a very soft toothbrush that has nylon bristles. To soften the bristles even more, soak the brush in hot water before brushing and rinse it with hot water during brushing. If the toothbrush hurts, use a Popsicle stick with gauze wrapped around it or a cotton swab instead. You can also get soft foam mouth swabs from the drugstore. Use a nonabrasive toothpaste. Whitening toothpastes can contain hydrogen peroxide, which can irritate mouth sores.
  - After use, rinse the toothbrush well in hot water and store in a dry place.
  - If you have dentures, remove and clean them between meals on a regular schedule. If you have sores under your dentures, leave your dentures out between meals and at night. Clean them well between uses, and store them

in an antibacterial soak. If your dentures fit poorly, do not use them during treatment.

- Gently rinse your mouth before and after meals and at bedtime with one of the following solutions: one teaspoon baking soda in two cups water or one teaspoon salt and one teaspoon baking soda in one quart water. (Stir or shake the solution well, swish it around in your mouth and gargle gently, then spit it out.)
- If you normally floss, keep flossing at least once a day unless you are told not to. Tell your doctor if flossing causes bleeding or other problems. If you do not usually floss, talk with your doctor before you start.
- Avoid store-bought mouthwashes, which often contain alcohol or other irritants.
- Keep your lips moist with petroleum jelly, a mild lip balm, or cocoa butter.
- Drink at least two to three quarts of fluids each day, if your doctor approves.
- If mouth pain is severe or makes it hard to eat, ask your doctor about medicine that can be swished fifteen to twenty minutes before meals or applied to painful sores with a cotton swab before meals. If this does not work, you might need pain medicine that you can take before eating.
- Sip warm tea slowly.
- Eat chilled foods and fluids (for instance, ice pops, ice cubes, frozen yogurt, sherbet, or ice cream).
- Eat soft foods that are moist and easy to swallow.
- Eat small, frequent meals of bland, moist, nonspicy foods. Avoid raw vegetables and fruits and other hard, dry, or crusty foods, like chips or pretzels.
- Avoid very salty or sugary foods.
- Avoid acidic fruits and juices, such as tomato, orange, grapefruit, lime, and lemon.
- Avoid fizzy drinks, alcohol, and tobacco.

Call your doctor or nurse if your gums start to bleed, if you have a fever, or if you are having trouble eating, drinking, or taking medicines for more than a day because of mouth or throat sores.

Nail Changes

During chemotherapy, your nails may become darkened, brittle, or cracked, and they might develop vertical bands. These changes will go away as the new nails grow in.

Caring for Your Nails

Consider the following ways to care for your nails:

- Keep your nails clean, short, and filed smoothly.
- Wear gloves when working in the yard or doing chores to protect your hands and nails.
- Use a cuticle cream to help prevent dryness, splitting, and hangnails.
- Do not use hand creams that contain alpha hydroxy or beta hydroxy acids.
- Do not cut or trim your cuticles.
- Nail polish can be used to cover discolored nails and to help keep nails strong. Always use a formaldehyde-free nail polish. Use a nail polish remover that does not contain acetone, sometimes called an oily nail polish remover. Do not use artificial nails.

Contact your doctor or nurse as soon as possible if a nail becomes infected.

Nausea and Vomiting

Nausea (queasiness) or vomiting (throwing up) can be caused by eating something that disagrees with you, by infections, by the cancer itself, or by radiation or chemotherapy treatments for cancer. Nausea and vomiting vary widely. Some people undergoing cancer treatments never have these symptoms. For others, just thinking about going to treatment can cause nausea or vomiting. Nausea can be accompanied by sweating, lightheadedness, dizziness, and/or weakness. Some people become very sensitive to smells during treatment.

Anti-nausea/vomiting medicines (called antiemetics) are the main treatment for nausea and vomiting. Antiemetics are commonly given with certain chemotherapy drugs. If you are getting chemotherapy drugs that are likely to cause nausea and vomiting, talk to your doctor or nurse about anti-nausea drugs to help control or prevent nausea and vomiting.

Some complementary methods have also been proven effective for combating nausea, such as self-hypnosis, progressive muscle relaxation, biofeedback, guided imagery, systematic desensitization, acupuncture, and music therapy. See chapter 12 for more information on complementary therapies. Along with these methods, there are other things you can do that might help control nausea and vomiting.

Tips for Eating During Chemotherapy

Consider the following tips during chemotherapy:

- **Eat according to your normal schedule** on the morning of your chemotherapy treatment. Do not skip any meals, and take medicines as scheduled.
- **Eat a light meal** and avoid greasy, fried, spicy, or acidic foods prior to treatment.
- **Do not eat your favorite meal** before chemotherapy; if you get sick from the treatment, you might associate those smells or flavors with nausea. As a result, you might not be able to eat that food again without feeling sick—at least for a while.
- **During the weeks you are having chemotherapy,** avoid eating big meals, and do not drink large amounts of fluids with your meals.
- **Eat foods that can be kept at room temperature** without spoiling—these foods tend to be mild and have very little odor.
- **You might not always feel like eating** when you are getting chemotherapy. Make the most of days when you do feel like eating. Try to eat regular meals and snacks, but listen to your body. Never eat if you feel full or force yourself to eat something that you don't want.
- **After eating, do not lie down** for at least two hours.
- **If you do not have side effects,** do not think that the chemotherapy is not working. Some people simply have fewer side effects than others.

Managing Nausea

Consider the following ways to help control nausea:

- Try starchy foods, such as dry toast, crackers, dry cereals, breadsticks, or rice.
- Eat bland foods, such as gelatin, cream of wheat, smoothies, and mild-flavored soups.
- If you have nausea only between meals, eat frequent, small meals and a snack at bedtime. Try eating small amounts of high-calorie foods that are easy to eat (such as smoothies, pudding, ice cream, sherbets, yogurt, and milk shakes) several times a day.
- Drink cold, clear liquids such as flat ginger ale, and sip them slowly. You can also try ice pops or gelatin.
- Suck on hard candies with pleasant aromas, such as lemon drops or mints, to help get rid of bad tastes.
- Avoid fatty, fried, spicy, or very sweet foods.

- Try tart or sour foods, which might be easier to keep down. (Do not try this if you have mouth sores.)
- After meals, try to rest quietly while sitting upright for at least two hours.
- Distract yourself with soft music, a favorite television program, or a visit with friends while eating.
- When you are feeling nauseated, relax and take slow, deep breaths.
- Take your antiemetic medicine at the first sign of nausea.
- Eat food cool or cold to decrease its smell and taste. Sometimes strong smells and flavors can make nausea worse.
- If nausea occurs just before chemotherapy or doctor visits, ask about medicines, hypnosis, relaxation, or behavioral treatment to lessen this problem.

Managing Sensitivity to Smells

- Foods with strong odors may cause nausea and loss of appetite. If the smell of food being cooked bothers you, ask others preparing food in your home to cook in a separate part of the house, to use a slow cooker or microwave on the back porch or in the garage, or to grill outdoors.
- Drink soups, broths, or nutritional supplements out of containers with lids, which will help block odors.
- Other people might not be aware that you are sensitive to smells. Don't hesitate to tell others which smells bother you, whether it is certain foods, perfumes or colognes, or air fresheners.

To Help Control Vomiting

Consider the following ways to help control vomiting:
- Request that medicines be prescribed in suppository form, if possible. Take medicine at the first hint of nausea to prevent vomiting. If your medicine for vomiting is prescribed to be taken on a regular schedule, take the medicine as prescribed, even if you do not feel bad when the medicine is due to be taken.
- When you are lying down, lie on your side, not on your back.
- Try liquids in the form of ice chips or frozen juice chips that can be sucked on slowly.
- Do not force yourself to eat or drink.

- After vomiting stops, start by sipping small amounts of cool liquid every ten minutes. If you are able to keep that down after an hour or so, gradually increase to larger amounts.

Call your doctor or nurse if vomiting continues for more than three hours, if you vomit blood or material that looks like coffee grounds, if you cannot keep food down for more than two days, or if you are not able to keep medicines down.

Pain

When you have cancer, you may have pain at different points in your illness—before your cancer diagnosis, during your treatment, or through your recovery. For some, a tumor might be pressing on an organ, nerve, or bone. For others, surgery might cause some pain for a time, and certain types of chemotherapy can cause nerve pain or aching in your bones and muscles. Although there are ways to control pain with medicine, some women suffer needlessly rather than ask their doctors to treat their pain or prescribe stronger medicines. Some even believe that pain is part of having cancer and something they just have to deal with.

Pain can affect your sleep patterns, appetite, work, and other daily activities, leading to a lower quality of life for you and your family. But it does not have to. Pain can be controlled, and you have a right to pain relief.

The goal of pain management is to prevent or stop pain whenever possible and to control pain that cannot be prevented. Doctors and other health care professionals who treat cancer pain match the severity of pain a person is having with the treatment they prescribe, being careful not to over- or undermedicate.

Describing Your Pain

Cancer pain depends on many things: the type of cancer, the extent of the disease, and your pain thresholds (the level of pain at which you become aware of it). It is important to remember that regardless of the cause, pain can almost always be relieved. You will need to describe your pain to your doctor or nurse. Pain is different for every person, and only you can tell them what you are feeling.

Health care professionals will need to know the following information:
- the location of the pain
- when it started
- whether it is constant or comes and goes

- what it feels like (dull, aching, stabbing, burning, etc.)
- how bad it is (for example, on a scale of 0 to 10)
- what makes it better
- what makes it worse
- how it affects your life

Types of Pain

As you become aware of any pain you are having, you will be able to say what the pain is like, what makes it better or worse, and how long it lasts. Your medical team can then determine what type of pain it is and how best to treat it.

Questions to Ask Your Medical Team About Pain

- **What kind of pain am I likely to have** during or after this treatment?
- **How will I know whether my pain** is "normal" or a sign of some other problem?
- **Will I need pain medicine?**
- **What kind of painkiller** will I need and what are the potential side effects?
- **Can I become dependent** on pain medicines?
- **What can I do** to reduce pain?
- **What options do I have** for pain control without medicine?
- **What kind of pain** should I watch for and report?

Chronic pain: Chronic pain can range from mild to severe and is present in some degree for long periods. Chronic pain can have many causes. The tumor might be pressing on nerves, organs, or bones, which can cause pain. Even stiffness from a lack of activity can be experienced as pain.

Acute pain: Acute pain lasts a relatively short time and is often severe. It is usually a signal that body tissue is being injured in some way, and the pain generally goes away when the injury heals.

Breakthrough pain: Breakthrough pain is a brief—and often severe—flare of pain that occurs even though a person is taking medicine regularly for persistent pain. It is called breakthrough pain because the pain "breaks through" a regular pain medicine schedule.

Neurologic (nerve) pain: Neurologic pain can be caused by tumors pressing on a nerve, or it can be a side effect of surgery or some chemotherapy drugs. When it's caused by a tumor, nerve pain may be felt in a circular pattern around the chest or abdomen and might shoot down the arms and legs. Breast surgery can sometimes cause nerve pain in the chest wall, armpit, and/or arm, and this pain may not go away over time. Chemotherapy-related nerve pain is more often felt in the hands or feet; this is called peripheral neuropathy. There might also be tingling and numbness in the area of the pain. Nerve pain often is not relieved by regular painkillers and might require other drugs, such as antidepressants.

Pain Medicines

Your medical team has many tools they can use to help treat pain.

Nonsteroidal anti-inflammatory drugs: Nonsteroidal anti-inflammatory drugs (NSAIDs) are mild pain relievers, many of which are sold over-the-counter (without a prescription). Examples are aspirin (Bayer) and ibuprofen (Motrin or Advil). These drugs can cause such side effects as increased risk of bleeding, stomach upset, and kidney damage.

Acetaminophen: Acetaminophen (Tylenol) is another mild pain reliever that is sold over-the-counter. It works differently from NSAIDs and can have different side effects, including liver damage.

Moderate pain opioids: Opioids are more potent than mild pain relievers such as NSAIDs or acetaminophen, and they are more effective for stronger pain. These are also known as narcotics, and they always require a prescription from a doctor. If mild pain medicines do not work, or if the pain is rated as moderate pain, then moderate pain opioids are used. Moderate pain opioids are often combined with an NSAID or acetaminophen. Examples of opioids and combinations used for moderate pain are codeine, hydrocodone plus acetaminophen (Lortab), or oxycodone plus acetaminophen (Percocet). It is important to take only the amount prescribed by your doctor, as these medicines can have side effects. For example, too much acetaminophen can damage the liver. Opioids can cause constipation and other side effects, such as drowsiness, itchiness, and nausea.

Severe pain opioids: These strong opioids control severe pain, and they can be short-acting or long-acting. Morphine and hydromorphone (Dilaudid) are two examples of strong opioids whose effects last three to four hours. Many pain medicines also come in sustained-release (longer-acting) forms that last eight to twelve hours. Examples include long-acting forms of morphine such as MS-Contin or Oramorph SR. Kadian and Avinza are even longer-acting forms of morphine that last up to twenty-four hours. Fentanyl (Duragesic) comes in a patch that delivers the medicine through the skin continuously for seventy-two hours.

Adjuvants: Adjuvants are medicines that are used to help enhance the effects of pain relievers, treat symptoms that can increase pain, and relieve certain types of pain. Examples include antidepressants such as amitriptyline (Elavil); anti-anxiety drugs such as lorazepam (Ativan); stimulants such as modafinil (Provigil); anticonvulsants such as carbamazepine (Tegretol), phenytoin (Dilantin), or gabapentin (Neurontin); and corticosteroids such as dexamethasone and prednisone.

Fear of Addiction to Pain Medicine

Addiction is a common fear for people taking strong pain medicines such as opioids. This fear can even keep people from taking the medicine or cause family members to encourage them to hold off as long as they can between doses.

Addiction is defined as uncontrollable drug craving, seeking, and continued use. When opioids are taken for cancer pain, they rarely cause addiction. If a person takes opioids for long periods, the body can get used to the medicine such that it might not relieve pain as well as it once did. This is called tolerance. Tolerance is rarely a problem with cancer pain treatment because your doctor can increase the amount of medicine you are taking or add other medicines. Some people are alarmed by tolerance because they are afraid it means they are addicted, but tolerance and addiction are not the same thing. Tolerance only means that your body has learned to adjust to the drug in your system over time.

When you are ready to stop taking opioids, the doctor will reduce the amount of medicine you are taking over the course of a few days or weeks. By the time you stop completely, your body has had time to adjust. Talk to your doctor, nurse, or pharmacist about how to take pain medicines safely and about any concerns you have about addiction.

Managing Pain

Consider the following tactics to help relieve your pain:

- Talk with your doctor or nurse about your pain—where the pain is, when it began, how long it lasts, what it feels like, what makes it better, what makes it worse, and how it affects your life. Rate your pain using a pain-rating scale, with 0 equaling no pain and 10 indicating the most severe pain. This will help you describe your pain to others.
- Make sure you take pain medicine exactly as prescribed, even if the pain is not severe at the time of the scheduled dose. Medicine for chronic pain should be

given around the clock on a schedule—not just when the pain is severe. Check with your doctor if you think your pain medicine schedule needs to be changed.

- Keep at least a one-week supply of pain medicine on hand. Most pain medicines cannot be refilled by phone, so you will need a written prescription.
- Be as active as the pain allows. When pain is relieved, increase your activity; as pain increases, reduce your activity.
- Some pain medicines can make you drowsy or dizzy. This often lessens after a few days, but you may need help getting up or walking. Do not try to drive or do anything dangerous until you know how the medicines you are taking will affect you.
- Ask the doctor for medicine to control nausea if you have this side effect.
- Ask your doctor about laxatives and stool softeners to combat constipation, which is a very common side effect of opioids.
- Do not crush or break your pain pills unless you have checked with your doctor, nurse, or pharmacist. If medicines are delivered in time-release form, taking broken pills can be dangerous.
- Do not suddenly stop taking all pain medicine; instead, reduce the dose slowly as the pain decreases. Talk with your doctor, nurse, or pharmacist before you taper off or stop any medicines, or if you have questions.

Call the doctor if any of the following occurs:
- You have new, severe pain.
- You become unable to take anything by mouth, including the pain medicine.
- Your pain is not relieved by the medicines that you have been prescribed.
- You become constipated, nauseated, or confused.
- You have questions about how to take the medicine.
- Your pain is accompanied by a new symptom (for example, inability to urinate).

Relief from cancer pain is available for everyone. If your doctor runs out of options, ask to be referred to a pain specialist.

Relieving Pain Without Medicine

Some pain can be relieved or lessened without using drugs. Methods such as relaxation, imagery, and distraction can be used to help ease pain. These techniques are sometimes referred to as complementary methods because they can also be used along with pain medicines.

Your Role in Pain Relief

A crucial part of your cancer treatment is controlling your pain, but this goal cannot be reached without your help. It is up to you to keep your medical team informed about the type and severity of any pain you are feeling. Talk to your doctor, rather than putting on a brave face and trying to deal with the pain. Not addressing pain sometimes worsens it in the long run; pain is easier to control in its early stages. Pain can also be a sign of a more serious problem, so talk to your doctor about your pain as early as possible to make sure it is not a sign of other problems.

Which Methods Work for You

It might be helpful to vary or combine pain relief methods to figure out which methods work best for you. Know yourself and your limits and capabilities. Be open-minded and willing to try new methods until you find those that help the most.

Keep a record of which methods help and which ones do not. Some medicines, such as antidepressants, can take two weeks or longer to work. Sometimes it takes time to determine the right dose for your pain. Ask yourself whether you are getting enough pain relief to do what is important to you and those you care about.

Factors That Can Increase Pain

Fatigue and emotions can increase pain; some of these are caused by cancer treatment and can be worsened by your natural concern about having breast cancer. You can control these factors to some extent.

Fatigue: Fatigue can make it harder for you to deal with pain. When you are tired, it can be harder to cope with pain than when you are well rested. Many people notice that pain seems to get worse as they get tired. It is important to get as much rest as possible, as lack of sleep can also increase your pain.

Anxiety, depression, and other emotional factors: Cancer can cause some women to experience a wide range of emotions. Some women feel hopeless or helpless. Others may feel alone, embarrassed, inadequate, angry, frightened, or frantic. These emotions can make dealing with pain more difficult for some women.

Try to talk about your feelings with others, such as doctors, nurses, family members, friends, or other people with cancer. It can be especially helpful to have the support of other women going through breast cancer treatment. If you need more support dealing with problems like anxiety or depression, you might want to talk with a counselor or a mental health professional. Another option is to ask your doctor about treating your anxiety and/or depression with medicine. Sometimes drugs such as antidepressants or anti-anxiety medicines can be helpful. Some of these medicines can help relieve pain in addition to their other effects.

Skin Changes

Radiation therapy can cause skin irritation on the breast, armpit and nearby areas. You might have skin redness that will fade over time, the way a sunburn fades to a tan. Skin changes usually go away after a few months. The pores in the skin of your breast might be enlarged and more noticeable after radiation therapy. Some women report that the skin on the breast becomes more sensitive, whereas others have decreased feeling. The skin and the fatty tissue of the breast might feel thicker and firmer than before your radiation treatment. Radiation can sometimes cause what's called a "moist reaction," where the skin becomes wet and very sore. This is more likely in areas where there are skin folds. Talk to your medical team about ways to prevent infection if this happens.

Sometimes the size of your breast also changes—it might become larger because of fluid buildup or smaller because of the development of scar tissue. Many women have little or no change in breast size.

Most breast changes from radiation therapy occur within twelve months of treatment. If you notice new changes in breast size, shape, appearance, or texture after this time, report them to your doctor at once.

Managing Skin Irritation

Consider the following ways to help with skin irritation:

- Go without your bra whenever possible or, if this makes you uncomfortable, wear a soft cotton bra without underwires.
- Wear loose clothing that is easy to put on and take off.
- Bathe or shower in lukewarm water using mild soap. Just let water run over the treated area—do not rub. Pat the skin dry. Limit bathing to once a day or less. Or try a sponge bath instead.
- Add baking soda to bath water to soothe sensitive skin and relieve itching.

- Try not to rub, scrub, or scratch any sensitive spots, as this can lead to infection, irritation, or soreness.
- Do not shave your armpit on the treated side unless your doctor tells you it is okay to do so.
- Do not put anything that's hot or cold, such as heating pads or ice packs, on your treated skin, unless your doctor tells you it is okay to do so.
- Ask your doctor or nurse before using any powders, creams, perfumes, deodorants, body oils, ointments, lotions, or home remedies on the treated area while you are getting treatment and for several weeks afterward. Many skin products can leave a coating on the skin that can cause irritation, and they can even alter the amount of radiation that enters the body.
- Drink plenty of fluids (two to three quarts) every day to reduce the risk of dehydration and help restore moisture to skin tissues.
- Avoid exposing the area to the sun during treatment and for at least one year after your treatment ends. Do not use tanning beds. If you expect to be in the sun for more than a few minutes, wear protective clothing (such as a shirt with long sleeves). Ask your doctor or nurse about using sunscreens.

Managing Hand-Foot Syndrome

Hand-foot syndrome is a side effect of some cancer treatments. The chemotherapy drug capecitabine (Xeloda) is the most common cause of this problem. This condition is marked by pain, swelling, numbness, tingling, or redness of the hands and feet. It is important to let your doctor know if you have any of these symptoms. Decreasing the dose you are getting can often improve symptoms. Treating hand-foot syndrome early can keep it from getting worse.

Consider the following tips for managing hand-foot syndrome:

- Elevate your hands and feet whenever possible. Avoid standing for long periods.
- Drink plenty of fluids to keep your skin well hydrated.
- Keep your hands and feet moisturized with mild skin creams. Avoid excess friction by patting the lotion dry.
- Avoid exposing your skin to heat for long periods, such as in a hot tub or sauna.
- Use ice packs wrapped in towels to cool burning hands and feet.
- Avoid activities that put pressure on your hands, such as using hand tools, and your feet, such as running or aerobics.

Sleep Problems

People who are being treated for cancer can sometimes tire more easily and may need more sleep than usual. They might also have the opposite problem and have trouble sleeping. Changes in usual sleeping habits can be caused by pain, anxiety, worry, depression, or side effects of cancer therapy, such as hot flashes.

Managing Sleep Problems

Consider the following ways to help deal with sleep problems:
- Sleep as much as your body tells you to.
- Try to exercise at least once a day. Schedule this activity at least two to three hours before bedtime.
- Drink warm, caffeine-free drinks, such as warm milk, before sleep.
- Avoid stimulants, such as coffee, caffeinated tea, or cola, especially before bedtime.
- Use a quiet setting to rest at the same time each day.
- If your doctor has prescribed sleeping medicines or pain relievers, take them at a regular time each night. Do not "hold off" on taking sleep or pain medicines. Do not take any other drug or supplement as a sleeping aid other than what your doctor prescribes.
- Have someone rub your feet and back before bedtime.
- Keep sheets clean, neatly tucked in, and as free from wrinkles as possible.
- Talk with your doctor about relaxation therapy or a referral to a hypnotherapist.

Long-Term Side Effects

Some side effects that occur during or after breast cancer treatment may persist for some time after treatment ends. Whether these side effects occur depends on the person and the treatment she receives. There is no way to predict who will get these side effects. Some problems, such as changes in the way you think and certain sexual problems, tend to be shorter in duration. Others, such as changes in fertility, may be permanent; and lymphedema, or the risk of it, can be a lifelong concern.

Changes in Memory and Concentration

Although it is not clear why, some people with cancer report memory and attention problems after chemotherapy. You may hear this called "chemo brain." People who have had high doses of chemotherapy might be particularly affected by chemo brain, but even those who have had standard doses sometimes notice these changes.

These effects may be noticed before, during, or after treatment. They can last a short time or go on for years. Usually, the changes that women notice are very subtle, and others around them might not notice any changes at all. Still, you may feel like you have lost the ability to think and focus the way you used to.

Other medicines, depression or anxiety, and menopause can also affect your ability to concentrate and recall things. Your doctor might be able to help in these situations.

Try not to become too distressed by minor memory lapses or lack of concentration. It can be upsetting, but there are steps you can take to help manage these problems.

Managing Memory Problems

If you notice memory problems after cancer treatment, you might find the following suggestions helpful:

- Use a detailed daily planner to keep track of your appointments and schedules, to-do lists, important dates, phone numbers and addresses, meeting notes, and even movies you would like to see or books you would like to read. Keeping everything in one place will make it easier to find the reminders you need.
- Exercise your brain. Take a class, do word puzzles, or learn a new language.
- Get enough rest and sleep.
- Exercise your body. Regular physical activity is not only good for your body, but it also improves your mood, makes you feel more alert, and decreases fatigue.
- Eat your veggies. Eating more vegetables has been linked to keeping more brain power as people age.
- Set up routines, and follow them. For example, pick one place for commonly lost objects and put them there each time. Try to keep the same daily schedule.
- Do not try to multitask. Focus on one thing at a time.
- Ask for help when you need it. Friends and loved ones can help with daily tasks to cut down on distractions and help you save mental energy.
- Track any memory problems. Keep a diary of when you notice problems and the events that are going on at the time. (You might keep track of this in your daily planner.) Taking note of any medicines taken, the time of day, and the situation you are in might help you figure out when you are most likely to have memory problems. Keeping track of when the problems are most noticeable can also help

you prepare. You will know to avoid planning important conversations or appointments during those times.

- Talk to your doctor about the problems you are having. Ask what might be causing them and whether he or she can offer anything to help you.
- If your memory and thinking problems keep causing trouble in your daily life, ask your doctor whether a neuropsychologist can help you. These professionals can test brain function and recommend ways to help you deal with the problems. Find out what your insurance will cover beforehand.
- Try not to focus too much on the problem. Accepting chemo brain can help you deal with it. As many people have noted, being able to laugh about things you cannot control can help you cope. And remember, you probably notice your problems much more than others do. Sometimes, we all have to laugh about forgetting to take the grocery list with us to the store.
- Make sure your symptoms are not caused by depression. Depression can affect memory. If you feel depressed, talk to your doctor.

Sexual and Reproductive Changes

Women being treated for breast cancer often notice decreased sexual desire. Physical side effects, such as upset stomach, tiredness, and weakness, might leave little energy or desire for sex. Some women also feel unattractive during or after treatment. Breast changes from surgery, as well as hair loss and weight changes from chemotherapy, can make it harder for you to have a positive sexual self-image. Over time, most women adjust to the changes in their bodies and enjoy their sexuality again. For more information on resuming intimacy after breast cancer treatment, see chapter 21.

Along with changes in energy levels, body image, and other factors that can distract from a healthy sex life, some treatments for breast cancer can directly affect your sexual organs. Both chemotherapy and hormone therapy can alter hormone levels in the body, which can cause physical changes to your sexual organs. As a result, you might experience the symptoms listed here.

Pain During Sex

Pain in the genital area during sex is a common problem for women getting chemotherapy and hormone therapy. It is often related to changes in the size or moisture level of the vagina. These changes can be caused by treatments that affect your hormones. Sometimes the pain sets off a problem called vaginismus, in which the muscles around the opening of the vagina become tense without the woman knowing it. This condition makes penetration difficult and sometimes impossible. Counseling and special relaxation training can be helpful.

Consider the following suggestions if you have genital pain during sexual activity:

- Let your doctor know about the pain. Several common problems can cause pain in the vulva or deep in the vagina. Medical treatments can often help. Do not let embarrassment get in the way of seeking medical care.
- Make sure you feel very aroused before you start intercourse. Your vagina expands to its fullest length and width only when you are highly excited. Also, the walls of your vagina produce lubricating fluid when you are aroused. As women go through menopause, either because of aging or cancer treatment, it might take more time and more touching to get fully aroused.
- Spread a water-based lubricating gel in and around your vagina before penetration. You can also use lubrication suppositories that melt in the vagina during foreplay.
- Let your partner know if any type of touching causes pain. Show your partner ways to touch you or positions that are not painful. Usually, light touching around the clitoris and the entrance to the vagina will not hurt, especially if the area is well lubricated.
- For intercourse, try a position that lets you control the movement. That way, if deep penetration hurts, you can make the thrusts less deep. You can also control the speed.

Even if you do not have pain in the genital area, pain elsewhere can make it more difficult to feel pleasure during sex or make sex less desirable. This could be soreness in the arm and chest after breast surgery or tingling and numbness in the hands and feet after some types of chemotherapy. If you are having pain outside of the genital area, the following tips might help lessen it during sex:

- Plan sexual activity for the time of day when you feel the least pain. If you are using pain medicine, take it an hour before planned sexual activity so it will be in full effect during sex. Try to find doses of medicine that offer pain relief without drowsiness.
- Find a position for touching or intercourse that puts as little pressure as possible on the sore areas of your body. If it helps, support the sore area and limit its movement with pillows. If a certain motion is painful, choose a position that

does not require it or have your partner help you. You can guide your partner on what you would like.

- Focus on your feelings of pleasure and excitement. With this focus, sometimes the pain fades into the background.

Vaginal Dryness

Chemotherapy and hormone therapy often reduce the amount of moisture your vagina produces when you are excited. You might need extra lubrication to make intercourse comfortable.

If you use a vaginal lubricant, choose a water-based gel with no perfumes or coloring; these chemicals can irritate your delicate genital tissues. Lubricants can usually be found in stores near the condoms or feminine hygiene products. Or you might want to use a vaginal moisturizer a few times a week; regular use may help keep your vagina moist all the time and at a more normal pH. This can help prevent yeast infections.

Doctors can prescribe local vaginal hormones (applied to the genital area) to help with vaginal dryness for women who do not have breast cancer. These hormones come in gel, cream, ring, and tablet forms. But it is not clear whether these products are safe for women with breast cancer, and they may raise the risk for breast cancer recurrence. Although the increased risk is not certain, many doctors are hesitant to recommend hormone use after a breast cancer diagnosis. Still, vaginal hormones might be something to discuss with your doctor if other methods of relieving vaginal dryness do not work.

> ### Questions to Ask Your Medical Team About Treatment and Sexuality
>
> - **Will this treatment** affect my desire for sex?
> - **Will I still be able** to have a normal sex life?
> - **How long** will any side effects last?
> - **What physical side effects** could I have that would affect my sex life?
> - **How can I deal** with pain during sex?
> - **How can I help my partner cope** with the treatment's effects on our sex life?
> - **How can I minimize** a treatment's effects on my sexuality?

Hot Flashes

In women who have not gone through menopause, chemotherapy or hormone therapy for breast cancer can cause menopausal symptoms such as frequent hot flashes, especially at night.

Female hormones (such as estrogen) in the form of a pill, shot, or patch can help with hot flashes. However, doctors do not generally prescribe them for women with breast cancer. These hormones enter the bloodstream and can travel throughout the body, and they might promote the growth of breast cancer cells (and can cause other health problems) in women who have had breast cancer. If you have questions about hormone replacement therapy, talk with your doctor or health care provider about the risks and benefits as they apply to you.

Nonhormone treatments that sometimes help with hot flashes include antidepressants called selective serotonin reuptake inhibitors (SSRIs), which include venlafaxine (Effexor), fluoxetine (Prozac), paroxetine (Paxil), and others. But it is important to talk to your doctor before taking these medicines, as some of them can affect the way tamoxifen acts in the body. Other drugs that might be helpful include clonidine (Duraclon) or Bellergal (a combination of ergotamine, belladonna, and phenobarbital). For some women, nonmedical treatments such as exercise, behavioral therapy, relaxation techniques, and acupuncture might help with hot flashes.

Dietary supplements and herbs have also been promoted to help relieve hot flashes, including black cohosh, red clover, and soy supplements. These compounds contain phytoestrogens—plant-based chemicals that can act like weak estrogens in the body. However, only a handful of studies have looked at their usefulness for treating hot flashes, and most have not found them to be very effective. In addition, they have not been studied extensively in women who have had breast cancer, so their safety is not well established. If you are considering trying one of these products, discuss it with your doctor first.

Fertility and Pregnancy After Treatment

For younger women dealing with a breast cancer diagnosis, an important question may be whether treatment will affect your ability to have children. Some treatments affect fertility, and for women whose fertility has not been affected, there is some debate as to whether pregnancy after breast cancer can affect the risk of recurrence. Studies have suggested that women with cancer are less likely to be given information about preserving their fertility than men. If you are interested in having children in the future, you may need to be the one to start this conversation with your doctor before treatment begins.

Some chemotherapy drugs affect fertility by damaging the ovaries and reducing the amount of hormones they produce. Whether infertility occurs and how long it lasts depend on many factors, including the type of drug, the dosage given, and the woman's age. Hormone therapy can also affect your ability to have a child. Surgery and radiation therapy in the chest area generally do not affect fertility.

These are a few important points to remember:

- **Periods do not always mean fertility:** Even if a woman's periods start back after cancer treatment has stopped, her fertility is uncertain. You may need a fertility expert to help you find out whether you are actually fertile.

- **Avoid getting pregnant during chemotherapy:** Many chemotherapy drugs can hurt a developing fetus, causing birth defects or other harm. You might be fertile during some types of treatment, even if menstrual periods are irregular or have stopped. You will need to use an effective form of birth control.

- **It can harm the baby to become pregnant too soon after chemotherapy:** Women are often advised not to get pregnant within the first six to twelve months after chemotherapy, as the medicines can damage the eggs that are maturing during treatment. If a damaged egg is fertilized, the embryo could miscarry or develop into a baby with a genetic problem.

Questions to Ask Your Medical Team About Fertility After Treatment

- **Will this treatment** have any short- or long-term effect on my reproductive system? If so, what kind of effect and how long will it last?

- **Can anything be done** to prevent infertility before I start cancer treatment?

- **Will any of the options to preserve** my fertility interfere with my cancer treatment?

- **If I become infertile,** what are my options for having a family, such as adoption, using a donor egg or sperm, or having a woman carry a pregnancy for me?

- **Are there steps I can take** to preserve some healthy eggs?

- **Can you refer me to a fertility specialist** before treatment?

- **Once I finish treatment,** how will I know if I am fertile or infertile?

- **How long should I wait** to try to become pregnant after cancer treatment?

- **Is my infertility** likely to be short-term or permanent?

- **Can cancer treatment damage** my ovaries so that I lose some or all of my eggs or go into early menopause?

- **Is my cancer treatment likely to damage my uterus,** heart, or lungs in such a way that I could have trouble carrying a full-term pregnancy?

Before you start cancer treatment, talk to your doctor or nurse about any concerns you have about your fertility. An open discussion with your doctor will help you plan your cancer treatment and know what to expect. Your oncologist may not be well informed about fertility problems, or may look at this issue as less important compared with saving your life with cancer treatment. But you have a right to get answers to your questions, even if it means asking for a second opinion or seeing a specialist. You can talk to an oncologist, surgeon, gynecologist, nurse, reproductive endocrinologist, or fertility specialist.

For women who are concerned about infertility after treatment, medically assisted reproductive techniques might be an option. The most common and successful method of preserving a woman's fertility is embryo cryopreservation (freezing fertilized eggs). Some women are able to have children using donor eggs or embryo donation. Several new fertility-preserving techniques are also being studied, but they are still experimental. Adoption is another possibility for couples who are infertile.

If you plan to have children after treatment, your doctor might advise that you wait for a time to conceive. As mentioned previously, you may be told to wait six to twelve months after chemotherapy before trying to get pregnant. This is because the medicines may have damaged the eggs that were maturing during treatment, and if one of these damaged eggs is fertilized, the embryo could miscarry or develop into a baby with a genetic problem. Your doctor may suggest that you wait at least two years after breast cancer treatment before becoming pregnant. This is because most recurrences of breast cancer happen during that time. Still, this waiting period is not based on strong scientific evidence, and earlier pregnancy might not be harmful.

Because of the link between estrogen levels and the growth of breast cancer cells, some doctors advise women who have been treated for breast cancer to avoid becoming pregnant indefinitely. However, most studies have found that pregnancy does not increase the risk of recurrence after successful treatment of breast cancer.

Talk to your medical team about your risk of recurrence and about how treatment might affect your chances for pregnancy. In many cases, counseling can help you sort through the choices that come with surviving breast cancer and planning a pregnancy.

Lymphedema

Some women who have been treated for breast cancer develop swelling of the arm, breast, and chest. This is called lymphedema, and the swelling can range from mild to severe. Lymphedema can start soon after surgery and/or radiation treatment or it can begin months or even years later. Both types are discussed here.

Most women who have had breast cancer will not develop this side effect. However, any woman whose breast cancer was treated with surgery and/or radiation is at increased risk for lymphedema. The risk of lymphedema also goes up with the number of lymph nodes removed and is higher in women who are obese.

Lymphedema is a buildup of lymph fluid in the fatty tissues just under your skin. It usually develops slowly over time. The body has a network of lymph nodes and lymph vessels that carry and remove lymph fluid, similar to the way blood vessels circulate blood to all parts of the body. During surgery for breast cancer, the doctor sometimes removes lymph nodes from the underarm area to see whether the cancer has spread. Some lymph vessels that carry fluid from the arm to the rest of the body are removed too, because they are intertwined with the nodes.

The removal of lymph nodes and vessels changes the way the lymph fluid flows within that side of the upper body, making it harder for fluid to drain from the arm and chest area. If the remaining lymph vessels cannot remove enough of the fluid in the breast and underarm areas, the excess fluid builds up and causes swelling, or lymphedema. Radiation therapy to the lymph nodes in the underarm also can affect lymph fluid flow in the arm, chest, and breast area by causing scarring and damage, further increasing the risk of lymphedema.

There is still a lot to be learned about lymphedema, but there are ways that you can care for your arm and breast area to reduce your chances of having future problems. Once lymphedema has started, it cannot be cured. But early and careful management can reduce symptoms and help keep it from getting worse. In fact, some women manage their lymphedema so well they become convinced they no longer have it. All women who have had episodes of lymphedema or are at risk for it should follow these guidelines and their doctor's instructions to avoid the return, worsening, or start of lymphedema.

How to Reduce Swelling After Surgery or Radiation

Right after surgery, the incision in the breast and underarm area may swell. This swelling is usually short-term and slowly goes away over the next six to twelve weeks. Some women also have swelling in the arm, which may go away on its own. But arm swelling after breast surgery can mean a higher risk of lymphedema later. Talk to your doctor or nurse about what you should expect and what you should do. These tips may help ease the swelling:

- Use your affected arm as you normally would when combing your hair, bathing, dressing, and eating.

- Put your affected arm above the level of your heart two to three times a day and keep it there for forty-five minutes. Lie down to do this, and fully support your arm. Place your arm on pillows so that your hand is higher than your wrist and your elbow is a little higher than your shoulder. While the arm is elevated, exercise the arm by opening and closing your hand fifteen to twenty-five times. This helps reduce swelling by pumping lymph fluid out of your arm through the undamaged lymph vessels.
- Talk to your doctor, nurse, or physical therapist before doing any other types of exercise. Exercise is an important part of fitness, but you need time to heal after surgery and should follow the advice of your medical team.

Keep in mind that radiation therapy after surgery may also cause some swelling in the arm, chest, and breast, especially toward the end of treatment. In most cases, this swelling will last only a short time and will slowly go away. However, this swelling can increase the risk of lymphedema later. During and after radiation therapy, you should do stretching exercises each day to keep full movement in your chest, arm, and shoulder muscles. Talk to your doctor or physical therapist to find out what kinds of stretching exercises are right for you. The tissue damage from radiation treatment continues over decades, so plan to make these simple exercises a long-term part of your daily routine.

Recent studies are trying to find lymphedema early and treat it right away to better control it. If you notice tingling or strange sensations in your arm after surgery, talk with your doctor, even if you have not noticed swelling. If you are concerned, consider asking your doctor to refer you to a specialist who is an expert in managing lymphedema.

Some doctors measure the arms before surgery, then remeasure afterward so that swelling can be detected and treated before it becomes obvious. You can ask your doctor to take these measurements or refer you to a physical therapist to have this done. If possible, ask to be referred to a certified lymphedema therapist (CLT).

For Women Who Have Had Surgery or Radiation Therapy

Any woman who has had surgery or radiation therapy is at risk for lymphedema. Having both surgery and radiation therapy increases your risk even more. At this time, there are no scientific studies to show that lymphedema can be prevented. Still, most experts say following some basic steps might lower your risk, delay the onset of lymphedema, or reduce its impact.

Signs of Lymphedema

If you have had lymph nodes removed or had radiation therapy, you should be alert for the signs listed below. These are some signs of lymphedema:

- Swelling in the breast, chest, shoulder, arm, or hand
- Feelings of fullness or heaviness in the arm, shoulder, chest, or hand
- Reddening of the skin, changes in the skin's texture, or feelings of tightness or hardness in the area
- New aching, tingling, or other discomfort in the area
- Less movement or flexibility in nearby joints, such as your shoulder, hand, or wrist
- Trouble fitting your arm into jacket or shirt sleeves
- Changes in how your bra fits
- Feelings of tightness in the fit of rings, watches, or bracelets, without weight gain

If you have had any type of breast surgery, radiation treatment, or had lymph nodes removed, get in the habit of looking at your upper body in front of a mirror. Compare both sides of your body and look for changes in size, shape, or skin color. Get to know your body and what's normal for you. This way you can spot changes and get treatment right away.

When to Get Help

Call your doctor, nurse, physical therapist, or lymphedema therapist if you notice any of the signs of lymphedema listed above or any of these changes:

- If any part of your affected arm, chest, breast, or underarm area feels hot, looks red, or swells suddenly. These could be a sign of infection or a blood clot, and you might need treatment right away.
- If you have a temperature of 100.5°F or higher (taken by mouth) that is not related to a cold or flu
- If you have any new pain in the affected area with no known cause

Regular checkups: Regular checkups should include screening for lymphedema. If you have been recording arm measurements, this may be part of the checkup. Talk to your medical team about how often you should be checked.

- **Report any changes.** After surgery, you will learn how your arm, chest, and breast should normally feel. Report any changes in size, color, temperature, feeling, or skin condition to your doctor right away.

- **Do not avoid mammograms.** At this time, there is no link between mammograms and the start of or worsening of lymphedema. Mammograms are a key part of breast cancer follow-up care and should not be avoided because of worries about lymphedema. If you notice breast swelling or soreness after a mammogram, talk to your doctor or lymphedema therapist.

Weight and lymphedema risk: Try to get to and/or stay at a healthy weight. We know that obese women are at higher risk for lymphedema. Talk to your health care team to determine a healthy weight for you, and get their advice on how to get to or stay at that weight.

Exercise: Using your affected arm for normal, everyday activities will help you heal properly and regain strength. This includes doing things like brushing your hair and bathing. Using your muscles also helps drain lymph fluid from your arms.

The challenge with exercise recommendations and their relationship to lymphedema risk is that there are risks both in exercising and not exercising. Certain types of exercise can reduce your lymphedema risk and can make lymphedema better. Avoiding exercise and allowing your arm to get out of shape may lead to lymphedema and episodes of swelling, sometimes called flare-ups. However, some kinds of exercise can actually increase your risk of lymphedema or make existing lymphedema worse. Overuse can result in injury and has been linked with the start of lymphedema in some women. It is important that you work with a well-trained fitness or health care professional to design a program that starts at a low level of intensity and progresses slowly enough to ensure that you are able to avoid the overuse that we know is bad for the lymphatic system.

If you have had surgery or radiation treatment, ask your doctor or nurse when you can start to exercise and what type of exercises you can do. It is a good idea to follow these tips:

- Use your affected arm as normally as you can. Once you are fully healed, about four to six weeks after surgery or radiation therapy, you can begin to go back to the activities you did before your surgery.
- Exercise regularly, but try not to overtire your shoulder and arm. Talk with your doctor, nurse, or physical therapist before starting any exercise. They can help you set goals and limits so that you can work at the level of activity that is right for you.
- If your arm starts to ache, lie down and raise it above the level of your heart.
- Avoid vigorous, repeated activities.
- Avoid heavy lifting or pulling.

- Use your unaffected arm or both arms as much as possible to carry heavy packages, groceries, handbags, or children.

Use of compression garments: Compression garments are fitted sleeves that can help control lymphedema. They can help prevent or reduce swelling by moving lymph fluid from the arm back into the body. The sleeve should be carefully fitted by a professional, and you should follow your health care professional's advice on use and care of the garment.

Compression garments are most often used by women who already have lymphedema. But if you are at risk for lymphedema, you might want to use one to lower your risk in certain high-risk situations. For instance, lymphedema has been linked with air travel, possibly because of air pressure changes, but there are pros and cons to using a compression garment on long or frequent airplane flights. Speak to your doctor or lymphedema therapist about your risk factors and whether you should be fitted for a sleeve to wear during air travel. You might also want to discuss ways to safely raise your arm above the level of your heart and

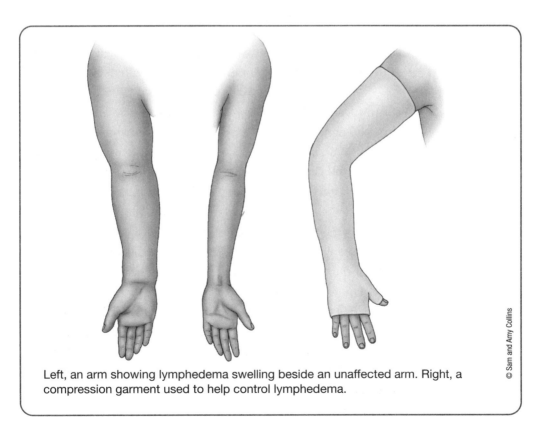

© Sam and Amy Collins

Left, an arm showing lymphedema swelling beside an unaffected arm. Right, a compression garment used to help control lymphedema.

exercise it during long flights. Do not use a poorly fitting sleeve under any circumstances, as this may increase your risk for lymphedema or make lymphedema worse.

You usually do not need a compression garment to prevent lymphedema during exercise. But if you have noticed swelling during exercise, talk to your doctor or therapist.

Avoid infection: Your body responds to infection by sending extra fluid and white blood cells to fight the infection. Removal of or damage to lymph nodes and vessels makes it harder for the body to move this extra fluid, which can trigger or worsen lymphedema. Good hygiene and careful skin care may reduce the risk of lymphedema by helping you avoid infections.

Follow these suggestions to help you care for the hand and arm on the side where you had surgery:

- Whenever you need to have blood drawn, blood pressure taken, and IVs started, make certain the unaffected arm is used. Have flu shots and vaccinations given in your unaffected arm or somewhere else, such as in the hip. Tell the doctor or nurse that you are at risk for lymphedema.
- Keep your hands and cuticles soft and moist by regularly applying moisturizing lotion or cream. Push cuticles back with a cuticle stick rather than cutting them with scissors.
- Keep your arm clean. Clean and protect any skin breaks caused by cuts, scratches, insect bites, hangnails, or torn cuticles. See the following section "How to Care for Cuts, Scratches, or Burns."
- Wear protective gloves with sleeves when gardening, doing yard work, working with animals that could scratch or bite, and when doing household chores that involve harsh chemical cleansers or steel wool.
- Wear a thimble when sewing to avoid pricking your fingers on needles and pins.
- Be extra careful when shaving your underarms, and use a clean razor on clean skin.
- Use an insect repellent when outdoors to avoid bug bites. If you are stung by a bee on the affected arm, clean and elevate the arm, apply ice, and call your doctor or nurse if the sting shows any signs of infection.
- Protect yourself against falls, fractured bones, and serious burns.

Watch for cellulitis: Lymphedema can increase your risk for cellulitis, a serious bacterial infection in the tissues just under your skin. Cellulitis can develop from an injury as minor as a mosquito bite or scratch. Signs of this problem include fever; flu-like symptoms; and redness, warmth, and pain in the affected arm and/or hand. The infection can begin as a small reddened area in the hand or arm and spread outward over the arm and/or hand. Report this urgent medical problem to your doctor right away. Cellulitis can lead to or worsen lymphedema, and if you already have lymphedema, your risk of cellulitis is higher. If cellulitis becomes a repeated problem, suppressive antibiotics may be used to keep it under control.

How to Care for Cuts, Scratches, or Burns

If you hurt yourself or break the skin on your affected arm, be sure to do the following:

- Wash the area with soap and water.
- Put an over-the-counter antibiotic cream or ointment on the area. Check with your doctor, nurse, or pharmacist if you are not sure what to use.
- Cover the area with a clean, dry gauze or bandage. Keep the area clean and covered until it heals. Change the dressing each day and any time it gets wet.
- For burns, apply a cold pack or cold water for at least fifteen minutes, then wash with soap and water and put on a clean, dry dressing.
- Be alert for early signs of infection: pus, rash, red blotches, swelling, increased heat, tenderness, chills, or fever.
- Call your doctor right away if you think you have an infection.

Avoid burns and extreme temperatures: Like infections, burns can cause extra fluid to build up and cause swelling when lymph nodes have been removed or damaged. Follow these suggestions to avoid burns:

- Protect your chest, shoulders, and arms from sunburn. Use sunscreen with a sun protection factor (SPF) of 30 or higher, and try to stay out of the sun between the hours of 10 a.m. and 4 p.m., when ultraviolet rays are strongest.
- Use oven mitts that cover your lower arms when cooking.
- Be careful when frying foods, boiling liquids, and removing food from a microwave oven.
- Avoid high heat, such as from hot tubs and saunas. If you use a heating pad or ice pack on the affected areas, limit the length of time you use it until you know how your body will respond. Both heat and cold can damage tissues and can increase fluid buildup. Some doctors may advise you to stay away from all sources of extreme temperatures.

Take Care of Yourself

It is important to take good care of your skin—especially in the affected area. Keep your skin clean and dry, and use moisturizers regularly to keep your skin from becoming dry, which can make it prone to cracking.

Taking care of your whole body is also important. Here are some good ways to stay as healthy as possible:

- **Maintain a healthy weight.**
- **Eat more servings of vegetables and fruits** each day (aim for at least two and one-half cups total).
- **Choose whole grain foods** instead of white flour and sugars.
- **Cut back on processed meats,** such as hot dogs, bologna, and bacon.
- **If you drink alcohol,** limit yourself to one drink a day (6 ounces or less).
- **Don't forget to get some type of regular exercise.** This is a key part of lymphedema management. Talk to your medical team about the types of exercise that are best for you. The challenge with exercise recommendations for women with lymphedema is that there are risks to both exercising and not exercising. This situation is much like exercising after a heart attack: Not exercising allows for further deconditioning (which is bad), but overexercising can cause harm. Trained health care professionals such as fitness trainers and physical and occupational therapists can help you learn how to exercise safely.
- **Try to reduce the stress** in your life and get enough sleep.

You also need people you can turn to for strength and comfort. Support can come in many forms: family, friends, cancer support groups, places of worship or spiritual groups, online support communities, or one-on-one counseling. You may want to get support from others with lymphedema. It helps to talk to people who understand what you are experiencing. Call the American Cancer Society at 800-227-2345, or contact the National Lymphedema Network at 800-541-3259 or www.lymphnet.org to find support groups in your area.

Avoid constriction: Constriction or squeezing of the arm may increase the pressure in nearby blood vessels, which can lead to increased fluid and swelling (much like water building up behind a dam). Some women have linked this with the onset of lymphedema. Consider following these precautions:

- Wear loose jewelry, clothing, bras, and gloves. Avoid anything that fits too tightly or puts pressure around your chest, arm, or wrist. Be sure compression garments fit well and are worn properly. Clothing and compression garments should be supportive and have smooth, even compression.

- Do not use shoulder straps when carrying briefcases and purses.
- Wear a loose-fitting bra with padded straps that do not dig into your shoulder. Make sure underwire bras do not put pressure on your breast or chest. If you have had a mastectomy and are using a prosthesis (breast form), try to choose a lightweight one. A heavy prosthesis may put too much pressure on the area.
- If you are having your blood pressure taken, have it done on the unaffected arm or, if both arms are affected, on your thigh. You can also ask that blood pressure be measured by someone using a hand pump and stethoscope rather than using a machine; the machines often use high pressures for a longer time.

For Women Who Have Lymphedema

If lymphedema develops, there are treatments to reduce the swelling, keep it from getting worse, and decrease the risk of infection. The treatment is prescribed by your doctor and should be given by an experienced therapist. Be sure to check with your health insurance to be sure the treatment is covered.

Mild lymphedema should be treated by a physical therapist or other health care professional who has had special training. Moderate or severe lymphedema is most often treated by a therapist with special training and expertise who will help you with skin care, massage, special bandaging, exercises, and fitting for a compression sleeve. This is sometimes known as complex decongestive therapy, or CDT. Manual lymphatic drainage, or MLD, is the type of massage used as part of CDT to manage lymphedema. The therapist will also teach you things like how to care for the lymphedema at home and how and when to wear the compression sleeve.

Although most insurance companies will pay for lymphedema treatment, some do not cover the cost of compression garments and dressings. Check with your insurance company about coverage for these therapies.

Seeking and getting treatment early should lead to a shorter course of treatment to control your lymphedema. Again, it is important to notice changes right away and get help as soon as possible.

CHAPTER 14

Staying Emotionally Healthy During Treatment

It may feel as if cancer is consuming everything in your life right now. But eventually cancer will become part of your life history—it will not devour your life itself or your ability to enjoy life. Just like other crises and other joys you've had in the past, cancer will be part of your life story, but it will not overshadow everything else.

Breast cancer often causes women to reevaluate their priorities. Other worries may seem insignificant compared to having cancer. Many women have said that breast cancer forced them to achieve their goals, assert themselves, become closer to their families, get organized, and do all the things they never made time for before. They did these things not because they were running out of time, but because they could now appreciate and use time in new ways.

Acknowledging Your Feelings

Going through a life-changing experience such as cancer can bring out a wide range of emotions. This is normal. You might feel anxious or depressed because of changes in your ability to perform family or work roles, loss of control over events in life, and changes in body image. You may fear death or a cancer recurrence, suffering and pain, and the unknown. You might feel angry that you have had to go through this experience, frustrated at not being able to "do enough," or stressed by all the unknowns, family upheaval, and other changes in your life. These feelings might last for several days to several weeks and can come up periodically throughout treatment and recovery.

These emotions are normal. It is important to give yourself permission to experience these feelings. It will take time to accept, understand, and face your diagnosis. However, there are things you can do to deal with these emotions and work through them.

Expressing Feelings

Research has not proven that a positive outlook prolongs survival. A positive attitude can certainly help people feel hopeful, but it does not mean that you will never feel sad, stressed, or uncertain. Trying to keep a hopeful, positive attitude often lessens the impact of cancer on you and those close to you and may make it easier to deal with problems that come up. But your attitude will not be the difference between illness and recovery. Similarly, any difficulty you have coping with your situation will not trigger a setback or recurrence. Those who believe that a positive attitude is the key to their survival might blame themselves if their cancer returns—this assumptionn is simply wrong. Cancer is a complex disease; people's attitudes do not cause or cure cancer.

Hiding feelings can actually prevent you from being able to feel hopeful, positive, and more in control of your life. If you keep emotions bottled up, they will continue to bother you and become unmanageable, potentially leading to serious problems, such as rage or depression. If you blame yourself or others for problems and focus only on the unfairness of life, you can be distracted from gathering the information you need to make important decisions. It can also keep you from getting the help you need from other people. For example, someone who is devastated about losing her hair because of chemotherapy might avoid the company of friends or family so she won't be seen. But those loved ones can give needed help and support during the difficult weeks of treatment. Acceptance can be a part of coping with your illness. People who cope well tend to be flexible and able to adapt to uncertainty and change. Those who can grieve their losses and accept change will also have a better quality of life than people who cannot accept change.

These are some other things you can do to deal with your emotions:

- Get spiritual support through prayer, meditation, or other practices that help you feel more at peace. You may want the guidance of a chaplain, pastor, rabbi, or other religious leader.
- Pay attention to your physical needs for rest, nutrition, and other self-care measures.
- Find ways to express your feelings, such as talking or writing in a journal.
- Allow yourself private time and space.

- Walk or exercise. Be sure to talk with your medical team about your plans before starting a new exercise program or activity.
- Find out what helped other patients and families cope with cancer, and/or talk with other people with the same type of cancer.
- Make changes at home to create a healthier environment; talk with your doctor about making healthy lifestyle choices.
- Ask for support from family, friends, and others. Just having someone who cares and will listen to you can be very helpful. If friends or family members are not able to be supportive, find others who will be supportive. Health care professionals (such as social workers, psychologists, or other licensed health professionals) and support groups can be extra sources of support.

If you have feelings of sadness that last weeks or months or that are getting in the way of day-to-day life, this can be a sign of clinical depression. About one in four people with cancer will develop clinical depression, which causes great distress, impairs functioning, and decreases one's ability to follow a treatment schedule. Signs of depression include a loss of pleasure in everyday activities and a persistent blue mood. Depression can also affect your appetite, causing significant weight loss or weight gain. You might have disruptions in your sleep schedule, either oversleeping or suffering from insomnia. You may also have little energy or have trouble focusing, remembering things, or making decisions. These symptoms are often accompanied by feelings of guilt, worthlessness, or helplessness that can escalate into thoughts of death or suicide.

If you have these symptoms and they are severe enough to interfere with your ability to function normally, talk with your doctor. Clinical depression can be treated with medicines, psychotherapy, and/or other specialized treatment. These interventions not only improve one's psychological well-being but also reduce suffering and enhance quality of life. Your doctor can refer you to a professional counselor who specializes in working with people who have cancer. Private counseling sessions offer the chance to express feelings and thoughts that you may not feel comfortable sharing in other settings. In individual therapy, you have the full attention of a professional who can offer feedback and suggest coping strategies. The confidentiality and objectivity of individual therapy can be valuable.

Managing Depression

Consider the following ways to manage depression:

- Seek help through counseling and/or support groups. Continue treatment until your symptoms improve (usually after several weeks). Seek different treatment if there is no improvement.
- Tell your doctor how you are feeling and talk with him or her about the possible use of antidepressant medicines.
- If you are taking antidepressants, avoid alcohol unless you check with your doctor or pharmacist.
- Talk about your feelings and fears with friends and family members—don't keep them inside.
- Engage in enjoyable activities.
- Use prayer or other types of spiritual support, if you find this helps.
- Try deep breathing and relaxation exercises several times a day (see chapter 12 on complementary therapies).
- Spend time with other people. Being around helpful, loving people can help take your attention away from negative feelings.
- Try journaling as an outlet for feelings. See page 292 for ways to get started.
- Remember that it is okay to feel sad and frustrated. Do not blame yourself for feelings of fear, anxiety, or depression. Look for the cause of these feelings, and then talk about it.

Call your doctor or nurse if you are having trouble eating, sleeping, or getting out of bed, or if you have any thoughts of death or suicide.

Asking for Help

Developing a support system is very important. Sometimes you just need to remind yourself to use the support you already have. You might feel reluctant to call on others for fear of being a burden. However, most of your family and friends will feel better knowing they can help you in some way. Seeking the support, assistance, and companionship of others is an important part of coping with cancer. People who have strong bonds with others tend to endure crises better than those who do not have that support.

One of the first things a friend or family member will often say is, "What can I do to help?" You may be tempted to say, "Oh, nothing right now. We're just fine." Maybe you don't really know what you need, want your privacy, or feel you have all you can handle without having more people around you.

However, remember that most people really do want to help, and it is likely that you will need extra help at some point during your cancer treatment. Your loved ones want to do things for you and support you. It helps them feel like they are part of your life. Allow them to help you. Be as specific as possible about the kind of help you need. Some people keep a list of things they need by the telephone. For example, you might need a ride to the doctor or help with housecleaning, yard work, or childcare. There will be times when you don't know what you need, but even just saying that will be helpful. It also gives your loved ones a chance to offer something they can do for you.

If you enjoyed walking or hobbies with friends before your cancer diagnosis, remind your friends that you still enjoy those things. But do not be afraid to say so if you don't feel up to talking or other activities. If you want to be asked again later, tell them that, and ask them to keep inviting you. A lot of people will be happy to do that for you. Let them know it feels good to be asked—even on the days you are not up to it.

Reach Out for Help

Reaching out to others and making use of the people in your life and support groups, advocacy organizations, and mental health professionals can help in the following ways:

- restore your sense of self-worth
- counteract fear
- reduce isolation
- keep your spirits up
- help you take care of yourself
- offer practical assistance and information

Rebuilding Self-Esteem

One psychologist who specializes in counseling adults who have had cancer has described self-esteem as a set of bank accounts. These accounts include the net worth of the following:

- your physical self—what your body can do and how you look
- your social self—how easily you get along with others and how much emotional support you can count on from others
- your achieving self—what you have done in school, work, and personal and family relationships
- your spiritual self—your religious and moral beliefs and the strength they give you

During your life, you make deposits into your accounts and add to your self-image, but when a crisis such as cancer arises, you must make withdrawals. Going through cancer treatment has costs. It takes time and might take away some of your physical

Feelings Journal

Consider keeping a journal. Writing down your experiences and your emotions can help you come to terms with your situation. A journal may help you understand how events have affected and changed you and how far you have come in processing your experiences. It is also a safe and healthy way to express any feelings of anger, confusion, joy, or guilt. If you have never journaled before, it can be helpful to have prompts to get you started. You might begin by completing the sentences below about your feelings.

- **When I first found out** I had cancer, I felt...
- **I wish** that I...
- **I can make this come true** by doing...
- **One of the things** I worry about most is...
- **What would make me** feel better is...
- **When I tell others** about my condition...
- **I feel closest** to people when...
- **Other people** see me as...
- **I would like other people** to see me as...
- **When I get** angry...
- **When things get to be** too much...
- **I would like** to handle things by...
- **I couldn't get along** without...
- **The best times** are...
- **What I like most** about myself is...

ability to function. It can harm your relationships with others, your career goals, and sometimes your faith. When funds from one of your accounts become low, you might need a "loan" from one of the others to balance your account.

Try to keep in mind the costs of cancer in your life and make an effort to make new deposits in the active accounts. By doing so, a drain in one area of your self-worth will not bankrupt you. If your cancer treatment has affected your looks, you might focus on the love, caring, and support you get from friends and family who react to you with a deep level of intimacy. If treatment interrupts your work, use some of your energy to enrich your social or spiritual life.

Although you might sometimes feel that all your accounts are getting low, a careful look can reveal some areas where "income" is still flowing in.

Strengthening Your Self-Esteem: Body Image and Other Factors

Feeling physically attractive is only one aspect of your self-esteem. Cancer and its treatment can greatly affect your feelings about how your body looks, how it works, and how you feel about yourself. Most women come to terms with their new body image, but learning to accept the changes takes time and energy. Those who cannot accept the changes right away should respect their own timetable and work on self-acceptance when the time is right for them.

Although many women focus on taking care of their bodies during treatment, it is also important to nurture the spirit. The following are suggestions for strengthening your self-esteem and relationships and preventing problems with body image:

- Learn as much as you can about how and why your body is changing and how to manage each symptom. For example, learn to spot the early signs of lymphedema or learn how to take care of your skin. Information and knowledge may help you feel less frightened and intimidated by physical changes. It also helps restore a sense of control over your body and life.

- Begin to touch and look at your scars if you had surgery. This is the new you, and you will need to adjust to how your body looks now. If it is too difficult to touch or look at your scars right away, don't worry. You might need more time to get comfortable with the changes.

- Shift your focus to another attractive part of your body. For example, if you are self-conscious about your chest but feel good about your legs, it might help you to wear skirts or tights to draw attention to that part of your body.

- Learn to value your body as a whole. Just because one part of your body has changed does not mean you are unattractive or less of a woman.

- You may become so absorbed with managing your physical challenges that you lose sight of who you are as a person. It might be hard to think of yourself as a whole person, not just a body part or a person with cancer. Remember that you have many positive traits and attributes that you and others value. You are more than a chart, a number, or an appointment time. Even though you are sick, you are still the same person, and you have things to offer.

- Talk about it. Open communication can help relieve stress and clear up misconceptions about what the cancer has and has not changed about you. For example, you might be worried about your partner's feelings about changes in your appearance. It is not unusual to find that your partner is less upset about any changes than you imagined. He or she is no doubt more grateful that you are alive than concerned about your mastectomy scar, for example. Your partner and other family members might be nervous about touching you because they don't want to cause you any pain, so you will have to let them know what's okay and what you need.

- Do something new and different. Find a way to do something that makes you feel capable and valued. You might want to take up a new hobby, start a journal, take a class, do volunteer work, or learn to play an instrument—anything that makes you feel competent and worthwhile.

- Shift your work expectations. If you cannot continue your career, turn your attention to something else, such as another kind of job or going back to school.

- Try to find some value in what has happened. This may take some real work and growth, but with some soul searching, you may be able to find a grain of something positive in what has happened.

- Look for hope. People who can focus on what they have rather than what they have lost often feel spiritually enriched, more involved in their daily lives, and more connected to others. You can learn to see something positive in most experiences. Try finding the smallest things that are worth living for. Set manageable short-term goals that you enjoy and can achieve, such as attending a child's or grandchild's recital or going to dinner with a friend.

- Don't pressure yourself or feel that you need to fake it. Be aware of any pressure you might feel from yourself or others to be positive and cheerful about what is happening. Keeping your true feelings bottled up and feeling guilty about them will make it much harder to cope with what is going on. It will also keep you from dealing with other people honestly and intimately and may keep you from getting the help you need.

- Try new activities with new people. If you cannot do something you used to do because of a cancer-related change, try something else. Volunteer with a friend at a community organization or join a book club—anything that helps you enjoy time with other people.

- Live in the present. Try to take one day at a time and live in the now. Focus on what is meaningful and enjoyable in the present, rather than on what you risk losing in the future. When you have a bad day, don't read too much into it. Everyone has a bad day once in a while.

- Be a problem solver. There are many ways to approach the problems that cancer and its treatment present. At one end of the continuum, there is the approach of "taking the bull by the horns"—getting information and opinions, evaluating options, setting priorities, considering pros and cons, and ultimately making choices. However, this approach does not work for everyone, especially if you are feeling ill, anxious, isolated, or drained of strength. Still, the other extreme—doing nothing and passively letting things happen—rarely works and usually creates more problems that become harder to resolve. Good problem solvers try to break down problems to a manageable size, ask for the help they need, and take things one step at a time.

Monitoring Self-Esteem

To safeguard your self-esteem during cancer treatment, it is important that you keep track of how you are feeling about yourself throughout the process. Evaluating different aspects of yourself and your life can help you focus on your strengths and recognize areas that need to be fostered.

The following chart can help you identify how you feel about yourself in various areas that can affect your self-esteem. Circle how well you feel in each area, with 1 indicating very poor and 5 indicating very good. You can make a copy of this chart for each month you are in treatment.

As you progress through treatment, compare the columns and note where there have been changes in your scoring. Think about why you feel lower in certain areas and what you can do to improve these scores. Though it sounds simple, just the act of physically taking note of how you are feeling can help you be more in tune with your feelings.

	Before Treatment	Treatment Weeks				After Treatment
		1	2	3	4	
Body image	1 2 3 4 5	1 2 3 4 5	1 2 3 4 5	1 2 3 4 5	1 2 3 4 5	1 2 3 4 5
Personal relationships	1 2 3 4 5	1 2 3 4 5	1 2 3 4 5	1 2 3 4 5	1 2 3 4 5	1 2 3 4 5
Work performance	1 2 3 4 5	1 2 3 4 5	1 2 3 4 5	1 2 3 4 5	1 2 3 4 5	1 2 3 4 5
Work relationships	1 2 3 4 5	1 2 3 4 5	1 2 3 4 5	1 2 3 4 5	1 2 3 4 5	1 2 3 4 5
Accomplishments	1 2 3 4 5	1 2 3 4 5	1 2 3 4 5	1 2 3 4 5	1 2 3 4 5	1 2 3 4 5
Self-respect	1 2 3 4 5	1 2 3 4 5	1 2 3 4 5	1 2 3 4 5	1 2 3 4 5	1 2 3 4 5
Spirituality	1 2 3 4 5	1 2 3 4 5	1 2 3 4 5	1 2 3 4 5	1 2 3 4 5	1 2 3 4 5

Coping Strategies

There are a number of strategies you can use to cope with the stresses of cancer and its treatment. Different people will respond differently to these techniques, but one or more of these strategies may help you deal with negative emotions.

Cognitive Restructuring

Cognitive restructuring is a way of changing the way you normally think. It involves identifying negative thoughts, feelings, or fears and replacing them with constructive or realistic ones that lead to positive action. This practice can help you review your usual ways of responding to stress and modify them by thinking through problems differently.

There are many cognitive restructuring techniques. Identifying critical thoughts and irrational beliefs is the key to understanding how to change negative thought patterns. You can teach yourself to develop an internal dialogue and change any automatic negative thinking into rational responses. One way to do this is to record your negative thoughts on paper, list how they make you feel, and write a rational response to the situation.

Cognitive Restructuring	
Situation: Explain what happened that was upsetting.	I was late and I missed my appointment.
Feelings: Describe how you felt after it happened and the intensity of the feeling (1 = weak, 10 = strong).	• Stupid (8) • Frustrated (6)
Thoughts: Write down any negative things you told yourself or thoughts you had.	I never do anything right.
Evidence: Is there any validity to the irrational beliefs? Provide examples.	That's not true; there are a lot of things I do right.
Alternate Response: Write down other things you can tell yourself to counterbalance the negative thoughts.	• I'm usually on time. • Next time I'll be on schedule.

Thought Stopping

Women experience many stresses and anxieties as they go from diagnosis through treatment. It is hard not to worry about everything from deteriorating health and medical expenses to family and work pressures. But constant worry can undermine healing efforts.

Thought stopping is a classic technique of behavioral therapy. It is a simple self-help tool for interrupting repetitive or unpleasant thoughts. First, identify the thought you want to stop (for instance, "How will I pay for the hospital bill?" or "What if I'm dying?" or "Poor me."). Then, every time you have this thought, visualize a big red stop sign (or another image that means "stop" to you) and say "Stop!" loudly and firmly. Practice the exercise until it is second nature. Over time, you can learn to shout to yourself without actually speaking aloud. Whenever the thought pops up, so will the image, and your inner voice will silently command the thought to stop.

Graded Task Assignments

Using graded task assignments is a way to identify a goal and then list small steps needed to achieve it. For example, the demands of treatment can make it hard to keep in touch with friends. When your treatment is over, you will want to resume these friendships but might feel overwhelmed by the task of trying to rebuild your life.

First, identify your goal: to reconnect with friends. Then give yourself graded task assignments—specific, manageable steps toward that goal. You might make a list of people with whom you have lost touch and then call one friend a day. The next tasks might be to make one lunch date a week, to go on that date, and to talk with a friend about how it feels to pick up the pieces after cancer. Step by step, you can reach your goal without exhausting yourself physically or emotionally.

Distraction

One of the easiest and most useful coping methods for handling short-term discomfort is distraction. If you have ever daydreamed in a meeting, counted sheep, worn headphones to avoid the boredom of exercise or a bus ride, or kept busy to avoid thinking about something unpleasant, you already know how to use distraction.

Distraction involves a wide range of techniques, from imagery and thought stopping to using music, movies, TV, and podcasts to occupy your attention. The goal is to direct your awareness away from the physical or emotional distress you are feeling. This technique does not require much energy, so it can be very useful when you are tired. Distraction can be used to manage anxiety, control nausea or vomiting, handle acute

Resolving Problems

When you have a lot on your mind, it can be hard to focus on one problem at a time. It often helps to write things down. Use the following questions to organize your thoughts and make decisions. Repeat steps three through ten for every problem on your list, in order of importance.

1. **What are the problems** I need to resolve now? *(List all that come to mind, in any order.)*
2. **How important are these problems?** *(Set priorities by numbering each item on your list, from most important to least important.)*
3. **Beginning with my highest-priority problem,** what are all the solutions I can think of? *(List all that come to mind, in any order.)*
4. **Do I need more information** about any of the options I've listed or about other possible solutions? *(If you answered yes, list what you can do or whom you can ask to find out more.)*
5. **What are the advantages and disadvantages** of each option I've thought of? *(List all that apply.)*
6. **Considering all the advantages and disadvantages,** which option seems to make the most sense and why?
7. **Whose help do I need** to implement this choice?
8. **What do I need to do now** to move forward with this decision?
9. **When will I take the first step?** *(Set a realistic schedule.)*
10. **I still can't seem to make up my mind** or take action. What's bothering me? *(Write down everything that comes to mind. Then relax and approach the problem again when you're ready.)*

pain, manage treatment-related phobias (such as fear of needles or MRIs), and stop repetitive, negative thoughts.

Any activity that occupies your attention can be used for distraction. If the mere smell of the infusion center makes you ill, you can distract yourself by taking along strong mints, a small bottle of perfume, or a scented oil to smell when you feel nauseated. Losing yourself in a good book might divert your mind. If you enjoy working with your hands, crafts such as needlework, model building, or painting might be useful. Going to a movie or watching television are also good distraction methods. Try math games, such as subtracting forty-seven from one thousand or counting back from a certain number. Slow, rhythmic breathing can be used for distraction and relaxation. You might find it helpful to listen to relatively fast music through a headset or earphones. To help keep your attention on the music, tap out the rhythm or adjust the volume.

Denial

The ability to proceed as if you have no problems can be either helpful or harmful, depending on the behavior it produces. Denial is destructive, for example, when a person with a lump or troubling symptom puts off getting medical help because "there's nothing wrong." This type of denial can have negative consequences during and after treatment, too, such as causing people to skip appointments, ignore important information, fail to participate actively in their health care or ask questions, avoid making plans, and suppress the emotions that are appropriate to their situation.

But the ability to keep fear at some distance can also be beneficial, as long as you do what needs to be done to take care of your mind and your body. Keeping your mind off the seriousness of your cancer diagnosis can help you focus on the things that need to be dealt with soon, such as getting second opinions, making arrangements at home and work, and deciding on a treatment plan. Going about your life at home or at work as normally as possible can minimize your fear and anxiety and contribute to your quality of life. Just be sure you address the real-life problems that will not go away no matter how much you ignore them.

Laughter

Humor can ease physical and emotional difficulties and can be a way to cope with illness. Humor cannot cure cancer, but it can improve your quality of life, lessen pain, encourage relaxation, reduce stress, and provide an overall sense of well-being. The use of humor can even lead to an increase in pain tolerance. It is thought that laughter stimulates the release of endorphins, special substances in the brain that help control pain. The physical effects of laughter on the body include increased breathing, oxygen use, and heart rate, which stimulate the circulatory system.

Many hospitals and ambulatory care centers have incorporated special rooms where funny materials—and sometimes people—are present to help people laugh. Materials commonly used include movies, CDs, books, games, and puzzles. Many hospitals have volunteer groups who visit patients to give them a chance to laugh.

Exercise

Physical activity can be another important part of coping with treatment. It can help you feel more in control of your body and build strength and endurance. If you feel up to it and your doctor agrees that you are ready, try activities such as walking, yoga, swimming, and stretching, all of which stimulate the muscles and circulatory system without stressing the joints. If your treatment involved surgery, certain exercises can help speed your recovery. Talk with your doctor about the exercise programs that are best for you.

Work

Being productive at work helps many women feel more in control of their lives, and the familiar routine of a job can provide stability. Many women want to feel as normal as possible after treatment and choose to return to work right away. Women undergoing lumpectomy for early-stage breast cancer, for example, typically do not have side effects that keep them from returning to work. They sometimes go back to work a few days after surgery and continue working during radiation treatment. Of course, not everyone will be physically or emotionally ready to work throughout treatment or so soon after surgery. Only you can be the judge of what you are ready to handle.

Complementary Therapies

Many complementary therapies, such as meditation, yoga, tai chi, or relaxation therapy, can help you cope, too. These methods fall into the area of mind-body medicine, which focuses on the interplay of thoughts, emotions, and health. Complementary methods can often be used both during and after treatment and are used along with conventional treatments. They can be helpful in dealing with the physical effects and mental stresses of having cancer, and they can be a welcome distraction from some of the emotions and physical hardships you might be facing. For more information on complementary therapies, refer back to chapter 12.

CHAPTER 15

Breast Reconstruction and Prostheses

In recent years, breast reconstruction has become an increasingly popular option for women facing the loss of a breast because of cancer. Breast reconstruction is surgery that can rebuild the breast mound so that it is about the same size and shape as it was before the surgery. The nipple and the areola can also be added. Breast reconstruction is not a cancer treatment, but many women elect to have reconstructive surgery to help restore the body's appearance after mastectomy.

Insurance plans can vary in how much they cover breast reconstruction procedures, so it is important to talk with your insurance provider before making a decision.

Considering Reconstruction

Having breast reconstruction is a matter of individual choice and can be an emotional decision, one that is often affected by society's association of breasts with femininity. Women will have different reasons for choosing reconstruction after mastectomy— because they want their breasts to look as similar as possible to the way they looked before surgery, because they want clothing to fit as it once did, or because they feel unbalanced with just one breast, for example. Some women feel that breast reconstruction helps them put their cancer experience behind them.

You should be realistic about the cosmetic results of reconstruction. Reconstruction cannot erase all signs that you have had a breast removed. The goal of reconstruction is to make your breasts similar to one another in size and shape so that you will feel comfortable about how you look in most types of clothing. Although breast reconstruction may improve a woman's body image and self-esteem, the difference between the reconstructed breast and the remaining breast can still be seen when a woman is nude. If tissue from elsewhere on your body (such as your abdomen, shoulder, or buttock) is used in the reconstruction, that area will also look different after surgery.

Some women are comfortable having one breast or no breasts and do not pursue reconstructive surgery. Some women use breast forms to fill out their bras and give the outward appearance of breasts and are not concerned about having two breasts when nude. Some women use breast forms permanently, and some use them while deciding about reconstruction.

The American Cancer Society's Reach To Recovery program matches trained volunteers, themselves breast cancer survivors, with women going through breast cancer. To contact an American Cancer Society Reach To Recovery volunteer who has undergone breast reconstruction, call 800-227-2345. You can also refer to the resource guide in the back of this book for information on groups that can offer information and support.

Who Can Have Breast Reconstruction

Breast reconstruction is most often an option for women who have had an entire breast removed. Almost any woman who has had a mastectomy can have breast reconstruction, regardless of her age, the type of surgery first performed, or the number of years since the surgery. However, some women are not candidates for reconstructive surgery because of other medical conditions. Other women decide against breast reconstruction because they do not want more surgery or are uncomfortable with having breast implants. These women might opt to use prostheses or nothing at all.

Timing of Breast Reconstruction

For most women, the breast can be reconstructed either at the same time as mastectomy (immediate breast reconstruction) or later (delayed reconstruction). Some women choose to have mastectomy and breast reconstruction done at the same time, to avoid being without a breast and to be able to heal from the mastectomy and the breast reconstruction at the same time. Although an immediate reconstruction might mean less surgery overall, several steps still might be needed to complete the reconstruction process. If you are considering immediate reconstruction, be sure to ask what will need to be done afterward and how long the reconstruction process will take.

Other women wait until after the mastectomy and the completion of cancer treatment to have reconstruction, giving themselves more time to make reconstructive choices. Women with health problems such as obesity and high blood pressure and

Questions to Ask Your Medical Team About Breast Reconstruction

- **Am I a candidate** for breast reconstruction?

- **When can I have** reconstruction done?

- **What types of** reconstruction could I have?

- **What is the average cost** of each type? Does insurance cover them?

- **What type of reconstruction** do you think would be best for me? Why?

- **How much experience** do you (plastic surgeon) have with this procedure?

- **What results** are realistic for me?

- **Will the reconstructed** breast match my other breast?

- **Can you show me pictures** of what each reconstruction procedure I'm considering will look like after healing?

- **How will my reconstructed breast** feel to the touch?

- **Will I have any feeling** in my reconstructed breast?

- **What possible complications** should I know about?

- **How much discomfort** or pain will I feel?

- **If I choose a tissue flap procedure,** will there be pain, scars, or other changes in the parts of my body from which tissue is taken?

- **How long** will I be in the hospital?

- **Will I need blood transfusions?** If so, can I donate my own blood?

- **How long** is the expected recovery time?

- **What type of care** will I need at home?

- **Will I have a drain** (a tube that lets fluid out) when I go home?

- **How much help** will I need at home to take care of my drain and wound?

- **When can I start** my rehabilitation?

- **How much activity** can I do at home?

- **What do I do** if I have swelling in my arm (lymphedema)?

- **When will I be able** to return to normal activities, such as driving and working?

- **Can you connect me** with other women who have had the same surgery?

- **Will reconstruction interfere** with chemotherapy or radiation therapy?

- **If I have a breast implant,** how long will it last?

- **What kinds of changes** to the breast can I expect over time?

- **How will aging** affect the reconstructed breast?

- **What will happen to the breast** if I gain or lose weight?

- **Are there any new** reconstruction options that I should consider?

women who smoke may be advised to wait before having breast reconstruction, and some of these women might not be candidates for reconstruction at all. Some oncologists prefer to delay reconstruction until after any necessary chemotherapy or radiation treatments are completed. You might simply want to wait until you feel rested and ready for another surgery.

If you are thinking about having reconstructive surgery, talk with your breast surgeon and a plastic surgeon experienced in breast reconstruction before your mastectomy. This will allow you to consider all reconstruction options. Your breast surgeon and your plastic surgeon should work together to come up with a treatment plan that will put you in the best possible position for reconstruction if you decide to pursue it, even if you choose to have delayed reconstruction.

Types of Breast Reconstruction

For women facing mastectomy, the main breast reconstruction options are to use breast implants to restore the shape of the breast or to have a flap procedure (also called a natural tissue reconstruction), in which doctors use tissues from other parts of your body to restore the breast shape. In some cases, both can be used. Nipple and areola reconstruction can be part of these procedures, as can surgery on the other breast to help match it to the reconstructed one.

Women who are considering breast reconstruction should talk with their doctors to help determine the technique that might best suit their situation. In general, which type of surgery is best will depend on the following:

- the amount of tissue removed from the breast during mastectomy
- the size of the woman's natural breast
- the amount of body tissue available for a flap (for example, very thin women might not have enough extra body tissue to make flap grafts)
- whether radiation therapy is part of the treatment
- the woman's general health, including whether she smokes or has diabetes or certain connective tissue disorders
- the woman's preferences (for example, implants might require less extensive surgery, but the result might not look or feel as natural as a flap procedure)

See the tables on pages 305 and 314–315 for comparisons of some of the major points of breast implants and flap procedures (natural tissue reconstruction).

Implants Versus Natural Tissue (Flap) Reconstruction

	Breast Implants (With or Without Expander)	Natural Tissue Reconstructions or Flap Procedures
Surgery	• Two separate, shorter surgical procedures (plus visits to fill expander) • Separate procedure to create nipple and areola	• One longer procedure • Separate procedure to create nipple and areola
Hospitalization	• Usually one to two days with mastectomy; one day if done later as a separate procedure	• Up to seven days with or without mastectomy (varies by procedure)
Scar	• Mastectomy scar and often breast crease scar	• Mastectomy scar, scar at donor site, and possibly breast crease scar
Recovery Time	• Shorter recovery (two to three weeks)	• Longer recovery (three to six weeks)
Initial Result	• Less natural shape and feel (often does not match opposite breast); might be firm	• Very natural shape; soft
Other Breast	• More changes usually needed	• Fewer changes usually needed
Potential Complications	• Breast hardening with shape changes or skin ripples due to capsular contracture • Implants might rupture • Implants will need to be replaced (most last at least ten years)	• Abdominal weakness or bulge (TRAM flap) • Partial breast hardening • Risk for flap "not taking"
Expense	Less expensive	More expensive

Source: ©2003 Memorial Sloan-Kettering Cancer Center. Adapted with permission.

Breast Implant Procedures

A breast implant is a flexible silicone shell filled with either saline or a silicone gel. It can help restore the shape of the breast. Saline implants are more common. Silicone gel–filled implants were not used for several years because of concerns that silicone leakage might cause immune system diseases. However, most recent studies show that silicone implants do not increase the risk of immune system problems. Some newer types of silicone implants use a thicker gel, called cohesive gel, which is less likely to leak, even if the implant ruptures. Saline and silicone implants are similar in many ways, but each type of implant has potential advantages and disadvantages. For example, silicone implants tend to feel more like natural breasts, but once they are implanted, their size cannot be changed without surgery to replace them. The type of procedure needed to put the implant in place will depend on how much skin is remaining over the breast after the mastectomy.

For women who still have enough skin over the breast, a one-stage immediate breast reconstruction can be done at the same time as the mastectomy. After the breast surgeon removes the breast tissue, a plastic surgeon places a breast implant where the breast tissue was removed or behind the chest muscles to form the breast shape.

Most women who get an implant will need a two-stage reconstruction. This type of reconstruction is done if your skin and chest wall tissues are too tight and flat to allow for immediate placement of an implant. It can be started at the time of the mastectomy or at a later time. For this procedure, the surgeon inserts a type of implant called a tissue expander beneath the skin and chest muscle. The expander is like a balloon. At regular intervals over the course of several months, the surgeon injects saline through a tiny valve mechanism beneath the skin, filling the expander. The skin and muscle will gradually stretch, just as they do over the abdomen during pregnancy. Once the skin over the breast area has stretched enough, the expander is typically removed in a second surgery and a permanent implant is put in its place. Some tissue expanders are designed to be left in place as the final implant.

You should consider several important factors when deciding whether to have breast implants. For example, problems can develop with implants. Scar tissue can sometimes form around the implant (called capsular contracture), which can make the breast harden or change shape so that it no longer looks or feels like it did immediately after surgery. Implants can also rupture or cause infection or pain. Your implants might not last a lifetime—up to half of all implants done for breast reconstruction need to be removed or replaced within ten years, which would require additional surgery.

Tissue expander

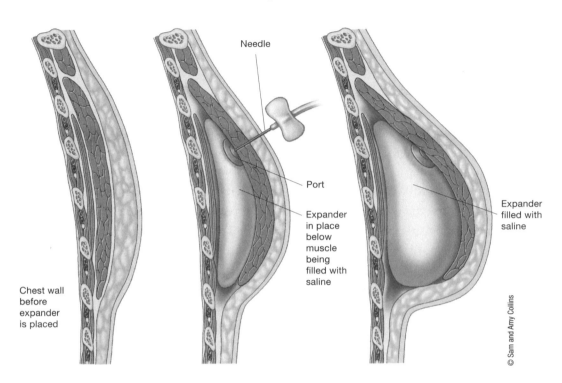

Needle

Port

Expander in place below muscle being filled with saline

Expander filled with saline

Chest wall before expander is placed

© Sam and Amy Collins

New Methods of Tissue Support

To reduce the need for a tissue expander (and the additional procedures it requires), some plastic surgeons now use a product made of donated skin tissue, known as acellular dermal matrix (such as AlloDerm and DermaMatrix). These products have had the skin cells removed, which reduces the risk that they carry disease or that the body will reject them. Acellular dermal matrix products are used to extend and support natural tissues and help them grow and heal. They allow the surgeon to create a pocket to support the implant and help create a larger breast mound. This can reduce the need to stretch the skin, which may shorten the time needed before the implant can be placed. In some cases, these products might allow the surgeon to place the implant without the need for an expander at all.

Acellular dermal matrix products are regulated by the US Food and Drug Administration (FDA) as human tissues used for transplant. These products are fairly new in breast reconstruction, and they have also been used in nipple reconstruction. Studies that look at outcomes are still in progress but have been promising overall. Potential risks associated with use of these products include a higher risk of implants having to be removed after surgery, higher rate of infection, fluid collecting in the surgical area, and the possibly of tissue flap death (in which the tissue that covers the implant dies and must be removed).

Natural Tissue Reconstruction or Flap Procedures

You might sometimes hear natural tissue reconstruction procedures called autologous or autogenous reconstruction techniques, which simply means that the surgeon is using your own body tissue to reconstruct your breast. Such surgeries use tissue from your abdomen, back, hip, buttock, or inner thigh to reconstruct the breast. Because blood vessels are involved, these procedures usually cannot be offered to women who smoke or to women with diabetes, connective tissue disease, or vascular disease.

These are the main types of natural tissue reconstruction techniques:

- the **transverse rectus abdominis muscle (TRAM) flap**, which uses tissue and muscle from the abdomen
- the **latissimus dorsi (LAT** or **LD) flap**, which uses muscle and skin from the upper back
- the **deep inferior epigastric artery perforator (DIEP) flap**, which uses tissue from the abdomen
- the **gluteal free** or **gluteal artery perforator (GAP) flap**, which uses tissue from the buttock
- the **transverse upper gracilis (TUG) flap**, which uses muscle and fatty tissue from along the bottom fold of the buttock extending to the inner thigh

TRAM and LAT flaps are the most common types of flap procedures. The other tissue flap reconstructions described here are more specialized and may not be available everywhere.

These operations leave scars both where the tissue is taken from the body and on the reconstructed breast. The scars will fade over time, but they will never go away completely. The possible complications of natural tissue reconstruction are similar to those of any major surgery and can include infection, blood clots, and accumulation of blood or fluid (called hematomas and seromas). There can also be problems at the donor tissue site, such as abdominal hernias and muscle damage or weakness. In some cases, the size and shape of the reconstructed breast might be different from your other breast.

In general, flap reconstructions behave more like the rest of your body tissue than implants do. For instance, they might enlarge or shrink as you gain or lose weight. There is also no worry about replacement or rupture.

Transverse Rectus Abdominis Muscle (TRAM) Flap

The transverse rectus abdominis muscle (TRAM) flap procedure uses tissue and muscle from the lower abdominal wall. The tissue from this area alone is often enough to shape the breast, but an implant might be needed as well. In this procedure, the skin, fat, blood vessels, and at least one of the abdominal muscles are moved from the abdomen to the chest. The flap of tissue is then shaped into the form of a breast.

The abdominal incision can result in significant discomfort for some time after the surgery. The TRAM flap can also decrease the strength in your abdomen and may not be possible in women who have had abdominal tissue removed in previous surgeries. One benefit of a TRAM flap, however, is that it results in a tightening of the lower belly, or a "tummy tuck."

Transverse rectus abdominis muscle or TRAM flap

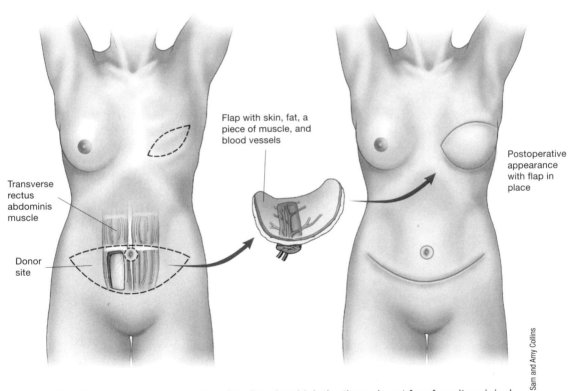

Flap with skin, fat, a piece of muscle, and blood vessels

Transverse rectus abdominis muscle

Donor site

Postoperative appearance with flap in place

© Sam and Amy Collins

The illustration above depicts a free flap, in which the tissue is cut free from its original location and reattached in the chest area.

There are two types of TRAM flaps: a pedicle flap and a free flap. A pedicle flap involves leaving the flap attached to its original blood supply and tunneling the blood supply under the skin to the breast area. A free flap is more complicated, because the surgeon cuts the flap of skin, fat, blood vessels, and muscle free from its original location and then attaches it to blood vessels in the chest area. This surgery requires the use of a microscope (microsurgery) to connect the tiny vessels and takes longer than a pedicle flap. The free flap is not done as often as the pedicle flap, but some doctors think that it results in a more natural breast shape.

Latissimus Dorsi Muscle (LAT) Flap

The latissimus dorsi (LAT flap) procedure moves muscle and skin from the woman's upper back. Extra tissue may be needed because the muscle over the chest wall has been removed, because the skin is too damaged by radiation to be stretched, or because there is not enough skin to cover a breast implant. The LAT flap procedure is most often used with a breast

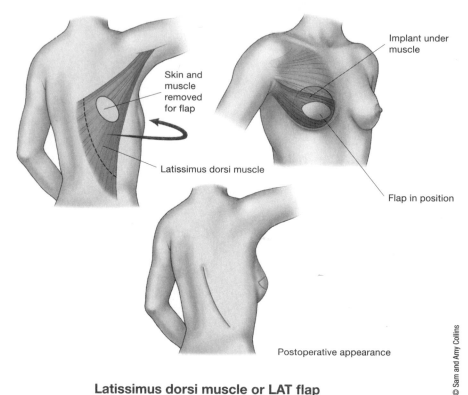

Skin and muscle removed for flap

Latissimus dorsi muscle

Implant under muscle

Flap in position

Postoperative appearance

© Sam and Amy Collins

Latissimus dorsi muscle or LAT flap

American Cancer Society

implant, although it may be done by itself for women with smaller breasts. The surgeon removes a fan-shaped section of muscle and skin from the woman's back, keeping the blood supply intact. This flap, named for the back muscle from which it comes, is tunneled under the skin, pulled out through an opening in the chest, and sutured in place over the site of the mastectomy. The flap is used to create a pocket for an implant. The surgeon then places the implant under the muscle to complete the reconstruction.

Though it is not common, some women might have weakness in their back, shoulder, or arm after this type of reconstructive surgery.

Deep Inferior Epigastric Artery Perforator (DIEP) Flap

A newer type of flap procedure, the deep inferior epigastric artery perforator (DIEP) flap uses fat and skin from the lower abdominal wall (the same area used in the TRAM flap) but does not use the muscle to form the breast mound. Like the TRAM flap, this procedure results in a tightening of the lower abdomen, or "tummy tuck." This method

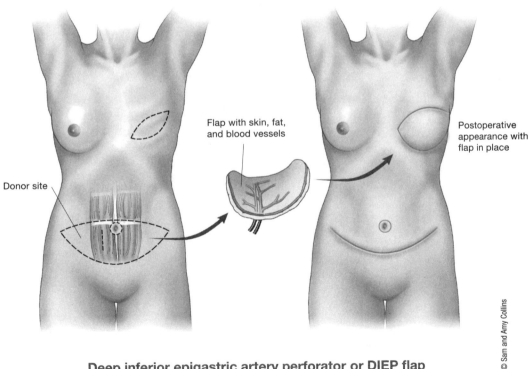

Flap with skin, fat, and blood vessels

Postoperative appearance with flap in place

Donor site

© Sam and Amy Collins

Deep inferior epigastric artery perforator or DIEP flap

uses a free flap, meaning that the tissue is cut free from the abdomen and moved to the chest, where blood supply is reestablished by connecting the tiny blood vessels. The procedure is more complex and takes longer than the TRAM flap. Because the underlying muscle is not disturbed, as it is with the TRAM flap, the DIEP flap may help avoid abdominal hernias and muscle weakness and allow women to recover more quickly.

Gluteal Free Flap or Gluteal Artery Perforator (GAP) Flap

The gluteal free flap or gluteal artery perforator (GAP) flap is a newer type of surgery and uses tissue from the buttock, including skin and fatty tissue over the gluteal muscles, to create the breast shape. It might be an option for some women who cannot or do not wish to use the abdominal sites due to thinness, a previous tummy tuck, or other reasons. The procedure is similar to the free TRAM flap. The skin, fat, and blood vessels are detached and then moved to the chest area. This, too, is a complex operation that requires microsurgery to connect the tiny vessels.

Gluteal free flap or GAP flap

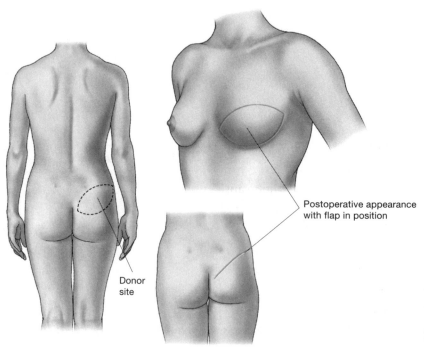

Postoperative appearance with flap in position

Donor site

© Sam and Amy Collins

Transverse upper gracilis or TUG flap

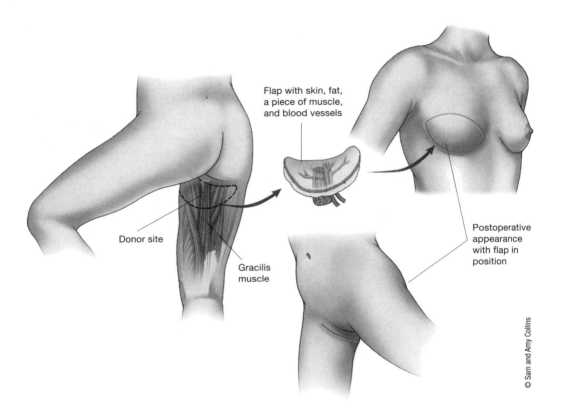

Flap with skin, fat, a piece of muscle, and blood vessels

Donor site

Gracilis muscle

Postoperative appearance with flap in position

© Sam and Amy Collins

Inner Thigh or Transverse Upper Gracilis (TUG) Flap

The inner thigh or transverse upper gracilis (TUG) flap is another new option for women who cannot or do not want to use tissue from the abdomen. This surgery uses muscle and fatty tissue from along the bottom fold of the buttock extending to the inner thigh. The skin, muscle, and blood vessels are cut out and moved to the chest, and microsurgery is used to connect the tiny blood vessels to their new blood supply. Women with thin thighs do not have much tissue in this area, so the best candidates for this type of surgery are women whose inner thighs touch and who need a smaller- or medium-sized breast. Sometimes there are healing problems because of the location of the donor site, but they tend to be minor and are easily treated.

Options for Breast Reconstruction

	Implants with Tissue Expander	Deep Inferior Epigastric Artery Perforator (DIEP) Flap
Where is the tissue coming from?	Not applicable	Abdomen
Length of surgery	One to two hours	Six to eight hours
Recovery time	One to two weeks (for each surgery)	Three to six weeks
Best if patient...	• Does not have enough fatty tissue in the back or stomach area • Has a good skin "pocket" for the implant • Prefers shorter surgery and recovery times • Wants a more perky-looking reconstruction • Willing to have surgery on other breast to help it match	• Is healthy enough to undergo a lengthy surgery • Has been pregnant • Has a body mass index of less than 35 • Has not had any other surgeries to the abdominal area (not including c-sections and laparoscopic procedures) • Has time for recovery
Advantages	• Less surgery and recovery time • Fewer scars • Satisfactory shape in clothing • Can augment the other breast for symmetry	• Patient's own tissue • May spare all or most of the abdominal muscle (so there is less risk of hernia later) • Along with TRAM flap, most natural-appearing reconstruction • May improve abdominal shape
Disadvantages	• Two steps for the procedure (i.e., tissue expander and implant), as well as many appointments for the expansion process • Hard to achieve nipple projection with nipple reconstruction • Often difficult to achieve appearance of a natural breast • Usually one scar* • Risks of implant problems: leaks, rupture, capsular contracture • Implants may need to be replaced periodically (every ten years)	• Challenging surgery that requires surgeon trained in microsurgery • Longer surgery and recovery • Usually two scars: mastectomy scar and scar at donor site (on stomach and around belly button)* • Risk of hernias and bulges on abdomen, but lower than with TRAM flap • Risk of partial or complete flap loss • Not always technically possible

*In some facilities, an extra breast crease incision may be made.

Adapted from *Reshaping You: Options for Breast Reconstruction* ©2009 The University of Texas MD Anderson Cancer Center, Patient Education Office, and used with permission.

American Cancer Society

Using Your Own Body Tissue (Flap Procedures)

Transverse Rectus Abdominus (TRAM) Flap	Latissimus Dorsi (LAT) Flap (May Use Implant)	Gluteal Free or Gluteal Artery Perforator (GAP) Flap	Transverse Upper Gracilis (TUG) Flap
Abdomen	Back	Buttock	Inner thigh
Four to eight hours	Three to six hours	Nine to twelve hours	Four to six hours
Three to six weeks	Two to four weeks	Two to four weeks	Two to four weeks
• Is healthy enough to undergo a lengthy surgery • Has been pregnant • Has a body mass index of less than 35 • Has not had any other surgeries to the abdominal area (not including c-sections and laparoscopic procedures) • Has time for recovery	• Is healthy enough to undergo moderate surgery • Wants a more perky-looking reconstruction • Has time for recovery	• Is healthy enough to undergo a lengthy surgery • Cannot get a TRAM or DIEP • Has enough buttock tissue to reconstruct a breast without leaving a large depression • Does not want implants • Has time for recovery	• Is healthy enough to undergo a lengthy surgery • Donor sites for other flaps (like abdomen and back) not suitable
• Patient's own tissue • Along with DIEP flap, most natural appearing reconstruction • May improve abdominal shape	• Patient's own tissue (except implant) • Less surgery and recovery time than other flaps • Better coverage over implant, which improves cosmetic result • One-time surgery, if implant is placed immediately	• Patient's own tissue • Less pain than abdominal tissue • Faster recovery than abdominal tissue	• Patient's own tissue • Improved thigh contour
• Challenging surgery that requires surgeon trained in microsurgery • Longer surgery and recovery • Variations in anatomy, leading to variations in amount of abdominal muscle and fascia taken • Usually two scars: mastectomy scar and scar at donor site* • Risk of hernias and bulges on abdomen • Risk of partial or complete flap loss	• Smaller volume of tissue for reconstruction, so often an implant is needed under the tissue • Risks of implant problems (leaks, capsular contracture, need for replacement) • Usually two scars: mastectomy scar and scar on back* • Possible weakness affecting movements that involve lifting the arm over head • Muscle will thin over time • May have fullness under arm where muscle was rotated	• Challenging surgery that requires surgeon trained in microsurgery • May cause a depression in the shape of the buttock • Usually two scars: mastectomy scar and scar on buttock* • Difficult to do bilateral reconstructions due to positioning on operating room table (may require two surgeries) • Risk of partial or complete flap loss	• Challenging surgery that requires surgeon trained in microsurgery • Smaller volume of tissue available, so reconstructed breast cannot be large • Risk of partial or complete flap loss

Nipple and Areola Reconstruction

Some women who have breast reconstruction decide to have their nipple and areola (the dark area around the nipple) reconstructed, too. Nipple/areola reconstruction is typically done a few months after the breast reconstruction, once the new breast has had time to heal.

Tissue for the nipple/areola is often taken from the woman's body. Most often, the surgeon removes a piece of skin from the upper inner thigh, transfers it to the reconstructed breast, and shapes it into a nipple. Alternately, small flaps of skin on the reconstructed breast might be raised and brought together to form the nipple. Once the skin heals, tattooing might be done to match the color of the nipple of the other breast and to create the areola.

What to Expect After Breast Reconstruction Surgery

You will probably feel tired and sore for a few weeks after implant reconstruction—longer if you have a flap procedure. Your doctor can give you medicines to control pain and other discomfort.

You should be able to go home from the hospital in one to six days. You might be discharged with a drain coming out of the surgery site. The drain is a flexible tube that is left in place to remove extra fluid from the site while it heals. Follow your doctor's instructions on incision and drain care. Also be sure to ask what kind of support garments you should wear. If you have any concerns or questions, call your doctor.

It might take six to eight weeks to recover from a mastectomy and reconstruction or from a flap reconstruction alone. For breast implants alone, your recovery time might be shorter. It may take up to eight weeks for bruising and swelling to go away. Try to be patient as you wait to see the final result.

Breast reconstruction restores the shape of the breast, but it cannot restore normal breast sensation. With time, the skin on the reconstructed breast can become more sensitive, but it may not give the same kind of pleasure as before mastectomy. Breast reconstruction often makes women more comfortable with their bodies, however, and helps them feel more attractive. It can help a woman enjoy sex more because of the boost it gives to her feelings of wholeness and attractiveness, even though it might not fully restore the physical sensation of pleasure she used to feel when having her breast touched. Most scars will fade over time, though it might take as long as one to two years. The scars will never go away entirely.

Follow your surgeon's advice about when to begin stretching exercises and when to go back to doing your normal activities. As a rule, plan to avoid any overhead or heavy lifting, strenuous sports, and sexual activity for four to six weeks after reconstruction.

Women who have reconstruction months or years after a mastectomy might go through a period of emotional readjustment when they have their breast reconstructed. Just as it takes time for a woman to get used to losing a breast, it also takes time to adjust to having a reconstructed breast. Talking with other women who have had reconstruction might be helpful. Talking with a mental health professional might also help you sort out anxiety or other distressing feelings.

For women who have silicone gel implants, some surgeons recommend regular MRIs of the implants to make sure they are not leaking. This follow-up is recommended because silicone implants can open up or leak inside the body without causing any noticeable changes or symptoms (unlike saline implants, which tend to "deflate" if they leak). You will likely have your first MRI about one year after your implant surgery and every two years from then on. Your insurance might not cover this test. Talk to your doctor about long-term follow-up.

> ## Questions to Ask Your Medical Team About Side Effects of Breast Implants
>
> - **What are my risks** for having capsular contracture?
> - **Do different types of** implants carry different risks?
> - **How will I know** if my implant is leaking and possibly affecting my health?
> - **Will I need any special** imaging tests to monitor my implant?
> - **Will my implant affect my risk** of recurrence? Or my overall cancer risk?
> - **Will the implant make it more difficult** to find a breast cancer recurrence on a mammogram?
> - **What other side effects** or risks are involved with implants?
> - **What complications** might affect me later?
> - **What types of complications** should I report to you?

Checking for Recurrence After Breast Reconstruction

If you are thinking about breast reconstruction, either with an implant or a flap, you need to know that reconstruction rarely, if ever, hides a return of breast cancer. This should not be a deciding factor if you are considering whether to have breast reconstruction after mastectomy.

After breast reconstruction, you can still practice breast self-examination (BSE) if you choose. Check both the remaining breast and the reconstructed breast at the same time each month. Learn what the reconstructed breast feels like. It will feel different.

The remaining breast may change, too, even if no surgery was done there. Your doctor or nurse can help you understand what's normal so that you can notice any changes and report them as quickly as possible.

Because breast implants are inserted behind any remaining breast tissue, they tend to push the tissue out so that it is close to the skin. This means that any cancer recurrence would likely be seen or felt during a physical examination. For this reason, most doctors recommend that women who get breast implants after mastectomy have regular physical examinations. Mammography is not likely to be as useful and is not typically recommended on the affected breast after a mastectomy (unless it was a nipple-sparing or skin-sparing mastectomy, which leaves behind some breast tissue). Mammography is still useful for the other breast.

Regular physical examinations are also important for women with tissue flap breast reconstructions. Mammograms are not usually recommended after flap reconstructions because reconstructed breasts can look fatty, and surgical clips and scars can show up on the mammogram. Still, breast changes or abnormalities can sometimes be seen, so some doctors still recommend them as a screening tool. Breast MRI might be another option, although it is much more expensive than mammography, and it is unclear how useful it is after reconstruction.

If you have had breast reconstruction, talk to your plastic surgeon and oncologist about which examinations and tests you should have and how frequently. See chapter 19 for more information about how and when to do breast self-examinations and when to have clinical breast examinations and mammograms.

Alternatives to Breast Reconstruction

If you choose not to have reconstructive surgery, you have other options. If your main concern is that your chest looks uneven under your clothes after a mastectomy, a breast form might be the right solution for you. Prosthetic breasts are becoming more and more natural looking, and some actually adhere directly to the body. Most breast forms are weighted to match the weight of your other breast. The weight of the form keeps the bra in place, helps your clothing fit better, and prevents backaches by balancing the weight of your other breast. Most women get used to the "heaviness" of the form in a short time.

Breast forms can be expensive, but prices vary considerably. High price does not necessarily mean that the product is the best for you. Similarly, because of different types of incisions, a prosthesis that feels good to a friend or relative might not fit you. Take time to shop for a good fit. Make sure to consider comfort and find a breast form that provides an attractive, natural appearance in your bra and under your clothing. Your clothes should fit the way they did before surgery. Some breast forms can be worn even while you are swimming or doing other strenuous activities.

The right bra for you might very well be the one you have always worn. It might or might not need adjustments. If you have tenderness during healing, a bra extender can help by increasing the circumference of the bra so that it does not bind the chest too tightly. Heavy-breasted women can relieve pressure on shoulder straps by slipping a shoulder pad under one or both straps.

If you decide to wear your breast form in a pocket in your bra, you can have your regular bras adapted. There are also special mastectomy bras with the pockets already sewn in. If the breast form causes any kind of skin irritation, use a bra with a pocket. If your bra has underwires, you might be able to continue to wear it, but be sure to clear this with your doctor first. If you want to wear your prosthesis under nightgowns but want something more comfortable than a regular bra, most department stores carry a soft bra, sometimes called a leisure or night bra.

A woman who has had lumpectomy, or a small-breasted woman who has had mastectomy, might be satisfied with a breast enhancer. Enhancers come in various sizes and shapes, are usually slightly weighted, and might be used inside a bra to make the affected breast match the natural breast.

Insurance coverage of breast prostheses can vary. Be sure to check with your insurance company to see what is covered and how you must submit claims. Also, ask your doctor to write prescriptions for your prosthesis and for any special mastectomy bras. When purchasing bras or breast forms, mark the bills and any checks you write "surgical." Medicare and Medicaid will pay for some of these expenses if you are eligible. The cost of breast forms and bras with pockets might be tax deductible, as might the costs if you have your regular bras altered. Keep careful records of all related expenses.

Some insurance companies will not cover both a breast prosthesis and reconstructive surgery. This can mean that if you submit a claim for a prosthesis or bra to your insurance company, the company might not cover reconstruction if you decide to have this surgery in the future. Make sure you get all the facts before submitting any insurance claims.

Prosthesis Tips

- **Check with your insurance company** to determine your coverage for prostheses and bras. Find out if your policy restricts you to a certain shop or manufacturer. You may need your doctor to write prescriptions for your prosthesis and any special bras for insurance reimbursement.

- **Call local shops** that carry prostheses and schedule an appointment with a trained fitter.

- **Choose a day that is relatively free** from other obligations when you shop for a prosthesis. Taking off and putting on your clothes and seeing your incision can be an exhausting and emotional experience.

- **Consider taking someone to the store with you** who will be completely honest about how different prostheses look.

- **When you shop for a prosthesis,** wear something formfitting that drapes nicely, like a silk shirt or fitted sweater, so you can get a clear look at the shape and contour of your breast. Wear something you enjoyed putting on before your surgery. Try on the prosthesis in a comfortable, supportive bra.

- **Be sure the prosthesis matches** your remaining breast as closely as possible from the top, bottom, front, and sides.

- **Comparison shop** to get a good idea of the different prostheses. Not all shops carry all brands or types. Don't buy the first one you see just to get it over with.

- **Not every woman needs a special mastectomy bra** with a pocket to hold the prosthesis in place. Ask your trained fitter which type of bra is best for you. Sometimes pockets can be added to existing bras. Many postmastectomy retailers offer pocket materials or precut pockets for this purpose. Many will sew the pockets into your bras for you.

- **A temporary breast form** can be washed by hand, then placed inside the foot of an old stocking and put into the dryer. You might need to reshape it after drying.

- **You can obtain prostheses and other products** for women with cancer through the American Cancer Society's "*tlc*"™ catalog (800-850-9445 or www.tlcdirect.org).

PART FIVE

Practical Matters: Work, Insurance, and Finances

With all of the physical and emotional challenges that come with cancer, it can be hard to spare the energy to deal with the necessary but sometimes mundane parts of life with an illness like cancer: paying bills, keeping up with insurance claims, and arranging time away from work. Yet these matters can be a challenging part of going through cancer treatment.

Cancer treatment is expensive, and insurance can be complex and difficult to navigate. Depending on your treatment and situation, you may have to take time off work. You may not be the primary person to deal with financial or insurance issues—a family member or friend may be able to help you deal with the paperwork and other issues that can come along with treatment—but either way, these issues can affect your breast cancer experience.

In the following chapters, we discuss some helpful tips for handling time away from work, explore the basics of what you need to know about insurance, and discuss managing your finances and some sources of financial assistance.

CHAPTER 16

Employment and Workplace Issues

Facing a cancer diagnosis can bring an increased sense of the importance of work in a person's life. Work can help you maintain your identity and keep a sense of normalcy. It can be a distraction from cancer and can even boost your self-esteem through daily successes. Having a role at your job that is uniquely yours can remind you that you are more than just a woman with cancer—you're a valued employee, a great boss, and/or a trusted coworker. You will also have regular contact with others when you go back to work. Cancer can be extremely isolating, and being around people can be a great comfort.

Telling Coworkers

Your coworkers might react to your cancer diagnosis and absences for treatment with understanding and helpfulness. Some people will be very supportive. Chances are, your supervisors and colleagues have had people close to them who have had cancer. Many women with breast cancer say they are glad they shared information about their illness with people at work. Think about what approach will work best for you at work. You may need to talk with your employer about options such as flextime, job sharing, or telecommuting, if these things will help you do your job.

Your cancer might cause some coworkers to feel uncomfortable around you. Employers and coworkers might react awkwardly out of a vague fear or uneasiness about cancer, thinking of cancer as some kind of lurking, unknown danger. Some people may see it as an unpleasant reminder of their own mortality. Coworkers might ask intrusive questions about your health or, on the opposite extreme, might avoid you. Your coworkers might also have to take on extra duties because of your absences, and they might resent this extra work.

How open you are with your coworkers about your health is a personal decision. In some environments, it will not benefit you to share details. For example, before opening up to your colleagues in a highly competitive and fast-paced work environment, it might help to decide first who is most likely to understand your situation. You can then confide in that person and ask for help in developing the best plan for telling others and for requesting time off.

Preparing for Time Away from Work

It can be helpful to make plans before an absence from work; it will make your return to work easier. You might want to make records of your usual work schedule and responsibilities and refer to them when planning time off and organizing any work you need to delegate to others. If you are going to be absent for a period, think about what others will need to know. Is information they need accessible? Are coworkers up-to-date on any projects or tasks they might need to handle in your absence? Document as much as possible.

Discrimination and Your Rights

Even though people's understanding of cancer is much improved over the past, some prejudices and wariness remain in the workplace, perhaps due to competitiveness, economic pressures, and people's fears. Some people with cancer face challenges related to employment and workplace discrimination issues.

Questions to Ask Your Medical Team About Work

- **Will I be able to work** during my treatment?
- **If I need to stay home** to recover from surgery or other treatment, how long will I be away from my job?
- **If I do return to work,** will I need a different work schedule?
- **Will any of my abilities to perform** my job be impaired because of treatment?
- **How will I know** whether I'm overdoing it at work?
- **Can I obtain documentation** from your office about my condition to provide to my employer in order to take time off from work?

Consider keeping records of your contact with office staff, including the names of the people with whom you spoke about your illness, the dates and places you spoke, and the information you received. It is also a good idea to keep copies of your job performance evaluations. Union officials are also good sources of information about illnesses and the workplace.

Your employer cannot discriminate against you on the basis of your cancer diagnosis. In fact, depending on your situation, laws may protect you from such discrimination. In many cases, you will be covered by the Americans with Disabilities Act (ADA), which prohibits discrimination resulting from myths and stereotypes about disability (many of the physical changes caused by cancer and its treatment meet the definition of "disability"). People are considered disabled if they have a physical or mental problem that substantially limits one or more major life activities, if they have a history of or are regarded as having a disability, or if they face discrimination because of a relationship with a person who has a disability (such as a child or parent). The ADA makes it illegal to discriminate in such employment activities as recruiting, advertising, applying, hiring, and training for jobs; work assignments; tenure; promotions; pay, benefits, and leave; firing; and other practices. For example, it would be illegal for a company to decide not to interview you because you have had cancer in the past—in other words, because they regard you as having a disability.

However, you must be qualified and able to perform the "essential functions" of the job. You must also satisfy the employer's job requirements regarding education, employment experience, skills, or licenses. Employers are not required to lower standards for a disabled employee, nor are they obligated to supply personal use items such as glasses or hearing aids. However, employers are required to make "reasonable accommodation" for qualified applicants or employees with disabilities unless they can show it would be an undue hardship to do so. A reasonable accommodation is any change or adjustment to a job or work environment that allows a qualified applicant or employee with a disability to participate in the job application process, perform the essential functions of a job, or enjoy the benefits and privileges of employment enjoyed by employees without disabilities. Examples of reasonable accommodations might include the following:

- providing or modifying equipment or devices
- restructuring a job
- offering part-time or modified work schedules
- reassigning an employee to a vacant position
- adjusting or modifying tests, training materials, or policies

- providing e-readers and/or interpreters
- making the workplace easy to get to and use by people with disabilities

The ADA does not completely protect your job just because you have a disability and are qualified for the job. The employer can still fire or lay off an employee with a disability for legitimate business reasons. For instance, a disabled worker would not be protected during downsizing. For general ADA information, answers to specific questions, free ADA materials, or information about filing a complaint, call 800-514-0301 or 800-514-0383 (TTY), or visit www.ada.gov.

Many states also have their own laws against discrimination. Although a vocational counselor can help with some of your job-related legal questions, you might want to look into which laws may apply to you and how you can deal with any problems. To find out more about job accommodation and the employability of people with functional limitations, contact the Job Accommodation Network at 800-526-7234 (www.askjan.org).

If you think you have been discriminated against at work on the basis of disability, you can file a complaint with the US Equal Employment Opportunity Commission (EEOC) within 180 days after the alleged discrimination (according to some state or local laws, you have up to 300 days). For more specific information about ADA requirements affecting employment, contact the EEOC at 800-669-4000 or www.eeoc.gov. You might also consider consulting an employment discrimination attorney.

The Family and Medical Leave Act

The Family and Medical Leave Act (FMLA) requires that employers with fifty or more local workers allow up to twelve weeks of unpaid leave to their employees each year. This leave can be used to take care of yourself, or a spouse, child, or parent can use FMLA leave to take care of you. To qualify, the employee must have worked for the employer at least one year and must have worked at least 1,250 hours over the previous twelve months. To be covered by the FMLA, you must tell your employer (and maybe your spouse's employer, if you are married) about your health condition. To file a complaint under this act, contact the US Department of Labor's Wage and Hour Division by calling 866-4-US-WAGE (866-487-9243) or visiting www.dol.gov/whd/.

Long-Term Disability Insurance

If you cannot work, find out whether you have a long-term disability insurance policy through your employer. This type of policy typically replaces 60 to 70 percent of your income. The amount of your income has nothing to do with whether you qualify for benefits.

Social Security Disability Income

You might qualify for Social Security Disability Income (SSDI) if you have been working for many years and have contributed to Social Security. Call the Social Security Administration (800-772-1213) or visit www.ssa.gov to find out how to apply.

The Social Security Administration's definition of disability is strict. If you are turned down the first time you apply, it is often useful to appeal. Some cases that are turned down the first time end up being approved after an appeal. If you are approved, benefits do not begin until the sixth month of disability.

If you qualify for SSDI, other family members might also be able to get payments. For instance, your children might qualify if they are under the age of eighteen. You can find out more about this from the Social Security Administration.

After getting SSDI for twenty-four months, you become eligible for Medicare coverage.

Life Insurance

If you have to leave work because of disability, your life insurance policy usually can be converted to an individual permanent policy without having to go through underwriting (proving that you are insurable). If you bought life insurance on your own, be sure to continue to make payments on time. If the policy has a waiver-of-premium rider, the insurance company will pay the policy's premium if you become totally disabled.

Supplemental Security Income

If you have not worked much or if your income was very low before you became unable to work, you might be eligible for Supplemental Security Income (SSI). To qualify, your income and assets must fall below a certain level and you must be disabled, over sixty-five years old, and/or blind. The amount of benefits you could get varies from state to state and from year to year. If you get SSI, you usually are eligible for Medicaid and the Supplemental Nutrition Assistance Program (SNAP), formerly known as food stamps.

You can get more information about SSI from your hospital's social worker or by calling the Social Security Administration (800-772-1213) or visiting www.ssa.gov.

CHAPTER **17**

Insurance and Your Rights

It is important that you understand your insurance coverage and your rights before you begin treatment. In chapter 6, we talked about the importance of talking with your insurance company early to get the details of your coverage. That information will be key as you plan for the expenses of cancer treatment.

Insurance options began changing quickly when the new Affordable Care Act (ACA) was signed into law in March 2010, and most of its requirements should be in place as of 2014. At that point, there will be more safeguards for the person with cancer. But even after that, the health care landscape may still be shifting for some time. Call the American Cancer Society anytime at 800-227-2345 for the most up-to-date information.

Keeping Records of Insurance and Medical Care Costs

It can be hard to keep track of all the bills, letters, claim forms, and other papers that begin flowing into your home after a cancer diagnosis. But keeping careful records of medical bills, insurance claims, and payments can help you and your family manage your money better and lower your stress level. You may already have a system for tracking your finances and records and only need to expand it and create new files. If not, you will need to come up with a plan to handle all of the paperwork.

Recordkeeping is also important for those who wish to take advantage of the deductions available in filing itemized tax returns. The Internal Revenue Service (IRS) has information and free publications about tax deductions for cancer treatment expenses. These rules change from time to time, so the IRS is the best source for current information.

Keep records of the following:

- medical bills from all health care providers, with the date they were received written on each one
- claims filed, including the date of service, the doctor, and the date filed
- reimbursements (payments from insurance companies) received and explanations of benefits (EOBs)
- dates, names, and outcomes of calls, letters, or e-mails to insurers and others
- medical costs that were not reimbursed, those waiting for the insurance company to process, and other costs related to treatment
- meals and lodging expenses
- travel to and from doctor's appointments, treatments, or the hospital (including gas, mileage, and parking for a personal car; and any use of taxis, buses, medical transportation, or ambulance)
- admissions, clinic visits, laboratory work, diagnostic tests, procedures, and treatments
- all prescriptions

Here are some ideas to help you with recordkeeping:

- Decide who in your family will be the recordkeeper or how the task will be shared. Get the help of a relative or friend, if needed. This may be especially important for people who are single or who live alone.
- Set up a file system using a file cabinet, drawer, box, binders, or loose-leaf notebooks.
- Review bills soon after receiving them and note any questions about charges.
- Check all bills and explanations of benefits (EOBs) paid to be sure they are correct.
- Save and file all bills, payment receipts, and EOBs. Talk to your bank or credit union about how to get copies of canceled checks if you need them.
- Keep a daily log of events and expenses; a calendar with plenty of writing space is useful.
- Keep a list of medical team members and all other relevant contacts with their phone and fax numbers and e-mail addresses.

Questions to Ask About Insurance

- Does my policy have a dollar limit on benefits?
- Will my policy cover a second opinion? Can I go outside the network for a second opinion?
- How is cancer managed in my plan? What are the plan's restrictions on my choices of doctors, including specialists?
- Which breast cancer treatments are covered? Are hospital stays covered?
- How do I find out whether a procedure is covered? Whom do I call?
- Does my policy cover all my chemotherapy or radiation expenses?
- Will I have access to a team of care providers in different disciplines—for example, medical, surgical, and radiation oncologists—to help with my treatment and recovery?
- Are my doctors or others in the network experienced in detecting and treating cancer in general, or my type of cancer in particular? Are they required by the plan to keep up with new developments?
- Does my plan allow my primary care physician to refer me to doctors outside the network or to specialized facilities if necessary?
- Does my primary care physician have to approve treatments, procedures, or tests, or can a specialist assume the role of principal care provider?
- What are the coverage limits on screening, diagnostic tests, and treatments?
- Does my policy offer coverage for clinical trials (investigational treatments)?
- Can I get coverage for rehabilitation, counseling, and supportive services if I need them?
- Does my policy cover breast reconstruction after mastectomy?
- Does my policy cover implant surgery, including the implant, anesthesia, and other costs?
- Does my policy cover treatments for problems that result from the implant or reconstruction?
- Does my policy cover the removal of implants?
- If I wait to have my breast reconstructed, will the reconstruction still be covered?
- Does my policy cover recurrence and its treatment?
- What is the insurance company required to pay for—what are the minimum standards of coverage?
- Is there any way I can appeal for additional coverage if I need it?
- What will I have to pay out of pocket?
- What programs can help me with the costs of traveling to and from treatment?
- Can the government help me?
- Do I qualify for any special benefits?
- Can I claim any of these expenses on my taxes?

Find out what expenses are tax deductible and be sure to keep the originals of those records. Many people go through times when they struggle to pay their bills on time. Most hospitals and agencies are willing to work with you to help resolve these problems. To keep a good credit rating, pay attention to notices that say the bill will soon be turned over to a collection agency. You want to avoid this if at all possible. Families can do the following:

- Explain the problem to the hospital or clinic financial counselor or the doctor's office manager.
- Work out a payment delay or an extended payment plan.
- Talk with the hospital social worker about sources of short-term financial help.
- Think about asking relatives or friends to help out with money on a short-term basis.

Sources of financial assistance are described in more detail in the next chapter.

Managing Your Health Insurance

Consider the following tips for managing your health insurance:

- DO NOT let your health insurance expire.
- If you are changing insurance plans, do not let one policy lapse until the new one goes into effect. This includes when you are switching to Medicare.
- Pay premiums in full and on time.
- Know the details of your individual insurance plan and its coverage. Get a copy of your plan's summary description (SPD), which tells you how the plan works, what benefits it provides, and how to get benefits or file your claims. If you think you might need more insurance, ask your insurance carrier whether it is available. If you do not understand your policy, call your state insurance commissioner for help. Do not rely on your benefits administrator or your agent.
- Submit claims for all medical expenses, even when you are not sure whether they are covered.
- Keep accurate and complete records of claims submitted, pending, and paid.
- Keep copies of all paperwork related to your claims, such as letters of medical necessity, explanations of benefits, bills, receipts, requests for sick leave or family medical leave (FMLA), and correspondence with insurance companies.
- Get a caseworker, a hospital financial counselor, or a social worker to help you if your finances are limited. Often, companies or hospitals can work with you to make special payment arrangements if you let them know about your situation.

- Send in your bills for reimbursement as you get them. If you become overwhelmed with bills or tracking your medical expenses, ask for help from the hospital social worker, financial planner, or case manager. Contact local support organizations such as the American Cancer Society for extra help. Often, payment arrangements can be worked out if doctors and hospitals are aware of your situation.

Getting Answers to Insurance-Related Questions

Questions about insurance coverage often come up during treatment. Here are some tips for dealing with insurance-related questions:

- Speak with the insurer or managed care provider's customer service department.
- Ask the hospital social worker for help.
- Talk with a financial counselor at your hospital or treatment center.
- Talk with the consumer advocacy office of the government agency that oversees your insurance plan.
- Learn about the insurance laws that protect the public. Call the American Cancer Society at 800-227-2345 for help.

Handling Claim Denials

Keep track of your bills and submit them as soon as you get them so you know when you have reached the limit for reimbursement. Hospitals, clinics, and doctors' offices usually have someone who can help you complete claims for insurance coverage or reimbursement.

It is not unusual for some claims to be denied or for insurers to say they will not cover a test, procedure, or service that your doctor orders. Still, there are things you can do when your insurance will not pay for a prescribed service. If this happens, it is important to have a working relationship with a customer service representative or case manager with whom you can talk about the situation. Before you appeal, you may want to take these steps: Ask your customer service representative for a full explanation of why the claim was denied. Ask how the appeals process works—that knowledge will guide your next steps. If your plan is through your or your spouse's employer, you may be able to contact your health plan administrator at work to find out more about the refusal. You may be able to speak with a supervisor with your health insurance company—sometimes these individuals have the authority to reverse the decision.

Ask the doctor to write a letter explaining or justifying what has been done or has been requested. Keep a copy of this letter in case an appeal is needed later. You can then resubmit the claim with a copy of the denial letter and your doctor's explanation, along with any other written information that supports using the test or treatment that has been denied. Sometimes the test or service will only need to be "coded" differently.

If questioning or challenging the denial in these ways doesn't work, you may need to file a formal appeal in writing, explaining why you think the claim should be paid. This internal appeal is done by the insurance company. Your medical team members (doctor, nurse, social worker) may be able to help with this process. You may need to put off payment until the matter is resolved. Request written responses to all communications. If necessary, resubmit the claim a third time and request a review.

Keep a record of dates, names, and conversations you have about the denial, as well as the originals of all letters you receive. Do not back down when trying to resolve the matter.

If your internal appeal is denied, you may be entitled to an independent external review, which is done by people outside of your insurance company. Call the US Department of Health and Human Services at 877-549-8152 for an external review request form, or visit www.healthcare.gov to learn more about internal and external appeals. You can also get a tracking form online to help you keep up with each step of the appeals process.

If you feel you have been treated unfairly by a private insurance company or private health maintenance organization (HMO), contact your state insurance commission. State insurance commissions monitor insurance companies and can force them to pay policyholders if needed. Some state insurance commissions might be willing to work with your health care providers and insurance company to help get coverage for procedures that are denied. Complaint forms are available on state insurance websites. For more information, visit the National Association of Insurance Commissioners' website at www.naic.org.

If you need to file a complaint about a federally qualified HMO, contact the Centers for Medicare & Medicaid Services at 800-633-4227 or www.cms.gov. If you need help filing a claim related to a private employer, union self-insurance, or self-paid plan, contact the Employee Benefits Security Administration at 866-487-2365 or 877-889-5627 (TTY) or online at www.dol.gov/ebsa. Medicaid complaints should be directed to your state department of social services or medical assistance services. Medicare complaints can be filed by calling 800-MEDICARE (800-633-4227) or by visiting the website:

www.medicare.gov/MedicareComplaintForm/home.aspx. Disputes regarding veterans' benefits are handled through the US Department of Veterans Affairs (877-222-8387 or www.va.gov).

Preexisting Conditions

Most insurance plans today have a pre-existing condition exclusion period. A preexisting condition is a health problem that you had before you joined your medical plan. In this case, you may have to wait up to a year before your plan pays the costs for treating that condition.

There are new rules about exclusion periods, and they might help you. If you have met the following, then an exclusion period does not apply to you:

- you have had medical coverage for eighteen months
- you have already met a preexisting condition exclusion period
- you have not been without health coverage for more than sixty-two days

As outlined in the Patient Protection and Affordable Care Act of 2010, a Preexisting Condition Insurance Plan provides new coverage options to adults who have been uninsured for at least six months because of a preexisting condition. States have the option of running this new program. If a state chooses not to do this, a federal program will be established in that state. This program serves as a bridge until 2014, when all discrimination against preexisting conditions in adults will be prohibited.

> ### The Women's Health and Cancer Rights Act
>
> The Women's Health and Cancer Rights Act (WHCRA) of 1998 (see page 429) requires all health plans that cover mastectomies to also cover breast reconstruction for women who have a mastectomy. This includes coverage of prosthetic devices, reconstructive surgery done to restore symmetry or balance, and coverage for any problems that result from mastectomy, including lymphedema. Coinsurance and deductibles might apply. For questions about this law, contact the US Department of Labor by calling 866-444-3272 or visiting www.dol.gov/ebsa/Publications/whcra.html.

Government-Funded Health Plans

Medicare

Medicare is federal health insurance for people who are at least sixty-five years old, have been permanently disabled, and/or have gotten Social Security disability benefits for twenty-four months. Medicare provides basic health coverage, but it does not pay all of your medical expenses.

Medicare is divided into four parts:

- Part A pays for hospital care, home health care, hospice care, and care in Medicare-certified nursing facilities. For most people, it is free.
- Part B covers certain doctors' services, outpatient care, medical supplies, and preventive services. You pay for it, but it is optional.
- Part C, also called Medicare Advantage, is a type of Medicare health plan offered by a private company that contracts with Medicare to provide you with all your Part A and Part B benefits. It is not available everywhere.
- Part D helps pay for prescription drugs. You pay for this part, too, but it is optional.

HMOs that have contracts with the Medicare program must provide all of the same hospital and medical benefits covered by Medicare. However, you usually have to use the HMO's network of health care providers. If you have questions about Medicare, call 800-633-4227, visit www.medicare.gov, or contact your Social Security office.

Medigap

If you are on Medicare, you might be able to add more coverage with a Medicare supplemental insurance policy, commonly called Medigap. Medigap policies are sold by private insurance companies to fill the "gaps" in standard Medicare coverage. Ten Medigap policies are offered, but the plans might not be the same in every state. The plans are identified by letters A through J. Insurance carriers offer different plans, so check with them for details of coverage.

Medicaid

Medicaid is another government program that covers the costs of medical care. To be eligible for Medicaid, your income and assets must be below a certain level. These levels vary from state to state. Not all health providers accept Medicaid. Some examples of groups eligible for Medicaid are low-income families with children, SSI recipients, and pregnant women whose income is below the family poverty level. Medicare beneficiaries who have low incomes and limited resources might get help paying for their out-of-pocket medical expenses from their state Medicaid program. For more information, contact your state Medicaid office.

Hill-Burton Program

Many hospitals and other medical facilities get funds from the federal government so they can offer free or low-cost services to people who cannot pay. This is called the Hill-Burton Program. Each facility chooses which services it will provide free or at lowered cost. Hill-Burton might cover services not covered by other government programs. Eligibility for Hill-Burton is based on family size and income. You can apply for Hill-Burton assistance at any time, before or after you receive care. To find out more information about this program, call 800-638-0742 or visit www.hrsa.gov/gethealthcare/affordable/hillburton/.

Veterans' Benefits

If you are a veteran, you might qualify for benefits from the government. Veterans' benefits change often, and the number of veterans' medical facilities is declining. To get the most accurate information, contact the benefits office of the US Department of Veterans Affairs at 800-827-1000 or www.va.gov.

Patient Assistance Programs

Some insurance plans may not pay for all your prescriptions, and these medicines can be very expensive. Patient assistance programs are available to help with these costs. These programs offer free or discounted drugs to people who need them but cannot afford them.

The Partnership for Prescription Assistance (PPA) helps people who do not have prescription coverage find assistance programs that are right for them. This program includes drug companies, health care providers, patient advocacy organizations, and community groups. PPA can help you access more than 475 public and private patient assistance programs, including more than 200 programs offered by drug companies. They also have information about free drug discount cards funded by private companies, which can help reduce your costs for certain brand name or generic drugs. For more information, call 888-477-2669 or visit www.pparx.org.

Needy Meds is another resource to help people with low incomes get needed medicines. It offers information on getting assistance from drug companies, but it also has its own drug discount card that you can print out free of charge. More information about Needy Meds can be found at www.needymeds.org.

You must meet certain requirements to participate in most patient assistance programs. You will need to complete an application and provide basic information, including the names of the drugs you need and information about yourself and your finances.

Most programs also require information from your doctor. Consider contacting the drug company directly to ask whether they have patient assistance programs and to learn about their eligibility requirements. Some companies prefer to speak directly with your doctor, so do not hesitate to discuss participation in these programs with your medical team.

Options for the Hard-to-Insure

The Health Insurance Portability and Accountability Act of 1996 (HIPAA) allows a person who has had health insurance for at least twelve months without a long break in coverage (no more than sixty-two days) to change jobs and be guaranteed other coverage with a new employer who also offers group insurance. This law also protects people from discrimination based on preexisting medical conditions. Because of HIPAA, many workers do not lose their insurance when they change jobs or move to a different state.

Risk Pools

Health insurance options are now available for hard-to-insure people. The Patient Protection and Affordable Care Act of 2010 created state-run or federally run high-risk pools in every state to cover people who have not had insurance for six months or more and have cancer or other preexisting conditions. These programs, sometimes called Preexisting Condition Insurance Plans (PCIPs), serve people who have known health conditions and have been denied or have had a hard time finding affordable coverage in the private market. People in these programs still must pay part of the monthly premium. For the most current information on health care coverage in your state, go to www.healthcare.gov.

As of 2014, exclusions for preexisting conditions will not be allowed. But until then, group plans can deny, exclude, or limit an enrollee's benefits for a preexisting condition for a waiting period of no more than twelve months from the effective date of coverage. However, some states waive waiting periods for people who show they have had continuous insurance coverage in the private market.

Risk-pool insurance generally costs more than standard insurance, but the premiums are capped by law in each state to protect people from excessive costs. Risk pools are not meant to serve the indigent or poor who cannot afford health insurance; they are designed to serve people who would not otherwise have the chance to buy health

Source of Health Care Coverage	Issues Involved
Medical Insurance	• Must continue paying premiums
COBRA	• 18- to 36-month extension of group health benefits • Must pay premium
Hill-Burton Program (low-cost or no-cost inpatient care)	• Must use Hill-Burton facilities (there are limited numbers of them) • Not all services are available • Eligibility is based on family size and income (income below current poverty guidelines)
Medicare	• Eligibility is based on eligibility for Social Security benefits or Railroad Retirement benefits and/or certain other health problems • Must pay for Part B of program
Medicaid (contact state office)	• Eligibility is based on family size, assets, and income
Veterans' Benefits (contact local office)	• Service-connected problems are generally covered • Might require low income for certain benefits • Might require some deductibles

insurance. The indigent can access coverage through state medical assistance, Medicaid, or similar programs. However, some state risk pools do have a subsidy for lower-income, medically uninsurable people.

Options for the Uninsured

For people who are not already insured, the following should be considered when seeking coverage:

Help from Independent Brokers

An independent broker might be able to help you find a reasonable benefits package. Group insurance is usually preferable to individual insurance.

Employment Benefits

Getting a job with a large company is the surest way to gain access to group insurance. The best type of plan is a guaranteed-issue insurance plan, one in which employees are eligible for benefits regardless of health history.

Health Maintenance Organizations

Health maintenance organizations (HMOs) or health care service plans in your community usually cover most expenses after a small copayment. Keep in mind that HMOs often limit your choice of providers to those within their approved network. Some offer a period of open enrollment each year, where applicants are accepted regardless of health histories.

COBRA

If you have been out of work for less than sixty days, you should be able to keep your medical insurance through COBRA (Consolidated Omnibus Budget Reconciliation Act). Your employer must tell you in writing about your COBRA option. You then can choose to keep your health insurance coverage at the employer's group rates, but you'll usually pay much more than you paid while employed. You can also keep the coverage you had for family members. In most cases, you can keep the insurance for up to eighteen months, as long as you pay your premiums on time. Some people can keep it even longer. COBRA is administered by the US Department of Labor; call 866-444-3272 or visit www.dol.gov/ebsa/cobra.html for detailed information about how it works.

Help from Professional Organizations

You might be able to apply for group insurance through fraternal or professional organizations (such as those for retired people, teachers, social workers, real estate agents, etc.). Look for a "guaranteed issue" plan.

If you are currently employed, do not leave your job until you have explored insurance conversion options through your current plan. Many group plans have a clause that allows you to convert to an individual plan, although premiums might be considerably higher than when you were an employee. You usually must apply for the individual plan within thirty days after you leave the job.

In looking at insurance options, know the differences in coverage. Ask about choices of doctors, protection against cancellations, and increases in premiums. Determine what the plan really covers, especially for severe illnesses. What are the deductibles?

(Remember, higher deductibles sometimes come with more complete coverage.) The Insurance Information Institute has "Ask the Expert," an online tool to help you get answers to questions about any type of insurance. You can find it at www.iii.org/services. It also offers some free publications. You can also get help by calling the National Insurance Consumer Help Line at 800-942-4242.

CHAPTER 18

Finances and Cancer Treatment

Cancer treatment is very expensive, and for many people, going through treatment can have a serious impact on their financial well-being. Many people worry that they will not be able to pay their medical bills. Financial resources are available to help people with cancer deal with the mounting costs that come with this disease. In this chapter, we will discuss the steps involved in making a financial plan, as well as how to locate sources of financial assistance.

Managing Your Finances and Staying Organized

Managing your finances at the same time that you are coping with cancer can be especially challenging. You might have a hard time keeping up with the direct and indirect costs of treatment. The easiest way to deal with financial issues is to tackle them one step at a time.

The major costs of a cancer diagnosis and treatment are for things such as time in the hospital, clinic visits, medicines, tests and procedures, home health services, and the services of doctors and other professionals. But families face many indirect costs and other expenses because of cancer and its treatment, along with their usual bills.

It is important that you keep careful records of medical bills, insurance claims, and other health care–related correspondence. This will make managing costs much easier and will also help prevent problems down the road. Organized financial records will also be useful if you have to demonstrate the need for financial assistance. Consider the following suggestions to help you cope with financial issues:

- Ask family and friends to help with organization and management of bills and statements. Have a helper open the mail and sort the bills into groups, such as medical bills, utility bills, credit card bills, and taxes. Rank the bills and pay them in order of priority. Make sure to look for benefit checks that may come in the mail so they do not get lost in the shuffle.
- Consider setting up a filing system just for health care–related paperwork. Save all bills, benefit statements, payment receipts, and canceled checks. Review all bills and benefit statements carefully to be sure they are correct. Make notes about any questionable charges or denials of claims. Follow up immediately with your insurer to resolve any disputes.
- Work with the staff member who handles billing for each provider so that you can be sure of what is owed to whom. The method of billing used by many hospitals is very complicated, and it can sometimes be difficult to keep track. Similarly, you will need to know whether office staff for different providers will be filing claims on your behalf or whether you are responsible for submitting claims to the insurer for reimbursement.

Using a Financial Planner

For some people, consulting a professional financial planner can be a helpful step. If you decide to use a financial planner, try to find one with experience working with people who have had cancer. Financial planners look at everything related to your finances, including your income, employee benefits, assets, investments, insurance, taxes, and expenses.

Ask at your treatment center whether financial counseling is available for patients. Some hospitals offer free financial counseling. Ask to speak with an oncology social worker, as well. They can be knowledgeable about financial issues and may be able to refer you to sources of financial aid. While not the same as a professional financial planner, they may be able to assist you with estimating expenses associated with cancer treatment and locating financial resources.

Making a Financial Plan

A sound financial plan requires planning for the worst and hoping it never happens. Planning can help give you peace of mind because you will know that you are prepared for whatever might happen in the future. Try to be honest about your current financial situation—that will help you create a plan that is helpful to you and your family.

To develop a financial plan, you will need to follow these steps: estimate your sources of income and benefits, estimate your medical and living expenses, manage your investments, plan your estate, and explore additional resources that might be available to you.

Estimating Your Income and Benefits

Life-threatening illnesses and the need for extensive medical care often lead to an immediate need for cash. As a first step, determine the sources of income and benefits you have at your disposal right now. Make sure to include all regular income and any assets that could be sold for cash. Next, think about what your sources of income and benefits would be if you had to stop working.

Consider the following sources of income and benefits and whether they are available to you:

- savings
- long-term disability insurance
- credit or other loans
- life insurance
- employee benefits
- government-provided medical programs
- other government programs

There are other possible sources of income you may not have considered. These can include home equity loans and conversions, family loans, retirement savings, viaticals (sale of an insurance policy for a percentage of its value), and living benefits. It is extremely important, however, that you carefully consider the advantages and disadvantages of using these options. These decisions can have tax implications, limit your eligibility for certain programs, and significantly impact your family's future finances. And, in some cases, these decisions cannot be reversed.

Home equity loans and conversions: Equity is the difference between the home's market value and any amount still owed on the mortgage loan. Equity increases as the mortgage is paid down and as the value of the property increases (appreciates). A home equity loan allows you to borrow against the value you have built up in your home. You might be able to convert part of your home equity into cash if you are at least sixty-two years old and own your home (or nearly own it).

Income and Expenses Worksheet

ESTIMATING YOUR INCOME AND BENEFITS

Include the following information in your financial plan:

- your salary
- your partner's salary or contributions to the household
- other regular income

Now determine what sources of income you would have if you stopped working because of your cancer treatment, such as short- or long-term disability, Social Security, or Supplemental Security Income. Calculate your total available financial resources while listing the worth of each asset that you would consider selling or liquidating:

- life insurance policies
- equity in your home
- stocks and bonds
- viaticals or living benefits
- other assets, including property, real estate, and investments

ESTIMATING YOUR EXPENSES

Refer to your insurance worksheet on page 119 for specific dollar amounts. For all of the expenses below, estimate for the highest possible expense. Consider the following types of expenses:

- insurance deductible
- copayments or coinsurance payments
- travel costs (flights, gas, cabs, rental cars, tolls, etc.)
- parking
- lodging
- food
- hospital stays and treatment sessions
- prescription drug costs
- experimental treatments that may not be covered by your insurance
- home health care costs
- lost wages
- services such as childcare, housekeeping, home/lawn maintenance, and meal preparation
- special garments, clothing, supplies, or equipment

Although your medical insurance might cover most treatment costs, out-of-pocket expenses can be a burden. There may be gaps in your coverage or you may find that you are incurring unexpected costs during your treatment and recovery.

The most common type of equity conversion is called a reverse mortgage. This is a loan against your home and does not have to be repaid for as long as you live there. The loan is repaid in the future—usually when the last surviving borrower dies or sells or moves out of the home. A reverse mortgage can provide cash to pay medical bills and other expenses, but as a loan, and interest charges and service fees apply. A reverse mortgage can also disqualify you from some government programs. Make sure to research this option carefully. Contact a financial advisor to find out whether a reverse mortgage would help you.

Family loans: Many people undergoing cancer treatment receive different kinds of support from extended family members. In some cases, family members can help pay some of your cancer-related expenses or bills. If you ask for a loan from a relative, make sure to outline a repayment period and an interest rate. Keep in mind that there are federal tax consequences if the person making the loan charges you an interest rate below the minimum federal rate. The tax laws in this area are complicated, so it is a good idea to first consult an accountant before agreeing to a family loan. And it is important to put your loan agreement in writing.

When considering family loans, be realistic. If you do not think you can repay the loan, ask for a gift instead. Anyone, including a relative, can give a tax-free gift of up to $14,000 each year. Married couples can make a joint tax-free gift of up to $28,000 per year. (These dollar amounts are for 2013.) In addition, anyone can pay the medical bills of someone else without being subject to the gift limit, if the payment is made directly to the medical facility.

Retirement savings: Some people use money from their retirement plan before they retire as a source of cash during cancer treatment, but you should weigh this option carefully. There are tax consequences, and this decision can significantly affect your family's future finances. You may qualify for hardship provisions in your retirement plan, and if you are under the age of fifty-nine and one-half, you may be able to avoid early withdrawal penalties if you meet the IRS's definition of disability. Read your benefits book so that you can fully understand your plan before making this decision. Contact a financial advisor or the human resources department of your employer for more information about this option.

Viatical settlements: A viatical is the sale of a life insurance policy for a percentage of its value. The process of selling a life insurance policy usually requires that the insured person be expected to live less than two years, and the life expectancy must be certified by a doctor. The payment given is usually between 60 and 80 percent of the policy's face value. Typically, the amount of money you could get is based on your life expectancy—the shorter it is, the larger the amount.

Sources of Cash	Issues Involved
Assets (sale of stock, real estate, etc.)	• Can create income tax debt • Can affect qualifying for government benefits
Home Equity Loan (can be lump sum or line of credit)	• Home is put at risk • Must have equity in home • Must make regular payments • Must pass credit check
Family/Personal Loan	• Requires repayment • Can strain family relationships • Can require collateral
Whole Life Insurance Policy Loan (from your life insurance company)	• Death benefit is reduced by the amount of the loan and accrued interest • Must have "cash value" type of policy • Must generally continue premium payments
Living Benefits (also called Accelerated Benefits)	• Must keep policy in force • Must be terminally ill (contact insurance company) • Can create income tax debt • Can affect qualifying for government benefits
Viatical Settlement (sale of life insurance policy for percentage of value)	• Can create income tax debt • Must own policy • Must meet definition of terminally or chronically ill • Can affect qualifying for government benefits

There are drawbacks to viatical settlements: heirs get no insurance money, the money received might affect government program benefits available to you, you might not make the best trade available, and the sale is usually not reversible. Before making a decision about your life insurance, think over your options very carefully. Talk about this matter with your partner, consult with a trusted friend, and/or get professional advice.

An alternative to a viatical settlement that is becoming more popular is called a "life settlement." This is another method of raising money by selling your life insurance policy, but it differs from a viatical sale in that the insured person does not have to be terminally ill. A life settlement company will consider the health of the insured, the age of the policy, and the premiums to be paid on the policy to determine a value. This amount might be higher than the cash value of the policy, but it will be less than a viatical agreement because the life expectancy of the insured is typically longer. Still, this should be considered only as a last resort, given that it will take away the life insurance death benefit for survivors.

Living benefits: Many insurance companies make it possible for life insurance policy owners to collect part of their death benefits early—before dying—to cover extraordinary expenses. These are called living benefits or accelerated benefits. In general, living benefits range from 25 to 95 percent of the death benefit. The payment will depend on your policy's face value, the terms of your contract, and the state in which you live.

Life insurance loans: You might be able to use your life insurance to get a loan from the insurer or a lender. A loan from the insurer will need to be paid off at death or when you surrender the policy. A loan from a bank will mean regular payments. The insurance that most employers offer to their workers is "term life insurance," not cash value insurance. Cash value (also known as whole or permanent) life insurance can be another source of emergency cash. If you have this type of policy, you might be able to get a loan on the cash value or even withdraw some of the cash. Talk with a financial planner for more information before pursuing this approach.

Cash Sources and Issues

As you consider sources of lump-sum cash, make sure you recognize the issues involved with the liquidation or sale of each asset. Consider implications such as tax obligations and the impact on your estate. Sometimes, financial resources can affect other benefits you receive.

Estimating Your Expenses

Try to estimate your current and future expenses in as much detail as you can. Looking back over your bills or bank records will help you estimate your day-to-day living expenses. But some of the medical costs associated with a breast cancer diagnosis may be hard to anticipate. You should plan on budgeting for out-of-pocket medical expenses, increased living expenses, and other special expenses. Consider talking to other women who have dealt with breast cancer diagnoses similar to yours. They may be willing to share practical information that can help you plan appropriately, in addition to providing you with emotional support.

Managing Your Savings and Investments

Dealing with a cancer diagnosis often means changing your priorities, including your approach to investing. Before you had cancer, you might have sought a high return on your investments. However, increased returns mean increased risk. During the time that you are undergoing treatment, try to keep your focus on your short-term needs and those of your family.

If you have money invested in certificates of deposit (CDs), Treasury bonds, mutual funds, or common stock, you might be able to convert some of these investments to cash. Some investments are easier than others to turn into cash. Remember that the profit from the sale of stocks and some bonds will become part of your taxable income. If possible, try to have six months' to a year's worth of estimated expenses available in investments that can be easily converted into cash. Avoid having your money in riskier (or growth-oriented) investments. Instead, choose short-term and limited-term investments that can provide income, such as money market accounts at a bank or a money market mutual fund.

Planning Your Estate

Estate planning is important for everyone, not just for people who have cancer. You may think that you don't have an "estate" to plan, but in fact you do. This is a commonly misunderstood term; everything you own is part of your estate. This includes your house, car, jewelry, and all other personal belongings. It also usually includes your life insurance policies, retirement funds, and savings.

But estate planning can be difficult for some people to face. Many people think that by planning their estate, they are giving up on life. However, estate planning can actually help you focus on treatment and recovery; you can be reassured that your wishes will be honored and that you will remain in control of your money and health care decisions, both now and in the future. Estate planning is an important part of making a financial plan. Take care of this part of your financial planning as soon as you feel ready. At a minimum, everyone should have the following estate planning documents prepared.

A Will

Your will directs how and to whom your assets will be distributed. Your will also names a guardian for any minor children and their assets. A will is especially important if you have children from a previous marriage. Depending on the state in which you live, if you do not have a will, your spouse could experience serious financial problems when your assets are distributed.

A Durable Power of Attorney

Naming a durable power of attorney is a way to plan for a time when you may be incapacitated or unable to make decisions regarding your business, finances, or health care. This document lets you name the person who will handle your affairs if you are unable to do so yourself. When selecting a durable power of attorney, choose someone whom you trust completely to carry out your wishes, even if that involves difficult decisions.

A durable power of attorney can be either general or limited. A general power of attorney lets your agent make any decisions that may be legally made by you. In contrast, a limited power of attorney can only make decisions in designated areas, such as health care, specific investments, and real estate transactions. A lawyer can help you customize a limited power of attorney that meets your specific needs.

A Health Care Proxy

A health care proxy lets you name a person who will make decisions about your health care if you cannot make them yourself. This document may be called a medical power of attorney or health care power of attorney in some states. This designation only applies to health care and not financial matters, but it is still an important part of your plans for the future.

A Living Will

A living will lets you specify the types of medical treatment you would or would not want if the time comes that you cannot communicate these choices directly to your care providers.

Using an Estate Attorney

If possible, talk to an estate attorney about your estate-planning needs. He or she can draw up the documents you need and customize them for your specific circumstances. Depending on your finances, you might need to set up trusts. Trusts can help protect your assets from taxes, probate costs, public disclosure, and can also help prevent family arguments. If your finances are simple, documents can be drafted by a legal clinic or nonprofit group. Contact the American Cancer Society at 800-227-2345 to find local resources that can help you. After your legal documents are in place, it is a good idea to review them from time to time to be sure the information is current and still reflects your wishes.

Locating Sources of Financial Help

You might be surprised by the number of organizations that provide financial assistance to people with cancer. Your hospital social worker, case worker, or doctor can refer you to organizations that provide such services as free or reduced airfare, transportation assistance, lodging for people going through treatment, and even meals or medicines. Make sure to ask for help early on and do not wait until you complete treatment. Some resources are available to people only while they are undergoing treatment.

Civic and religious organizations may offer financial help or services for people with cancer and their family members. Groups such as the Salvation Army, United Way, Lutheran Social Services, and Catholic Social Services are listed in the phone book under "Social Service Organizations," and most have websites, too. Churches and synagogues might also be able to help with transportation, childcare, home maintenance, and home care services, which could reduce your out-of-pocket costs. The Federal Citizen Information Center (FCIC) offers information about managing debt; government information, benefits, and services; and many other helpful topics. You can reach them at 800-FED-INFO (800-333-4636), TTY 800-326-2996, or online at www.usa.gov.

The National Endowment for Financial Education and the American Cancer Society have developed an easy-to-use financial management program for people with cancer in any stage of treatment. For more information about this program, called Taking Charge of Money Matters, please call the American Cancer Society at 800-227-2345 or visit www.cancer.org.

The American Cancer Society offers free lodging for people with cancer and their caregivers at some locations. Contact the American Cancer Society at 800-227-2345 to learn about Hope Lodges in your treatment area, as well other programs offered that could be of help.

Help for Senior Citizens

Contact your local office on aging for assistance. The National Association of Area Agencies on Aging (NAAAA) partners with the US Department of Health and Human Services' Administration on Aging to maintain the Eldercare Locator, a nationwide directory of services geared toward older adults and caregivers. This database, at www.eldercare.gov, has links to state and local agencies that offer information and assistance on transportation, meals, home care, housing alternatives, legal issues, and social activities for older people. You can also call 800-677-1116 to get information about Eldercare.

Nutritional Assistance

Contact your county board of assistance; Women, Infants, and Children (WIC) program; and the Supplemental Nutrition Assistance Program (SNAP; formerly called the Food Stamps Program) for more information on what additional help might be available to you and your family. These programs are run by the US Department of Agriculture. You can learn more about what is covered by SNAP and how to apply by calling 800-221-5689 or visiting www.fns.usda.gov/snap.

Paying Your Bills

Request payment plans with your utility companies, mortgage or rental managers, doctors, and other medical providers. If you have a good history of paying your bills on time, most businesses and creditors will allow you to arrange a payment plan. Try to be understanding of your creditors' positions and cooperate with them. They are more likely to work with you if you try to make arrangements before you are behind on payments.

If credit card debt is becoming unmanageable, move any credit card balances to the card with the lowest interest rate. People often pay for out-of-pocket expenses with credit cards during treatment, and it is easy for these bills to add up quickly, to the point that paying minimum payments is difficult. If this happens to you, call your credit card company. If you explain your situation, the company will usually try to make arrangements with you. Making small regular payments is better than making no payments at all. You also might be able to negotiate for lower payments, a lower payoff amount, or a lower interest rate.

Consider credit counseling to help you consolidate your bills. Creditors will often agree to accept smaller payments or a nominal monthly amount. The National Foundation for Credit Counseling (NFCC) is a national nonprofit service that offers free, confidential financial counseling. They help people set up budgets and make repayment plans. Their counselors are certified and often offer appointments on a same-day basis in their local offices. Call 800-388-2227 or visit www.nfcc.org to be referred to local Consumer Credit Counseling Services or to get more information.

Bankruptcy

If you try but cannot make ends meet, filing for bankruptcy may be an option. Bankruptcy is a complicated area of law that can affect you and your family for a long time, so get professional help if you are considering this option. It is best to work with an attorney who specializes in bankruptcy law and can help you understand all the issues involved with filing for bankruptcy. Legal aid clinics and other nonprofit agencies can also offer advice and guidance in this area.

SPECIAL CAREGIVER'S SECTION

Supporting the Woman with Cancer

Life changes when a woman is told she has breast cancer.
But life also changes for the caregiver. The caregiver—whether it be a spouse, part-ner, adult child, or friend—also participates in the experience, filling a role that is crucial to the physical and emotional well-being of the person with cancer.

Over the course of treatment, the caregiver may take on responsibilities that just a short time ago were reserved for trained health care professionals. Caregivers and patients themselves have the responsibility of monitoring medications, managing side effects, and reporting conditions and situations that require professional intervention. The caregiver may feed, dress, and bathe the person with cancer, in addition to arranging schedules, managing insurance issues and finances, providing transportation, keeping the household running, and providing emotional support to the woman with breast cancer.

Caring for someone with cancer can be fulfilling, but it can also be demanding. There is almost always too much for just one person to do. It is important that you take care of yourself, as well. Enlist the support of those around you, such as your family and friends. Allowing others to help will relieve some of the pressures of caregiving and allow you to recharge.

You may not be sure how to cope with your loved one's breast cancer diagnosis and the emotional and practical challenges it has raised. The support you give her will be essential throughout her diagnosis, treatment, and recovery. There are many things you can do—large and small, physical and emotional—to help. The most important thing you can do is let her know you care.

Caregiving involves solving problems. You have been solving problems your whole life; the only difference now is that many of the challenges that come with a cancer diagnosis are new to you and your loved one. You do not know what's in store, either for you or your loved one. The best thing caregivers can do is learn as much as possible about what is happening now and what might happen in the future. This knowledge can reduce any fear you might have of the unknown and help you plan realistically for the future. Talk with health care professionals and with other people who have cared for someone with cancer. Ask questions. You may also want to read other parts of this book to learn more about breast cancer. In this chapter, we talk about the many ways you can help support your partner throughout this experience.

Supporting Your Loved One

An illness such as breast cancer can be stressful to a marriage and family. Try to focus on what you will need to do to get through the treatment period with as little stress as possible. There are many different kinds of support—both emotional and practical. And you will need other people in your arsenal. Begin looking to those around you as you think about what types of help you may need. You may be the caregiver, but building a support network for both you and your loved one will be an invaluable part of being the best support you can.

Talking About Cancer

The strain of dealing with a cancer diagnosis can make communication between friends and family members difficult, even when you are used to being open with one another. You might be reluctant to talk about the illness with your loved one and with other people in your lives. You may not want to upset or depress her, and you certainly don't want to pry or say the wrong thing. Here are some tips on how to approach talking to your loved one:

- **Start slowly.** It is always hard to talk about important issues. Do not feel like you have to rush. And do not let silence scare you away. It can be hard to find the right words to describe your feelings. Start by opening up lines of communication, maybe by asking, "What are you feeling?" or "How do you feel about…?" Starting this way shows that it is okay for your loved one to open up to you emotionally. It also shows that you want to know how she is really feeling.

- **Listen without judging.** Avoid saying, "You shouldn't…" or "Do not say that." Allow your loved one to express herself, and don't downplay her feelings. If you are uncertain about what she means, ask for clarification. Repeat what you heard back to her in your own words, so she knows you understand what she has said.
- **Be honest.** Discuss real and possible changes and share your emotional reactions to them. Do not pretend that you do not feel upset or fearful if you do.
- **Express your feelings.** Saying, "I'm afraid of losing you" is one way to express your concern that your loved one might die. Let her know how much you care.
- **Resist the urge** to reassure your loved one with statements such as, "You'll be fine," "Everything's going to be okay," or "Don't worry." These statements may be untrue, and she knows it. Saying such things might indicate to her that you don't want to think about the unpleasantness of cancer and that she cannot confide in you.
- **Understand that people communicate in different ways.** Make allowances for differences in communication styles and in how your loved one likes to be supported.
- **Remember that you do not have to agree** with your loved one. Two people are not always in the same emotional state or at the same level of acceptance at the same time. There is no simple answer to many problems, especially long-standing problems.
- **Think about getting help** from an uninvolved party such as a therapist, clergy member, or someone else with whom you feel comfortable, and allow that person to guide conversations that are difficult for you.

Support During Diagnosis

A woman with breast cancer needs to be sure she can count on the emotional support of those around her. She will want to be sure that they will be there for her when she needs them. When a woman first receives a diagnosis of breast cancer, you can do many things to support her.

- **Show her that you will be there** for her whenever she needs you. Let her know that you will love her no matter what she says, what mood she's in, or what she looks like. Your emotional support will help her face the cancer diagnosis and the treatments to come.

- **Allow her to express her emotions** in any way she wants, without judging her. Hold her hand, sit next to her, or hug her. Don't be afraid to touch her. This affection shows that you're going to stand by her and that you love her.
- **Pay attention to the good stuff.** Make an effort to notice and talk about pleasant things that happen during the day. Be sure to talk about everyday things—not just cancer. The uncertainty and loss of control that comes with a new cancer diagnosis can be overwhelming. Try to remind her that other things are still important.
- **Sharing doesn't always mean talking.** She may feel more comfortable writing about her feelings or expressing them through an activity rather than discussing them. She may express feelings in other nonverbal ways, such as with gestures or expressions, touching, or just asking that you be with her. Sharing silence with someone can be a privilege.
- **Respect her privacy.** Although you might feel that she needs to share her feelings with you, sometimes she may just need to be alone. Make sure she knows you are there to listen if and when she wants to talk.
- **Help by being a spokesperson for your partner.** Retelling details over and over again can be emotionally exhausting. Talk to her about how you can help. You might look into websites designed for people dealing with serious illnesses where friends and family can get updates. Some people send out group e-mails every few days to update friends and family whenever something changes.
- **You can offer practical support** by going to the doctor with her and being an active participant, as needed. Cancer brings new people, places, and medical language into her life. Collect information and take notes on conversations so you can sort through them together when she is ready and better able to take in new information and start making decisions.
- **Help her prepare to put her normal activities "on hold"** while getting treatment. For instance, arrangements for work or childcare may be needed, and taking care of these things ahead of time can help her better focus on dealing with treatment.

Support During Treatment

During treatment, there will be many practical ways in which you can help your partner. However, one of the best things you can do is simply be there for your loved one. This may mean going with her for appointments and tests, but most of all, it means being there emotionally: listening, not judging, and responding to her needs at the moment.

As a caregiver and member of your loved one's support team, you should know the planned course of treatment, the physical and emotional side effects that could result, and what your responsibilities as a caregiver will be. Always write down any instructions you get from doctors. Before you leave the hospital or treatment center, make sure you understand exactly what needs to be done to provide care for your loved one at home and what problems or symptoms you should report right away—no matter what time it is. These problems could include fever, new pain, or other new or recurring symptoms. You can also ask in which circumstances it would be okay to wait until the next day or the next appointment. Be sure you know how to contact the doctor after office hours, on holidays, and over the weekend.

Keep the lines of communication open. You can help her just by listening as she expresses her feelings. Encourage her to explore some of the specifics of her situation and her feelings of anger or anxiety and try to find the causes of these feelings. She may just need you to act as a sounding board—someone to listen, react, and absorb her words. Whether it be her feelings about her illness, her job situation, or other concerns, she may not necessarily need you to "do" anything in order to be helpful. It can be very helpful just to listen and acknowledge her feelings.

Asking for Help

Sometimes, people with cancer are reluctant to ask for help. You can make caregiving and supporting your loved one easier by accepting offers of help from others in your life. Connections with others in your family and community can also help you and your loved one feel supported and cared for during this difficult time. Do not think that you have to shoulder the responsibility of caregiving all by yourself.

The support of friends and family is important both to the person with cancer and the caregiver. When others offer to help, accept their offers and give them options for specific things they can do. Friends cannot help if they don't know what to do. Try making a list of the ways in which people can help, whether picking up kids from school or practices, picking up groceries or dry cleaning, helping to supply meals, or helping to provide rides to treatment. Some people find it useful to post a list near the phone so that ideas are available if someone calls asking how they can help.

Family members' roles will probably need to change so that your loved one can focus on treatment and getting better. She may have side effects and probably will not be able to do all the things she normally does. Find others to help during this time, and divide responsibilities according to each person's strengths, interests, and personalities. For instance, some people are better at dealing with paperwork than providing a soothing presence at the bedside. Some might be good at dealing with medical personnel and taking notes. Others can run errands and cook meals. Friends and family members who may not be able or willing to contribute time might be able to help financially.

Even casual acquaintances can help support your loved one. Knowing that other people care is extremely important for a woman going through cancer treatment. Encourage others to reach out to her, whether by writing notes, making short calls, or visiting.

Transitioning to Recovery

Recovering from treatment can be challenging for some women. Your loved one will begin to transition to a new routine that focuses on healing and recovery. She will spend less time at her treatment center and will see her doctors less frequently. It may take a while for her to get used to this change. Without frequent appointments, some women feel less supported by their health care providers and may need additional emotional support. For some women, dealing with the uncertainty that comes after treatment ends is especially challenging—there is no way to know whether or when the cancer might come back, even if the doctor says there is "no evidence of cancer."

Maybe the doctor has given her the "all clear" to go back to work. Or maybe she needs to slowly increase her work duties—the timing will depend on her physical condition and her line of work. When your loved one starts working a more normal schedule, there may be days when she feels fatigued and needs your help. It might take some time to get past this phase, and, during this time, you may still need your support network so that you, too, can start getting back to a more normal schedule.

As a caregiver, you might find yourself continuing to do the things you did while your loved one was in treatment. But, over time, she will need to start doing the things she can and should do on her own. This may take place over a period of months as she gets stronger. Check in every few weeks to see what you have been doing that she can start doing, either alone or with a little help. If there are things that she cannot quite do, talk with the doctor about referral to a physical therapist or occupational therapist. These professionals may be able to maximize her abilities by helping build muscle strength and/or offering assistive devices.

You can help by continuing to offer support and allowing her to return to her normal life and daily routines slowly. Bolster hope and energy for her by celebrating her strengths and achievements. Celebrate what she means to everyone in your family and circle of friends. You may want to start new traditions and create new memories of family gatherings, outings, or celebrations, which will help reaffirm how vital she is to your family and friends.

Intimacy: For Spouses and Partners of Women with Breast Cancer

Partners of women with cancer face unique opportunities and challenges as they look toward their loved one's recovery. Hair loss, weight loss or gain, and breast changes can make it harder for your partner to have a positive sexual image of herself. Coping with both physical and emotional changes after breast cancer treatment can be challenging for many women. As your partner begins to look and feel better, different issues will come up regarding your emotional and physical relationship.

Losing a breast or both breasts can be very distressing for a woman. The most common sexual side effect from breast surgery is feeling less attractive. In our culture, breasts are often viewed as a basic part of beauty and womanhood. If a woman's breast is removed, she may feel less secure about whether her partner will accept her new appearance and still find her attractive.

Some women have sexual problems linked to breast surgeries such as mastectomy and lumpectomy. While there is no physical reason for surgery or radiation to the breast to decrease a woman's sexual desire, some women have difficulty resuming intimacy after cancer treatment ends. Breast surgery can interfere with the pleasure a woman experiences from having her breasts touched, but it doesn't change a woman's ability to feel sexual pleasure. It does not lessen a woman's ability to produce vaginal lubrication, feel or enjoy normal genital sensation, or reach orgasm.

Cancer treatment can impact a woman's feelings about her body. She may feel less attractive or avoid having certain parts of her body seen or touched. Breasts and nipples are sources of sexual pleasure for many women and their partners. Touching the breasts is a common part of foreplay and can add to sexual excitement. After treatment, some women still enjoy being stroked around the area of the healed scar. Others dislike being touched there and may not enjoy having the remaining breast and nipple touched, either. Some women who have had breast surgery feel self-conscious being the partner "on top" during sex. This position makes it easy to notice that the breast is missing or different.

A few women have long-term pain in their chests and shoulders after radical mastectomy. (This type of surgery removes the breast and the chest muscles underneath and is rarely performed anymore.) It may help to support her chest and shoulder with pillows during sex. It may also help if you avoid positions where weight rests on her chest or arm.

If surgery removed only the tumor (segmental mastectomy or lumpectomy) and was followed by radiation treatment, a woman's breast may be scarred. It also may be different in shape, feel, or size. Some women have areas of numbness or decreased sensation near the surgical scar.

Managing Medications

Keep a list of all medicines your loved one is taking, including prescription and over-the-counter medicines and any vitamins, herbs, or other supplements. This list should include the following information:

- name of each drug
- dose (number of milligrams [mg] per pill; this is usually on the medicine bottle)
- schedule (what times of day and which days of the week she takes the drug)
- reason(s) for taking each medication
- name of the doctor who prescribed the drug (if she sees more than one doctor, other doctors might not know what medications have been prescribed)

Don't forget the medicines she takes every now and then or "as needed"—for instance, for pain, fever, nausea, itching, or to help her sleep.

Keep this list and take it to each of her doctor appointments. Have the doctor's office make a copy and be sure to update it each time a medicine is added or taken away or if a dose changes. Share the new medication schedule with each doctor on the next visit. Also have it handy if you call the doctor about a problem. Some caregivers make lists or spreadsheets and keep copies posted on the refrigerator. That way the list is handy when someone comes in to help. Placing a second copy in your loved one's wallet might be useful, too.

As the person's condition changes, ask about the need to continue medicines. For example, if she loses weight, some blood pressure medicines may no longer be needed. If treatment for cancer is stopped, other drugs might be able to be stopped, too. Stopping medicines when they are not needed anymore can lower expenses and reduce the chance of drug interactions and side effects. You will also have fewer medicines to manage.

If Treatment Causes Early Menopause

Some of the hormone therapies used during breast cancer treatment and some chemotherapy drugs can cause symptoms of menopause. These symptoms include hot flashes and interruption of the menstrual cycle. Lower hormone levels also can cause the lining of the vagina to become thin, tight, or dry. These symptoms can be helped by water-based lubricants or vaginal moisturizers. If these lubricants do not work, a doctor can often prescribe a hormone cream to treat these problems. In spite of these changes, most women will eventually feel sexual desire and reach orgasm much as they did before cancer treatment.

Reestablishing Intimacy

Physical intimacy can be an important part of maintaining your sense of closeness with your loved one, but you may worry that having sex will be uncomfortable or hurt your partner. You might also feel awkward because you think that bringing up sex will be insensitive if your partner isn't ready, or maybe you are afraid that a sexual advance might come across as a demand. You might also be coping with your own upset feelings about the physical changes in your partner's body. Initiating physical intimacy may be difficult for both partners. And even though you don't mean to, you may withdraw because you are afraid of losing the woman you love. If your partner has withdrawn from you, try to prevent the cycle of misunderstanding by reaching out gently and repeatedly. Reassure her that cancer cannot destroy your love or your intimate relationship.

The following are suggestions for reestablishing intimacy with your partner:

- **Open communication is most important.** Try to bring up the topic of sex in a healthy, assertive way. It is usually not helpful to accuse, "You never touch me anymore!", or demand, "We simply have to have sex soon. I can't stand the frustration!" Instead, try to state your feelings positively. For example, you could say, "I really miss our sex life. I'd like to talk about what is getting in the way of our being close."
- **Don't be upset if your partner** does not seem interested in physical intimacy right away. Sometimes women initially shy away from physical closeness and have low energy levels for a while after cancer treatment ends.
- **Touching, holding, hugging,** and caressing are important ways to express acceptance and caring crucial to your partnership. This expression shows love and lets her know that you still find her desirable.

- **Your willingness to look at the changes** in your partner's body and willingness to touch her can contribute greatly to her self-acceptance and self-confidence.
- **If you need more help,** a professional counselor can help you work out your feelings toward your partner and the disease or any resentment about the responsibility that has been placed on you.

The Challenges of Caregiving

Caring for someone with breast cancer can be rewarding, but it can also be difficult. It often helps to explain your thoughts and fears to an understanding person, whether a friend or a therapist. Talking to a sympathetic person will show you that other people understand and appreciate how you feel and will help you work through your feelings and make sense of them.

Balancing Caregiving and Your Other Responsibilities

Caregiving is a big responsibility. To make time for caregiving, you might have to juggle your professional and personal responsibilities and cut back on your commitments. You might have to delay or postpone life plans, such as starting a new career or retiring. Although you are trying to be supportive of your loved one, it is normal to have some thoughts about your own personal losses. Your needs are important, too, and it is important to deal with your feelings. Consider these suggestions:

- **Get help from a support group,** a therapist, or member of the clergy before you allow conflicts over future plans to lead to guilt or anger. Talking to someone with an outside perspective can provide a welcome relief.
- **Focus on short-term accomplishments** or tasks and set manageable goals for yourself and your family.

Balancing Caregiving and Your Job

Being a caregiver can be a full-time job. The time demands of caregiving can lead to work-related issues, such as missed days, low productivity, and work interruptions. Some caregivers even need to take unpaid leave, turn down promotions, or lose work benefits as a result of the responsibilities of caregiving. The stress of caring for someone, in addition to worries about keeping your job, can be overwhelming. Dealing with these issues promptly is important.

Caregivers are likely to face even greater demands at certain times, such as when cancer is diagnosed and at the start of treatment. You might need to take more time off, and this can cause additional stress and financial strain, especially if you are a freelancer, consultant, or entrepreneur. In these types of fields, if you do not work, you are not paid. If you have a traditional job in a larger company, however, there might be benefits to help you take time off and still keep your job.

Some caregivers find that no one else can provide care for the person with cancer, and they have to cut back to working part-time. Some feel that they must quit their jobs entirely to be effective caregivers. If you need to keep your job, but the interruptions and time off are creating problems, you might want to consult your employer to determine whether you could work a different schedule during the times your loved one needs you most. Some companies let you take paid leave if you are caring for a spouse or close relative. You may be able to work half-days or split shifts, or take one day a week off for doctor visits, for example.

A federal law, the Family and Medical Leave Act (FMLA), guarantees up to twelve weeks off per year to take care of a seriously ill family member (spouse, parent, or child). It applies only to employees of larger companies, however, and you must meet certain criteria to be eligible for it. FMLA does not require that the leave be paid, though you can keep health insurance benefits if you are covered by your employer's health plan. Call the American Cancer Society at 800-227-2345 or talk to someone in the human resources department of your workplace to learn more about FMLA.

Even if you do not qualify for legal job protection, you might still explain your situation and ask your employer whether you can adjust your schedule to allow you to give care without leaving your job. Some employers are flexible in these cases. You will need to think ahead and be ready to spell out what you can keep doing and for how long you will need extra time off.

Taking Care of Yourself

Caregiving can be stressful and exhausting. Taking over responsibilities, changing habits and routines, and worrying about what might happen can wear you out. Caregiving takes emotional, spiritual, and physical strength. Caregivers often feel tired, isolated, depressed, or anxious and may find it difficult to reach out for help. Caregiving has also been linked to an increased risk of other physical problems, such as heart disease, high blood pressure, sleep problems, infections, depression, and fatigue.

Caring for the Caregiver

Consider the following ways to take care of your own needs and feelings:

- Plan things that you enjoy. There are three types of activities that you need for yourself:
  - activities that involve other people, such as having lunch with a friend
  - activities that give you a sense of accomplishment, such as exercising or finishing a project
  - activities that make you feel good or relaxed, such as watching a funny movie or taking a walk
- Make an effort to notice and talk about things you do as they happen during the day. Cancer should not be all you talk or think about. Watch the news, read the paper, or check out a news website. Set aside time during the day, such as during a meal, when you do not talk about your loved one's illness.
- Join a support group for caregivers or consider using counseling services. Talk with a nurse or social worker or contact the American Cancer Society at 800-227-2345 to locate services in your area. Many cancer organizations have ways for caregivers to connect to educational and support resources online.
- Reach out to others. Caregiving alone for any period of time is not realistic. Don't try to do it all yourself. Involve others in your life and in the care you provide for your loved one.

The demands of caregiving often do not leave time for caregivers to take care of their own needs. You may find that the needs of your loved one conflict with your own needs and those of your family. Many caregivers forget to eat, don't get enough sleep or exercise, and ignore their own physical health concerns. Caregivers may feel that they are pulled in too many directions at once to meet everyone's needs.

You are more likely to have a positive outlook and a healthy body when you take time to take care of yourself. Be sure to make and keep your own doctor appointments, get enough sleep, exercise, eat healthy foods, and keep your normal routine as much as you can. It is important not to feel guilty or selfish when you ask for help or take time for yourself. The more you can care for your own needs for rest, nutrition, enjoyment, and relaxation, the better a caregiver you will be.

Consider the following suggestions for caregivers:

- **Get help if you feel overwhelmed** by the changes in your family or the responsibilities suddenly placed upon you. Ask a nurse, doctor, social worker, or member of the clergy for help or for a referral to someone who can help you cope. You can also contact the American Cancer Society at 800-227-2345 or refer to the resource guide on pages 443–472 for information about organizations that offer support for caregivers and families.

- **Join a support group for caregivers.** Support groups and counseling for families address concerns, fears, worries, and practical problems. It can be very helpful to talk with other caregivers who have had similar experiences. They will usually understand how you feel.
- **As much as possible, maintain a sense of normalcy** within your family. Keep up your regular activities (such as watching movies or visiting friends) without feeling guilty.
- **Take care of children's needs.** Caregivers need to figure out how to take care of children's needs while they are caring for the person with cancer. Juggling children's schedules and keeping their lives as normal as possible often requires a lot of help from friends and family members.
- **Ask for help.** One of the most important things you can do as a caregiver is enlist support from family and friends. Don't try to do it all alone.

Adjusting to Life After Cancer

Adjusting to life after cancer can take time for both you and your loved one. You may experience a wide range of feelings after treatment ends. Caregiving can be stressful, but providing care for your loved one can also bring about feelings of satisfaction and confidence. After such an experience, you might feel closer to your family members and better understand how important your family is to your overall well-being. Assuming such an important role in your family during a crisis also may have opened doors to new friends and relationships as you talked to people who faced similar problems, or you might have been drawn closer to distant relatives as you shared updates and tasks. Facing cancer with loved ones can deeply enrich personal relationships and bring some people closer. A health crisis can challenge people to tap into their personal strengths and provide them with new opportunities to show their love and appreciation.

As your loved one begins to look to the future and the rest of her life, you can begin to focus more on your future, too. You can start setting new goals, such as taking a postponed vacation or developing your career. You and your loved one can make new plans for yourselves and your family. These plans may differ from the ones you had before breast cancer came into your lives. But you can still look forward to setting new goals, enjoying new experiences, and creating special family memories together.

Consider the following suggestions for looking at life beyond breast cancer:

- **As your partner or loved one changes her lifestyle,** which might include changes in diet and exercise, you may want to join her. Your participation will not only show your continuing support but will also help you look to your own future health and reduce your cancer risk.
- **Give yourself the opportunity** to think about what has changed in your life since you began your supportive role. Although you might have endured hardships along the way, focus on the things that have had a positive outcome and have brought you closer to your partner, family, and friends. Recognize the experiences that have given you greater joy in life.
- **If you find it difficult to move beyond** your loved one's experience with cancer, seek out a support group where you can feel free to share your experience with others who have gone through it, too.

PART SIX

Life After Cancer

Completing treatment can be both stressful and exciting. You may be relieved to finish treatment but find it hard not to worry about cancer coming back. For some people, emotions that were put aside during cancer treatment come flooding back all at once, and they feel overwhelmed with sadness, anger, or fear. All of these feelings make sense. You have just been through a difficult time. Your body has been assaulted by cancer and its treatment. Your outlook and your whole way of life have changed, at least for a time.

More and more people today live long and healthy lives after cancer treatment, and key to that is taking care of yourself. Good follow-up care is essential after cancer and will be a permanent part of life now. It is also important for you to do what you can to stay physically and emotionally healthy. Your body may have changed as a result of cancer treatment. Now that treatment is finished, you or your partner may be hesitant to talk about being close.

You might feel the need to refocus your energy by volunteering or getting involved somehow in your community. Finding positive outlets for your energy may help you feel better about yourself and more relaxed and encouraged about the future.

Every person who has had cancer lives with the possibility that the cancer will come back. In chapter 22, we discuss recurrence, how it is treated, the importance of keeping follow-up appointments, and what you can do to stay as healthy as possible.

CHAPTER 19

Taking Care of Yourself After Cancer: Health and Wellness

The way breast cancer affects your body and your life is unique. Some women feel fine after treatment. Others do not fare as well and react poorly to various aspects of cancer treatment. Your recovery depends on many things, including the type of cancer you have, the type of treatment used, how healthy you were before treatment, how quickly your body heals, and many other factors. Let your body set the pace for how quickly you return to your usual activities. Many women find that slowly going back to normal routines helps put them on the path to recovery.

There is a lot to look forward to after cancer treatment ends. But keep in mind that recovery takes time, and just like every other part of the cancer experience, each woman recovers in her own way at her own pace. This chapter will focus on developing a wellness plan so that you can concentrate on staying well, maintaining a healthy lifestyle, and taking good care of yourself for the rest of your life.

Creating a Wellness Plan

For the past few months, you have probably thought a lot about what it means to be sick. But have you thought much about what it means to be well?

Wellness is not just the absence of illness. It is a state of good physical and mental health. It is maintained by healthy lifestyle choices, proper diet, and good exercise habits. You might not have been able to control your cancer, but there are things you can do to improve your health and well-being after cancer. By taking a proactive approach to wellness, you can improve your overall quality of life.

What Is a Wellness Plan?

A wellness plan is a set of health-minded and life-enriching goals you would like to achieve. These goals do not have to be lengthy, complicated, or difficult to accomplish. The plan should be reasonable, meaningful, and—especially in the cases of exercise and weight loss—crafted under the guidance of your medical team. A complete wellness plan might address your physical well-being, your mental/emotional health, and your spiritual life. In this chapter, we will address factors related to physical well-being, and in the next chapter, we will focus on mental/emotional health and spiritual issues. For example, possible goals might be to control your weight, exercise regularly, manage stress more effectively, eat a healthy diet, or protect your skin from the sun. It can help to then break your goals down into specific, measurable steps and challenges (as shown in the Sample Wellness Plan on the next page).

Long-Term Follow-Up Care

Although your treatment has ended, you may still be coping with its effects on your body. You might be wondering how your body should feel during this time and what to expect. Every woman's body needs a different amount of time to get over the effects of cancer treatment. Your experience will depend on your overall health before treatment, the types of treatment you had and, of course, your body's response to treatment. Talk to your medical team about what you should expect and about setting up a plan for follow-up care.

Tips for Sticking with Your Wellness Plan

Use these tips to help you stick with your wellness plan:

- **Be specific and realistic.** Instead of saying, "I'm going to lose weight," resolve to lose one pound every two weeks. The latter goal is specific, realistic, and measurable.
- **Prompt yourself to stay on track.** Remind yourself constantly that you have goals in mind and that you are working to reach them. Write your goals down and post them where you'll see them throughout the day.
- **Choose wisely.** Don't make a hundred resolutions; instead, make two or three that you can reasonably accomplish. Decide on a few that are especially meaningful to you and that you know will improve your quality of life if you stick to them.
- **Rededicate yourself.** If you get off track, don't punish yourself. Reward yourself for the things you have accomplished and recommit to your goals.

A Sample Wellness Plan

Focus on one aspect of your wellness, such as your medical care and physical well-being after treatment. Using this format, you can actively work toward your wellness goals.

Wellness Goal	Plan of Action	Challenges and Resolutions
Eat a healthy, well-balanced diet.	Measure portions and log all meals and snacks consumed each day.	It is difficult to measure portions at catered weekly staff meetings. I plan to eat a sack lunch before the meeting.
Take steps to control my weight and get to a healthy BMI (body mass index).*	Attend weight loss management group each week.	I am not motivated to get up early on Saturday morning. I will carpool with Julie so I can't back out.
Locate a primary care doctor who understands the needs of women who have had breast cancer.	Get recommendations for a new primary care doctor from my oncologist's office.	Office staff has not yet returned my call. I will call again tomorrow or ask for the recommendation at my next follow-up appointment.
Promptly schedule regular mammograms and follow-up appointments.	Schedule mammograms on my birthday each year and schedule follow-up appointments at the end of the previous appointment.	I don't know my schedule that far in advance. Tentatively schedule these appointments and make a note to verify appointment times one month in advance.
Participate in physical activity every week.	Register for yoga class on Tuesdays and Thursdays.	Some nights I have to work late and miss class. I will find classes on the weekend.
Take precautions to prevent lymphedema or other complications from treatment.	Carry heavy handbags on my left side and use a rolling cart instead of my laptop briefcase.	Annual book fair requires parent volunteers for set-up. Ask to be assigned a job that doesn't involve heavy lifting.

*Information on how to calculate your BMI can be found online at www.cdc.gov/healthyweight/assessing/bmi.

Questions to Ask Your Medical Team About Follow-Up Care

- **Which doctor should I see** for follow-up visits?
- **How often should I see** the doctor for routine visits?
- **What follow-up tests,** if any, should be done? How often?
- **Are there symptoms** I should watch for?
- **If any of these symptoms develop,** whom should I call?
- **Will my insurance** cover my follow-up care?

At each visit, talk to your doctor about the following concerns:
- symptoms that you think might be a sign of cancer's return
- any pain that troubles you
- any physical problems that get in the way of your daily life or that bother you, such as tiredness, trouble sleeping, loss of sex drive, or weight gain or loss
- any medicines, vitamins, or herbs you are taking and any other treatments you are using
- any emotional problems you have, such as anxiety, worry, or depression
- any changes in your family medical history
- things you want to know more about

Follow-up care means visiting your doctor for regular checkups. These checkups will give you a chance to discuss your mental and physical health and address any changes or concerns. During these visits, your doctor will see how you are recovering from treatment and treatment side effects. The doctor will also check to be sure the cancer has not returned or spread to another part of your body. Follow-up care can help your doctor spot other illnesses or side effects of treatment, which can sometimes develop years later. You will have follow-up appointments with your oncologist for many years after treatment. Over time, the visits will become less frequent.

Mammograms

Mammograms are important diagnostic tools and should be a regular part of follow-up care after breast cancer. The American Cancer Society recommends that all women get mammograms annually starting at age forty. Women at increased risk for breast cancer (such as those with past breast cancer, a known breast cancer gene mutation, or a strong family history of breast cancer) should talk with their doctors about the benefits and limitations of starting mammogram screening earlier; having additional tests, such as MRI, done along with their mammograms; or having more frequent examinations.

Breast cancers found by mammography are typically less advanced than those felt by a woman or her doctor. When breast cancer is found when it is small, women have more treatment options and better treatment outcomes.

Doctors and scientists at the American Cancer Society and at all major US medical and public health organizations that have issued statements about breast cancer screening support the value of mammograms. Following the American Cancer Society's guidelines for the early detection of breast cancer improves the chances that breast cancer can be diagnosed at an early stage and successfully treated.

The mammogram log on the next page can be a helpful tool in keeping track of your mammograms. Particularly in the first few years after your treatment for breast cancer, you may need to have more frequent mammograms.

Mammograms After Breast Surgery

Regular mammograms are needed after breast surgery. This is very important, because women who have had one breast cancer are at higher risk for breast cancer to develop in the other breast.

Women who have undergone total mastectomy, modified radical mastectomy, or radical mastectomy for breast cancer do not need to have routine mammograms of the affected side(s). But mammograms should still be done on the unaffected breast every year. One type of mastectomy that does require follow-up mammograms is nipple-sparing or areola-sparing mastectomy. In this procedure, a woman keeps her natural nipple and the tissue just under the skin; enough breast tissue is left behind to require a yearly screening mammogram. If you are not sure what type of mastectomy you had, ask your doctor for clarification and ask how often you should have mammograms.

Women who have had lumpectomy and radiation therapy need a mammogram six months after surgery, another one six months later, and then mammograms of both breasts at least every year. Some doctors prefer that women have a mammogram of the treated breast every six months for two to three years.

Mammogram Log

Type and amount of breast cancer treatment received:

Treatment started on:

Treatment ended on:

First follow-up mammogram:

Date of Mammogram	Results Received	Comments	Next Scheduled Test

Mammograms After Breast Reconstruction

Most of the time, mammograms of the affected breast are not recommended after breast reconstruction, unless you had a nipple- or skin-sparing mastectomy, which leaves behind some breast tissue. Mammography is still useful for the other breast. However, your doctor may recommend a mammogram if there is an area of concern or if you are at high risk for local recurrence. The need to continue screening and the types of tests to be done should be discussed with both your plastic surgeon and your oncologist.

If screening mammograms are recommended on the affected breast and you have had reconstruction using silicone gel or saline implants, you should get your mammograms done at a facility with technologists trained in moving the implant to get the best possible images of the rest of the breast. Pictures can sometimes be impaired by implants, particularly silicone implants. These women should talk with both their plastic surgeon and their oncologist about the types of tests needed and the best schedule to follow.

Mammograms After Radiation Therapy or Chemotherapy

Radiation therapy and chemotherapy both cause changes in the skin and breast tissues that can make mammograms harder to read. Because these changes are most evident about six months after treatment is completed, most radiologists recommend a mammogram of the treated breast at that time. This mammogram helps establish a baseline image; future mammograms will be compared with this one to follow healing and check for recurrence. The next mammogram can then be performed six months later, when the woman is due for her yearly mammogram of both breasts. After the second follow-up mammogram, some doctors prefer that women have mammograms of the treated breast every six months for a total of two to three years, but others suggest that annual mammograms are enough. You should continue to have yearly mammograms of the unaffected breast. Talk to your doctor about the mammogram schedule that is best for you.

Mammogram Regulation

In the United States, the US Food and Drug Administration (FDA) must certify each mammography facility (except those of the Department of Veterans Affairs). It is illegal to perform mammograms in the United States without an FDA certificate. Visit www.fda.gov to search for FDA-certified mammography facilities.

Tips for Mammograms

The following are useful tips for getting a good-quality mammogram:

- **Discuss any new findings or problems** in your breasts with your doctor or nurse before having the mammogram.

- **Ask to see the center's FDA certificate,** which is issued to facilities that meet standards of safety and accuracy for mammography. (It's often posted near the receptionist's desk.)

- **Use a facility that either specializes in** mammograms or does many mammograms a day.

- **If you are satisfied** that the facility is of high quality, continue to use it so your mammograms can be easily compared from year to year.

- **If you change facilities,** ask for your old mammograms to take with you to the new facility so they can be compared with the new ones.

- **If you have sensitive breasts,** schedule mammograms when your breasts will be least tender. Try to avoid having a mammogram the week before your period. This will help lessen discomfort.

- **On the day of the mammogram,** do not wear deodorant, powder, or cream under your arms. These substances can appear as white spots on the x-ray and can interfere with the quality of the mammogram.

- **Describe any breast symptoms** or problems to the technologist doing the mammogram. Also tell the technologist about any related history, such as previous surgeries, biopsies, hormone use, or other treatments, and any family or personal history of breast cancer.

- **A mammogram might be uncomfortable** for a few moments, but it should not be painful; speak up if you are in pain. Tell the technologist, so she can try to make the compression more comfortable for you.

- **Bring a list** of all mammograms, biopsies, and other breast treatments you have had and the dates and facilities where they were performed.

- **If you do not hear from your doctor** within ten days, do not assume that your mammogram was normal—call your doctor or the facility and request your results.

Clinical Breast Examination

A clinical breast examination (CBE) is an examination of your breasts by a health care professional such as a doctor, nurse practitioner, nurse, or physician assistant. A CBE should be part of a woman's periodic health examination and should be done at least every three years for women under age forty and annually for women aged forty and older. Women who have had breast cancer will likely have a CBE every year.

For this examination, you undress from the waist up. The health care professional will first inspect your breasts for changes in size or shape. Then, using the pads of the fingers, the examiner will gently feel your breasts. Special attention will be given to the shape and texture of the breasts, location of any lumps, and whether such lumps are attached to the skin or to deeper tissues. The area under each arm will also be checked. The CBE is a good time for the health care professional to teach breast self-examination if you do not already know how to do it. Ask your doctor or nurse to teach you and watch your technique.

Breast Self-Examination

A woman can notice changes in her breasts by being aware of how her breasts normally look and feel and by feeling her breasts for changes (breast awareness) or by choosing to use a step-by-step approach and using a specific schedule to examine her breasts (breast self-examination). Ask your doctor about the benefits and limitations of breast self-examination (BSE). The American Cancer Society suggests that BSE is an option for women starting in their twenties. But regardless of whether women choose to do BSE, they should be aware of any changes in their breasts and report these changes to a doctor right away. This self-awareness might be accomplished with BSE or simply by being alert to any changes in your breasts.

If you choose to do BSE, consider these suggestions:

- Lie down and place your right arm behind your head. The examination should be done while you are lying down, not standing up. When you are lying down, your breast tissue spreads evenly over the chest wall and is as thin as possible, making it much easier to feel all the breast tissue.
- Use the finger pads of the three middle fingers on your left hand to feel for lumps in the right breast. Use overlapping dime-sized circular motions of the finger pads to feel the breast tissue.
- Use three different levels of pressure to feel all the breast tissue. Light pressure is needed to feel the tissue closest to the skin, medium pressure to feel a little

deeper, and firm pressure to feel the tissue closest to the chest and ribs. It is normal to feel a firm ridge in the lower curve of each breast, but you should tell your doctor if you feel anything else out of the ordinary. If you are not sure how hard to press, talk with your doctor or nurse. Use each pressure level to feel the breast tissue before moving on to the next spot.

- Move around the breast in an up-and-down pattern starting at an imaginary line drawn straight down your side from the underarm and moving across the breast to the middle of the breastbone. Be sure to check the entire breast area going down until you feel only ribs and up to the neck or collarbone. Do it the same way each time, check the entire breast area, and remember how your breast feels from month to month. There is some evidence to suggest that the up-and-down pattern (sometimes called the vertical pattern) is the most effective pattern for covering the entire breast without missing any breast tissue.

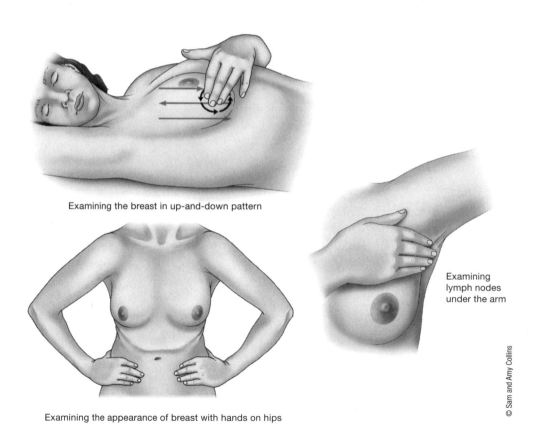

Examining the breast in up-and-down pattern

Examining lymph nodes under the arm

Examining the appearance of breast with hands on hips

© Sam and Amy Collins

- Repeat the examination on your left breast, putting your left arm behind your head and using the finger pads of your right hand to do the examination.
- Stand in front of a mirror with your hands pressing firmly down on your hips, and look at your breasts for any changes in size, shape, contour, dimpling, or redness or scaliness of the nipple or breast skin. Pressing down on the hips contracts the muscles of the chest wall and enhances any breast changes.
- Examine each underarm while sitting or standing and with your arm only slightly raised. Raising your arm straight up tightens the tissue in this area and makes it harder to examine.

If you notice any of the following changes, see a doctor or nurse as soon as possible:
- development of a lump or swelling in your breast or underarm area
- skin irritation or dimpling
- nipple pain or retraction (turning inward)
- redness or scaliness of the nipple or breast skin
- a spontaneous nipple discharge other than breast milk

Ask your doctor or nurse to teach you how to do breast self-examination or to watch your technique to be sure you are doing it correctly. Also, talk to your doctor or nurse if you are having trouble checking a breast that was treated with radiation or has been reconstructed. Your breast will feel different than it did before, and they can help you understand what is normal in the treated area.

Questions to Ask Your Medical Team About Breast Care After Cancer

- How often will I need to have mammograms after my treatment ends? (Be sure to ask about both the unaffected breast and the affected breast—the schedules might be different.)
- Do I need to have any other tests done with my mammograms? How about an MRI?
- What happens if something is found on a mammogram?
- Whom do I contact to get my mammogram results or if I have a problem getting them?
- Who should perform the clinical breast examination?
- What should I look for when I'm examining my own breasts?
- If I notice something different with my breasts, how should I contact you to discuss it with you? (By phone, by appointment, by e-mail?)

Maintaining Your Health and Making Positive Lifestyle Changes

Following a healthy diet, exercising, reducing your intake of alcohol, and quitting smoking can help speed your recovery and even reduce your future cancer risk. An improved lifestyle can benefit your family, too. As you make healthier eating choices in your own diet, you can also help your family eat better. You can also model positive lifestyle behaviors, such as exercising regularly. Your behavior might lead family members to follow suit, lowering their cancer risk.

Nutrition, Breast Cancer, and General Health and Wellness

Nutrition plays an important role in the management of cancer. In fact, research has suggested that people who eat well during cancer treatment can better manage the side effects of treatment. Proper nutrition can also help you stay at a healthy weight, which, along with regular physical activity, may reduce the risk of recurrence, as well as the risk of another cancer.

Even after your treatment ends, nutrition continues to play an important role in maintaining your strength and overall well-being. Fruits and vegetables contain a wide variety of helpful substances. Researchers have identified some of these vitamins and other compounds, but many remain unknown. Taking in nutrients and vitamins naturally by eating these foods is better than using dietary supplements.

A healthy, balanced diet can not only help reduce your risk for certain cancers, but it is also good for your general health. It can help prevent other conditions, too, such as heart disease, osteoporosis, and diabetes.

Maintaining a Healthy Weight

For a woman who has had breast cancer, getting to and/or staying at a healthy weight might be one of the most important things she can do. Studies have found that women who are overweight or obese when they first receive their diagnoses are more likely to have their disease come back and are more likely to die of breast cancer.

Excess weight increases levels of estrogen and insulin in the blood, which can stimulate cancer cell growth, so eating well and staying physically active should be an important part of your wellness plan. If you are overweight, create a plan with your doctor to lose weight after treatment.

Limit your intake of foods that are high in saturated fat: Studies of the relationship between dietary fat and breast cancer survival suggest that low levels of fat in the diet might be linked to lower recurrence rates and better survival, but this is not certain. Still, diets high in saturated fat (found in red meat and full-fat dairy products) tend to be high in calories, too, and this might add to obesity.

Most of the fat in your diet should come from monounsaturated sources such as olive or canola oil, avocados, and nuts and seeds—not from animal sources. Selecting nonfat and low-fat products such as skim milk or low-fat yogurt is a healthy step. You can also try replacing butter or lard with healthier vegetable oils whenever possible. If you are eating packaged, snack, or restaurant foods, try to look for low-fat versions. Don't forget, however, that a lot of fat-free cakes, cookies, snack foods, and desserts are still high in calories. If you do eat high-fat foods, try to limit your portion size, because foods high in fat also tend to be high in calories.

Limit your intake of red meats, especially processed meats (such as hot dogs, bacon, and deli meats) and those high in fat. Instead, focus on foods rich in omega-3 fatty acids, such as fish. If you do eat red meat, consider eating lean cuts in smaller portions and using meat as a side dish rather than the main dish. Beans, seafood, and poultry can also be healthier alternatives to beef, pork, and lamb. Preparation methods are important, too. Baking and broiling rather than frying reduces the overall amount of fat in food.

Choose most of the food you eat from plant sources: Try to eat at least two and one-half cups of fruits and vegetables a day. Studies suggest that a higher intake of vegetables may have a helpful effect on recurrence or survival for breast cancer, but this is not definite. Scientists do not know which of the compounds in vegetables and fruits are most protective, so the best advice is to eat different kinds of colorful vegetables and fruits each day.

Foods from plant sources tend to be high in fiber, and although the relationship between dietary fiber and breast cancer is not clear, a diet high in fiber might reduce estrogen levels, which might in turn reduce the risk for recurrence. Fruits and vegetables are also rich in vitamins and minerals and are either entirely fat-free or low in fat. Although fruits and vegetables are an essential part of a healthy diet, most people don't eat enough of them. It's easy to make these plant sources a part of your normal eating routine by substituting them for other snacks and including them in every meal. This will help you reach the recommended amount of two and one-half cups or more per day.

Try to eat other foods from plant sources, too, such as breads, cereals, grain products, rice, pasta, or beans. A healthy diet should focus on whole grain, plant-based foods. Eating whole grains is better for your health than refined (processed) grains. Whole grains are higher in fiber and certain vitamins and minerals than refined flour products.

Beans are excellent sources of vitamins, minerals, protein, and fiber. They are especially rich in nutrients that may protect against cancer and can be a useful low-fat, high-protein alternative to meat. Although soy products get a lot of attention, there is conflicting scientific evidence about whether they might be beneficial or harmful for women with breast cancer. Until more is known, the American Cancer Society recommends that women who have been treated for breast cancer consume soy as part of a healthy plant-based diet, and avoid high levels of soy found in pills, powders, or supplements.

Given the high level of interest in the relationship between foods and specific cancers, nutritional research gets a lot of publicity. No one study is the last word on any subject, and it is easy to become confused by what seems to be contradictory or conflicting advice. These stories often do not put new research in its proper context. It is rarely, if ever, advisable to change your diet based on a single study or news report, especially if the data are reported as "preliminary." The best advice is to follow the American Cancer Society guidelines, talk with your doctor before you make any major dietary changes, and use common sense.

American Cancer Society Guidelines on Nutrition and Physical Activity for Cancer Survivors

Achieve and maintain a healthy weight.
- If overweight or obese, limit consumption of high-calorie foods and beverages and increase physical activity to promote weight loss.

Engage in regular physical activity.
- Avoid inactivity and return to normal daily activities as soon as possible following diagnosis.
- Aim to exercise at least 150 minutes per week.
- Include strength training exercises at least two days per week.

Achieve a dietary pattern that is high in vegetables, fruits, and whole grains.
- Follow the American Cancer Society Guidelines on Nutrition and Physical Activity for Cancer Prevention (see page 441).

Physical Activity

Regular physical activity offers many benefits and can be especially helpful for women who have had cancer treatment. If you exercise regularly and build muscle tissue, your stamina and muscle strength will increase, giving you more energy—something you might be lacking after cancer treatment. Exercise helps you get to or stay at a healthy weight, too. It strengthens your heart and improves circulation while elevating your mood, which can help you live not only a healthier life but also a happier one.

Moderate exercise can help you fight fatigue and keep your muscles in good condition. Stretching, yoga, walking, and swimming are a few kinds of exercise that can help combat fatigue. Regular exercise can also help improve the range of motion in joints like your shoulder, which can be diminished after surgery. Good range of motion is essential to preserving general physical strength.

Not all the positive effects of exercise can be seen and felt. Exercise also benefits your mind and your emotional state. Regular exercise can carry emotional benefits such as helping you feel relaxed and optimistic. It might help combat depression, too. Exercise has a calming effect on many people.

For many people, exercise provides a sense of accomplishment and control. It might improve your sense of being in touch with your body. Taking on a challenging activity might also move you beyond changes in your body. You might find it gives you renewed self-worth, not to mention stronger muscles, a fit body, and more energy.

Aerobic exercise (such as walking, jogging, cycling, and swimming) increases the blood flow to your heart and the amount of oxygen your lungs take in. Regular aerobic exercise can lower your blood cholesterol level, strengthen your bones, increase your metabolism, and increase your endurance. Aerobic exercise might also improve immune function when done in moderation.

Some form of weight training (anaerobic exercise) is generally recommended along with aerobic exercise to preserve lean body mass and maintain strength and freedom of movement. Anaerobic exercise is essential for developing muscles, strength, speed, and power. It involves short bursts of intense activity such as weightlifting or sprinting. However, be sure to talk to your doctor before engaging in any weight-bearing activities—there may be special precautions you should take or certain exercises you should avoid.

The American Cancer Society recommends that adults get at least 150 minutes of moderate-intensity activity or 75 minutes of vigorous-intensity activity, or an equivalent combination, each week. This activity should preferably be spread throughout the week. You can accomplish this goal by walking briskly (three to four miles per hour), jogging, swimming, gardening, doing housework, or dancing at a level of intensity equivalent to brisk walking. However, doing any physical activity above your usual activities can have many health benefits.

Which exercises are best for you and how to get started: It is important to talk with your doctor before starting any exercise program, especially if you are restarting after a long break or if you have never exercised regularly. If you have never exercised or have been inactive for a while, you need to start slowly. You might want to start by walking five to ten minutes several times a day and work your way up from there. Over time, your endurance and stamina will increase. When exercising, try to maintain a positive attitude; set reasonable, reachable goals; and stick to a regular schedule.

Your ideal exercise program should combine aerobic and anaerobic exercises. For example, if you enjoy a half-hour walk every day (aerobic), you might add a light strength-training session two or three times a week (anaerobic). Warming up your muscles helps prepare them for exercise. Briefly stretch the muscles in your arms, legs, and the rest of your body. As circulation to the muscles increases, pick up the pace. Toward the end of your workout, slow down your exercise movements gradually. This cooling-down period allows your muscles to relax and helps prevent cramps. You should always stretch before and after you exercise.

Your doctor should be able to recommend an exercise professional or physical therapist to help you get started. You can also check with your local YMCA or American Heart Association for suggestions. Be sure you tell exercise instructors about your history of breast cancer treatment. This way, they can be sure you do exercises that are appropriate and safe. You might want to ask your doctor about the physical activities listed here and whether they're right for you.

Walking: Most people can start walking right away. Walking is an excellent exercise for people with cancer because it increases lung function, stimulates bone growth, and strengthens leg and back muscles. It is a safer alternative to running because it does not jar the joints. If you are concerned about putting strain on your joints, you can walk in a swimming pool and still stimulate your heart and lungs, building endurance.

Swimming: Swimming is a fun way to get aerobic exercise. It is not stressful to your joints, and, if you swim far and fast enough, you will increase your aerobic capacity. Swimming stretches your muscles and increases the amount of air you inhale and exhale. It also strengthens your muscles as you move against the water's resistance.

Strength training: Strength training by lifting weights (or using weight resistance machines) is sometimes recommended for people with cancer because it helps build muscle and bone. Women who have been treated for breast cancer are at higher risk for lymphedema, so you should start a strength-training program under the supervision of a doctor or physical therapist. Consider seeking out an experienced trainer who understands the needs and possible limitations of women who have had breast cancer.

Stretching and yoga: Stretching and yoga promote flexibility and relieve muscle tension. Stretching and yoga are gentle movements designed to extend and tone muscles that may have become shortened because of prolonged inactivity. Stretching also produces a feeling of well-being and increases blood circulation.

Physical limitations and conditions: If you exercised before your cancer diagnosis, you can probably go back to it after treatment, depending on the type of treatment you had. But avoid intense exertion. You don't want muscle strain or extreme fatigue.

Before you start an exercise program, take into account your preferences and physical health so that you can tailor your program to your needs. Pushing yourself too hard might be discouraging or even harmful and can end up making you feel worse. Know, too, that some types of treatment affect physical ability; for example, some chemotherapy drugs might affect organs in ways that limit physical activity. Make sure that you talk with your doctor and understand the types of exercise that are best for you right now and how active you can be without overdoing it. Listen to your body when exercising. Watch for signs that you are overexerting yourself, and be conscious of conditions that make certain activities inappropriate for you.

Dehydration: Never exercise in extreme heat, and always drink plenty of fluids. If you sweat a lot, you might want to try a sports drink that will replace your electrolytes (salt and potassium).

Bone stress: People with cancer are at special risk for bone fractures. If your cancer has spread to the bone, strength training is not recommended for you. You also should avoid activities like basketball, tennis, or jogging, which can be stressful to your joints.

Anemia: Anemia can make you feel very tired and short of breath, so if you are anemic, you may want to avoid physical activity that is tough on your body, such as running or aerobic step classes. Walking and yoga might be easier for you.

Nerve damage: If your brain or nerves have been affected and you are unsteady or have decreased feeling in your hands or feet, do not exercise by yourself. You might want to plan walks with a friend. You could also see a physiatrist or physical therapist to learn ways of dealing with your particular situation.

Advanced illness: Some form of physical activity is beneficial to everyone, even someone confined to bed. Range-of-motion exercises and general stretching can be done in bed. In fact, pain medicine combined with stretching exercises is one of the best solutions for keeping comfortable when confined to bed.

Physical activity will help you maintain mobility and relieve muscle tension, providing a temporary psychological boost. Talk with your medical team about what exercise program might be best for you.

Smoking

Studies have suggested a link between smoking and breast cancer, but this is still not certain. Still, smoking damages overall health and increases one's risk of heart disease, stroke, and other cancers. Do not use any form of tobacco, and avoid secondhand smoke. If you use tobacco and need help quitting, contact the American Cancer Society at 800-227-2345. Getting help increases your chances of quitting and staying tobacco-free.

Alcohol

Drinking alcohol increases the risk of breast cancer, as well as cancers of the mouth, esophagus, pharynx, larynx, liver, rectum, and colon. Cancer risk increases with the amount of alcohol consumed. The American Cancer Society recommends that women limit their intake to no more than one drink a day.

You can take an active role in making sure that the quality of your life is as good as or even better than it was before your cancer diagnosis. You might have suffered some difficult blows to your finances, your career, or your love life, and you have endured physical hardships during treatment, but your most important goal right now is moving forward and facing the future.

Remember, wellness is more than just the lack of illness. As you plan for a future of wellness, you can take small, measurable steps toward healthy habits. In the next chapter, we discuss ways to work toward emotional and spiritual health after cancer.

For more information on nutrition and physical activity related to cancer recurrence, see chapter 22.

CHAPTER 20

Emotional Wellness After Treatment: Moving On

In the previous chapter, we talked about building a wellness plan for your future. Looking after your body is an important part of wellness after cancer. But do not neglect your mind and soul. Being healthy means actively pursuing wellness in all parts of your life.

Once treatment is finished, you may find that you are ready to focus on your emotional recovery. Most women with breast cancer have mixed feelings about the end of treatment—another time of transition and changing routines. During the period of diagnosis and treatment, you established a routine for clinic visits and medical appointments and developed relationships with your medical team. Things that may have seemed extremely disruptive at first soon became an ordinary part of life. Visiting your doctor reminded you that your health was being monitored. This routine might have become familiar and even comforting and reassuring.

It might be hard for you to explain to others your uncertain feelings about the end of treatment, especially when people tend to view this as a time of celebration and victory. But like riding a bicycle for the first time without training wheels, you might find yourself worrying about potential falls. Give yourself time. You will work through these challenges in your own way.

Life After Breast Cancer

Each woman has her own way of coping with life after breast cancer, and the best method is the one that works for you. Many women find it helps to talk about their feelings with other women who have had breast cancer. Some find comfort in talking with friends or joining support groups. Some draw strength from solitude, taking long walks, meditating, listening to music, or soaking in the tub. This is a time to rebuild a positive self-image, make new plans, and reestablish priorities. Many of your fears and concerns will fade as you return to routine activities and start making plans and setting goals for the future.

In the previous chapter, we talked about creating a wellness plan—a set of health-minded and life-enriching goals you set for yourself. Just as you can set goals for yourself in regards to nutrition and physical activity, you can set goals for your mental health and spiritual life. In this chapter, we discuss ways to deal with some of the mental and emotional reactions you may have to finishing cancer treatment.

> ### Getting on with Your Life After Treatment
>
> Consider the following tips for getting on with your life after treatment ends:
>
> - **Celebrate.** You've made it through treatment!
> - **Reward yourself.** Do something special just for you. Get a massage or a manicure, take a walk in beautiful surroundings, or use some quiet time to relax.
> - **Take one day at a time,** and make sure to cherish everything around you.
> - **Let your loved ones know how much they mean to you.** Tell all the people who have supported you how much their thoughtfulness and caring have helped. This expression of gratitude will make you feel better, too.
>
> Now is the time to reassess what is truly special in your life. Put your priorities in order.

Feeling Alone

After treatment ends, you may miss the support and attention you got from your medical team. The family and friends who were there to support you during treatment might not be as present when treatment ends. For many weeks, you have had many different people telling you what to do. You may suddenly feel like you are facing the future alone.

Seek Support When You Need It

As during all other stages of your illness and treatment, it can be helpful to talk about your feelings, whether to a close friend, family member, chaplain, doctor, nurse, social worker, psychologist, or support group. When you share your feelings, you might find that you come away with a renewed spirit, awareness that you are not alone, and feeling better informed and hopeful.

Some women find support groups particularly helpful. In support and self-help groups, you can share knowledge and strategies that can promote effective coping. A support group gives you the chance to express your concerns with other women who have experienced this disease. For many women, a support group offers a safe place to say negative things, too—a place to let down the brave front that others might expect from you.

Support groups can have many social and emotional benefits, and they are not just for people undergoing cancer treatment. Research has shown that joining a support group improves quality of life and enhances survival. Some support groups are for women only, for breast cancer "survivors" only, or for those whose breast cancer has recurred. Some support groups meet face-to-face; others meet online. If you enjoy being part of a group, are ready to talk about your cancer experience, and would like to offer or listen to advice on coping with cancer from others who have "been there," you might benefit from a support group.

Revisit chapter 5 for more information on building your support network, including information on the American Cancer Society's Reach To Recovery program and the American Cancer Society Cancer Survivors Network®. The resource guide starting on page 443 also has more information on organizations that can offer support.

Improving Quality of Life

Come up with a list of things to do that would improve your overall quality of life. These might be things you always wanted to do that you never quite got around to doing. Now that you've faced a serious illness, these things might seem more important to you. Consider the following examples:

- Eat dinner as a family three nights a week—no TV in the background!
- Call my mother once a week.
- Volunteer at the community garden one Saturday a month.
- Learn to knit.
- Travel to a foreign country.
- Take an hour of "me time" once a week to do whatever I want.

Staying Emotionally Healthy

After dealing with breast cancer, you may feel mentally and emotionally weary. Your emotional state affects you on a daily basis and affects the choices you make, too. There are may ways to boost your emotional well-being.

Keep a Sense of Humor

A good laugh can dissolve both physical and emotional tension. Laughter is an activity (along with sex and exercise) that causes the release of endorphins, the body's natural opiates.

Nourish Your Mind

Read a book, enroll in a class, pick up a new hobby, or resume an old one.

Express Yourself

Try drawing or painting, writing in a journal, singing, dancing, or pursuing some other creative activity to channel your emotions.

Make Time for Yourself

Set aside time to focus on meeting your own emotional needs.

Do Nice Things for Yourself

So often, we equate being good to ourselves with buying things. But you can treat yourself without spending a lot of money. Check out books from the library, rent or download a funny video, feed ducks at the lake, ask your partner to give you a foot massage, or take a hot bath.

Let Some Things Go

Let go of old, rigid ways of living. Turn your back on trying to be perfect. If the house isn't in tip-top shape, say, "Who cares?" Learning to let go helps reduce stress.

Choose Your Battles

Decide what really matters, and let go of the small stuff.

Confide in Someone

It helps to confide in someone who can handle whatever emotions you might express. Find someone you feel completely safe with—a partner, friend, sister, religious leader, or counselor—and really let it all out.

Tap into Your Faith

Every religion offers comfort to help endure life's trials. You might want to join a prayer group or take a class at your house of worship. It can also help to read inspirational books and/or scripture. Find favorite prayers and say them often.

Set Limits

Take an inventory of your work duties, household tasks, and social commitments, and then set some limits. Cut back on activities and commitments until you are doing only the things that matter most and bring the most rewards.

Dealing with Stress

After your diagnosis, you may have put certain issues aside for a while, such as concerns about family, work, or finances. Now that treatment is over, these issues will begin to resurface—when you are too tired or might feel that there is already too much to handle. There is no research showing that stress causes cancer, but stress can cause other health problems. Finding ways to reduce or control the stress in your life will help you feel better.

Exercise

Exercise is a known way to reduce stress and feel less tense—whether you've had cancer or not. See your doctor before making an exercise plan, and be careful not to overdo it.

Dance or Movement

People can act out their feelings about cancer in classes using dramatic and/or dance-style body movements. Other class members talk about the issues the "performer" was trying to express.

Sharing Personal Stories

Telling and hearing stories about living with cancer can help people learn, solve problems, feel more hopeful, air concerns, and find meaning in what they have been through.

Music and Art

Even people who have never sung, painted, or drawn before can find these activities helpful, relaxing, and fun.

Dealing with Depression and Anxiety

After treatment, you might still feel angry, tense, sad, or blue. For most people, these feelings go away or lessen over time. But for up to one in four people, these emotions can become severe. If these painful feelings do not improve, and they get in the way of your daily life, you might be suffering from clinical depression. Sometimes cancer treatment even contributes to this problem by changing the chemicals in the brain.

Women who have dealt with breast cancer do not appear to be at increased risk for developing severe depression compared with the general population. But if you do feel very depressed, ask your health care provider for a referral to a mental health professional. Make sure it is someone who is knowledgeable about the effects of cancer and cancer treatment.

Strengthening Your Spirit

Dealing with a serious illness can affect a person's spiritual outlook, regardless of whether that person feels connected to traditional religious beliefs. People who have been treated for cancer often report that cancer causes them to look at their faith or their spirituality in new ways. For some, it might get stronger or seem more vital. Others may question their beliefs.

After treatment, you and your loved ones might struggle to understand why cancer came into your lives. You might wonder why you had to endure such a trial. At the same time, many people find that their faith, religion, or spirituality is a source of strength as they face life after cancer treatment. Many say that through their faith, they have been able to find meaning in their lives and make sense of their cancer experience.

Faith or religion can also be a way for people who have had cancer to connect to others in their community who might share similar experiences or perspective or who can provide support. Religious gatherings can offer a social outlet and be a valuable source of support through a trying time. For some, religion also can be an important part of both coping with and recovering from cancer.

The way cancer affects one's faith or religion is different for everyone. Some turn away from their religion because they feel it has deserted them. For others, seeking answers and searching for meaning in spirituality helps them cope.

Consider the following ways you might find comfort and meaning through your faith or religion:

- read spiritual materials that are uplifting and can help you feel connected to a higher power
- pray or meditate
- talk about your concerns or fears with a spiritual leader
- attend religious gatherings to meet new people
- talk with others at your place of worship who have had similar experiences

- find resources at a community center or place of worship for people dealing with illnesses such as cancer

Channeling Your Energy

Women who have dealt with breast cancer often express the need to understand what the experience means to their lives now. In fact, many find that cancer causes them to look at life in new ways. They might reflect on the purpose of life and what they value most. Many women find a surprising and positive aspect of the otherwise difficult and painful experience of having breast cancer: they come through it with a new wisdom and strength and, in many cases, the resolve to help others.

You have probably been thankful for the laws and services that exist to help women with breast cancer. These measures have been brought about by others' time, energy, and/or donations—people who care about the issue of breast cancer and the women who have it. You have benefited from the efforts of other women who had breast cancer and the efforts of their loved ones. Now, as you evaluate the priorities in your personal life, you might want to consider giving back to others. There are a number of ways you can make a difference in your own life and the lives of other people with cancer.

Volunteering

You needed others' help to get through your breast cancer diagnosis and treatment, and now you may be able to help others. Although you might not want to dedicate your life to eradicating breast cancer, you can apply your knowledge and experience in plenty of ways. Something as simple as looking for opportunities at work can make a difference. For example, one woman with breast cancer used her job as a pharmacist to make sure no one would suffer through breast cancer alone as she had—she put a Reach To Recovery information card in with every tamoxifen prescription she dispensed.

Why Volunteer

Volunteers are the backbone of many services for people who have cancer. They make possible much of the progress that nonprofits and other organizations make toward their goals. You might want to volunteer to show your commitment to a cause or belief or to have an impact. You might want to learn new skills, gain valuable work experience, increase awareness, or help save lives. Volunteering for others can help you stay active, maintain social connections and friendships, and feel valued and needed.

Where to Volunteer

When you consider where you might want to volunteer, think about your interests, skills, goals, and time. There are volunteer opportunities all around you. Hospitals, libraries, and churches regularly need volunteers, as do daycare centers; schools; halfway houses; community theaters; drug and alcohol rehabilitation centers; retirement centers and homes for older persons; Meals on Wheels; museums, art galleries, and monuments; prisons; neighborhood parks; youth organizations, sports teams, and after-school programs; shelters for battered women and children; and historical restoration groups.

Your skills can also help determine where to volunteer. If you enjoy talking to others, working in the garden, setting up websites, or teaching, for example, you might want to volunteer in a capacity that uses these skills. If you would like to learn new skills, you might seek out an opportunity where you could be trained in new skills or learn new skills on the job.

If you already donate to an organization, you might want to explore volunteer opportunities there. If you are interested in a cause and cannot find an organization that addresses it, you might start one yourself. That's how organizations begin. With enthusiasm, time, and effort, you can make the changes you envision.

You may be looking for an experience that's different from any you've had before, and you would like to find an organization that works with other cultures or other socioeconomic groups' concerns. Consider whether you want a long-term assignment or a temporary project. You might also want to begin working for an organization a few hours at a time until you get a feel for whether it is a good fit.

If you want to volunteer with any of the cancer programs and services listed in the back of this book, contact the organization for specific information and opportunities.

Advocating for Change

By being an advocate for people with cancer and supporting cancer-friendly legislation, you can bring about change and make a valuable contribution to the fight against cancer. There are several things you can do to advocate for change:

- Communicate with lawmakers and policymakers. Policymakers at all levels of government make decisions every day that affect the lives of millions of people who have had cancer, their loved ones, and all people who might receive a cancer diagnosis some day. To find out what legislation is currently in process, you can contact the American Cancer Society (800-227-2345 or www.cancer.org) or the

American Cancer Society Cancer Action Network (www.acscan.org). To look up and contact your state and federal legislators, visit www.usa.gov.

- Keep cancer issues in the media. You can help by writing to newspapers, magazines, and websites about cancer-related issues and participating in radio, television, and web-based call-in programs.
- Support cancer-related initiatives. The American Cancer Society and other organizations work on many fronts to fight cancer. Go to www.cancer.org to learn more about American Cancer Society efforts and the American Cancer Society Cancer Action Network.
- Talk about the issues and encourage others to join the fight. Make sure your family, friends, and coworkers know about cancer-related legislation and encourage them to get involved in supporting such legislation. Start a blog, "phone tree," or e-mail list to alert friends and coworkers as cancer-related legislation moves through the process.

Facing Your Future

Sometimes, having cancer causes people to take stock of their lives. You might find that you do not worry as much about minor problems anymore and that you are rearranging your priorities. For example, maybe now you let the housework go and work less so you can spend more time with loved ones. You might see the importance of your work, pleasure, and relationships in new ways and begin weeding out trivial distractions and superficial people.

You may find that you are more optimistic now, more independent-minded, and more compassionate. You may be more confident and proud of yourself. You may also emerge from your fight against cancer more assertive and braver than ever, and you may dare to take chances you would not have considered before your cancer diagnosis.

People who have faced cancer share a unique understanding of time and the desire to make every day count. Before you find yourself immersed in daily commitments and routines, with your resolutions in danger of fading into the background, write down the goals most important to your happiness and satisfaction. Use your newfound energy to take stock of your life and reevaluate your goals and desires, then resolve to take steps to achieve them.

You may have once believed that you would always have enough time to do what you wanted, so you were in no rush to change anything. Cancer may have robbed you of these blissful beliefs, but in return, it can present you with the realization that your life has meaning and that each day is a precious gift to be spent wisely. Making each day count is up to you.

CHAPTER 21

Intimacy After Cancer Treatment

In chapter 13, we discussed how cancer treatment can affect fertility and sexuality. Now that you have finished your treatment, you may be thinking about resuming the level of physical intimacy you enjoyed before treatment—the level of intimacy you will hope to maintain for years to come.

Reestablishing Intimacy with Your Partner

Many women need time to reestablish the physical and emotional intimacy they had with their partner before their cancer diagnosis. The love between a woman and her partner and the desire to be intimate can survive cancer treatment—even growing deeper because of it. If you were sexually active before your cancer diagnosis, you can be sexually active now. Most women can have fulfilling sexual experiences after cancer treatment.

You or your partner might be reluctant to make love, and you both might need time to get used to being physical again. It is important for both of you to take the time you need to get comfortable with any changes that have taken place. It is also important that you communicate your needs to each other.

Cancer and its treatment can change your appearance and how you feel about yourself, and it can affect your sexual desire. Some treatments for breast cancer, such as chemotherapy and hormone therapy, can change a woman's hormone levels and can negatively affect sexual interest and response. Physical changes to your breast or body after treatment can lead to concerns about resuming sexual activity. Hair loss, discomfort, disability, changes to your body, and skin changes can affect your sense of sexual attractiveness. And, although you know that sexiness is about more than just anatomy, if you feel unattractive, you are more likely to avoid being physical with your partner.

Keep in mind that your partner might be afraid to appear overeager and insensitive to your situation. You might need to be the one to show a desire to be physically intimate and tell your partner when you are interested in hugging, touching, kissing, and making love.

After treatment—especially surgery—it is common for both women and their partners to be concerned about how to express their love physically and emotionally. In this chapter, we give some suggestions to cope with your post-treatment frame of mind and health status.

Adjusting to Body Changes

The keys to feeling good about yourself and having a positive self-image after treatment are focusing on your positive features, your energy, and your sense of well-being. Becoming comfortable with your body again after treatment can be an important part of this process. Some psychologists suggest the following mirror exercise to help you adjust to body changes.

Find a time when you have privacy for at least fifteen minutes. Be sure to take enough time to really think about how you look. Try this exercise first dressed, then in more intimate clothing, and, finally, nude.

- Study yourself for at least fifteen minutes, using the largest mirror you have. What parts of your body do you look at most? What do you avoid looking at? Do you catch yourself having negative thoughts about the way you look? What are your best features? Has cancer or its treatment changed the way you look?
- What do you see when you look at yourself in the mirror? Many people notice only what they dislike about their looks. When they look in the mirror, they see pale skin, hair loss, or skinny legs. They fail to see a classic profile, expressive eyes, or a nice smile.
- First, try this exercise when dressed as a stranger on the street would see you. If you normally wear clothing or special accessories to disguise any body changes caused by cancer treatment, wear them during the mirror exercise. Practice this two or three times or until you can look in the mirror and see at least three positive things about your looks.
- Once you are comfortable seeing yourself as a stranger might see you, try the mirror exercise when dressed as you'd like to look for your partner. For example,

you may want to wear a sexy nightgown. Look at yourself for a few minutes, repeating the steps in the first mirror exercise. What's most attractive and sexy about you? Pay yourself at least three compliments on how you look.

- Finally, try the mirror exercise in the nude, without disguising any changes made by the cancer. If you have trouble looking at a scar, bare scalp, or missing breast, take enough time to get used to looking at the area. The changes to your body may seem ugly at first, but with time, you will become more comfortable with them. They are part of you now. If you feel tense while looking at yourself, take a deep breath and try to relax all your muscles as you exhale. Do not stop the exercise until you have found three positive features, or at least remember the three compliments you paid yourself before.

The mirror exercise might help you feel more relaxed when your partner looks at you. Ask your partner to tell you things that are positive about the way you look or how you feel. Tell him or her that these positive responses will help you feel better about yourself. Remember them when you are feeling unsure of yourself. This might help you become comfortable with intimacy again.

Sexuality

You might have lost interest in sex during cancer treatment, at least for a time. Many women find that they are not interested in sex during treatment. After all, you are dealing with the effects of cancer and cancer treatment. Sex can be far down on your list of needs right now.

Cancer treatment can affect your emotional attitude toward sex and cause side effects that have an impact on your ability to have or fully enjoy sex. However, these feelings are usually temporary.

How Depression Can Affect Sexuality

Some women find it difficult to adjust to life after treatment and become depressed, which in turn affects sexuality. Staying physically active is one good way to reduce stress and reduce your risk of becoming depressed. As long as you do not overdo it, exercise will help you feel healthy and more energized during and after treatment. Ask your doctor about the kinds of exercise that are right for you.

If depression lasts more than a couple of weeks, talk to your doctor. What doctors call clinical depression can have several symptoms. These include the following:

- lack of interest in sex or other things that usually give you pleasure
- being unable to feel pleasure at all
- problems sleeping
- changes in eating habits (besides those related to cancer treatment)
- fatigue or tiredness (besides tiredness caused by cancer treatment)
- trouble concentrating
- feeling worthless and hopeless

Depression can be treated with medicine, counseling, and other methods that can improve your sleep, appetite, energy, and ability to feel pleasure. In turn, this can help your self-esteem and desire for sex. Talk with your doctor if you think you might be depressed.

If you are given medicine to treat depression, be aware that some antidepressants, such as selective serotonin reuptake inhibitors (SSRIs), can make it harder to reach orgasm. If this is a problem for you, talk with your doctor about it. Other antidepressants might not have this effect.

Getting Back on Track with Your Partner

The most important part of keeping a healthy sexual relationship with a partner is good communication. Many people react to cancer by withdrawing. Each feels their partner will feel burdened if they share their fears or sadness. But when you try to protect each other, you both suffer in silence. No couple gets through cancer diagnosis and treatment without some anxiety and grief.

Learning and talking about each other's thoughts and feelings can lead to physical intimacy, just as physical closeness can lead to emotional intimacy. Expressing your needs openly and honestly will help both the physical and emotional aspects of your relationship. Good communication is the basis for a fulfilling sex life. Establishing trust, respect, and understanding in this area will help you through this process.

If your partner has been depressed and distant, you might be afraid that a sexual advance will come across as a demand. You can bring up the topic of sex in a healthy, assertive way. It is usually not helpful to accuse ("You never touch me anymore!") or demand ("We have to have sex soon. I can't stand the frustration."). Instead, try to state your feelings in a positive way. ("I really miss our sex life. What's getting in the way of our touching?")

Many couples believe that sex should always happen on the spur of the moment, with little or no advance planning. But sometimes you are dealing with a cancer-related change or treatment side effect that makes it impossible to be as spontaneous as you would have been in the past. The most important thing is to start the discussion and ensure that you have some relaxed time together, which can mean scheduling that time. Couples need to restart their lovemaking slowly. When you feel ready to try sexual touching with your partner, start with plenty of time and privacy. Plan for a time when you are not too tired and any pain is well controlled. Try creating a relaxed environment. For example, you could light the room with candles or put on some soft, romantic music. Although you might feel a little shy, let your partner know that you would like to have some time to be physically close. You could even make a date for this purpose. You might say, "I feel ready for sex again, but I'd like to take things slowly. Would you be in the mood tonight to try a little touching? I can't promise that it will go perfectly, but we can have fun trying."

Tips for Rebuilding Self-Esteem and Intimacy

Consider the following tips for rebuilding self-esteem and intimacy:

- **Come to terms with changes** in your body and body image by looking at and touching yourself, seeking others' support when you need it, seeking intimacy after treatment, and openly communicating your feelings, needs, and wants.
- **Find support groups for couples** dealing with cancer, which can be helpful even with intimacy problems. Sympathetic and experienced confidantes can offer you practical and tested guidance. Women who have discovered how to maintain or recapture closeness and intimacy throughout their cancer diagnosis and treatment may be able to help as you work toward restoring intimacy with your partner.
- **Be patient with yourself.** Many women who have had their breasts altered or removed find that their biggest struggle is coming to terms with the emotional impact of these changes. Some women cope better by reminding themselves that a woman does not need breasts to live well. You don't need a breast to breathe, eat, walk, talk, or have sex. The process of dealing with a change to your body takes time.
- **Explore your fears about intimacy** with your partner. This is usually the best way to overcome them. If you admit that you feel uncertain and insecure, it is more likely that you will get support and affection to help you lay your doubts to rest.
- **Feel free to be open, candid, and honest** with yourself and others about how you're feeling.

Many couples don't talk much about sex. But after cancer treatment, your sexual routine might need to change. This is not the time to let embarrassment silence you; you and your partner need to communicate openly. Be sure to let your partner know—either in words or by guiding with your hand—the kind of touching you enjoy. Try to express your desires in a positive way. For example, you might say, "You have the right place, but I'd like you to use a light touch," rather than "Ouch—that's too rough!" Wait to have sex until you both feel emotionally and physically ready for it.

If you have pain or feel weak from cancer treatment, you might want to try new sexual positions. Many couples find a favorite position and rarely try a different one. After cancer treatment, though, other positions might be more comfortable. No one position is right for everyone. Have fun with your partner, experimenting to find what's best for you. Pillows can help provide support. A good sense of humor can come in handy, too.

Rekindling the Flame

You might not have had any interest in sex lately. But almost everyone has sexual thoughts every now and then, even if sometimes we ignore or forget about them. Your sexual thoughts can be used to improve your sex life.

Writing down any sexual thoughts you have might help you recall what you find sexually exciting or stimulating. Designate a notebook or journal as your "Desire Diary." Every day for a week, take it with you wherever you go. Whenever you have a sexual thought or feeling, write it down, along with the time of day you had the thought and whether you were alone or with someone else at the time. If you do anything about the thought, write that down, too. Sometimes just keeping track of your desires will make the number of sexual thoughts and feelings that you notice grow. Maybe you mainly think about sex when you are relaxed at night, or when you are at work, or when you wake up in the morning. Once you have noted some patterns, you can work at recreating this sexual mood.

You might feel more sexual after you exercise, during a relaxed evening out with your partner, or when you make a special effort to look and feel sexy. Think about the things that helped get you into a sexy mood before cancer. Try looking at erotic pictures, reading erotica, or watching a movie with a romantic or sexual plot. Fantasize about a sexual encounter. Picture the scene as you would like it to be. How can you make your daydream come true? Although you can work at feeling more sexual by yourself, at some point you will want your partner's help. Discuss any fears either of you has about

Desire Diary

You might increase your sexual desire if you recognize the thoughts you are already having. Jot down your sexual thoughts and when and where you were when they came to you. Note anything about the situation that made you feel excited about sex, and make note of what you'd like to incorporate into your physical intimacy with your partner. Write down as many details as you want.

- What were your most frequent sexual thoughts? Jot down the situations and events you found arousing.
- Where were you when you had these thoughts? At work? At home? Daydreaming in the car? What time of day was it? At night? First thing in the morning?
- What were the thoughts you found most exciting? Why? Because of the intimacy you experienced? Because of the environment where the sexual situation took place? What details make the thought most arousing?
- What elements, timing, or surroundings help you feel more sexual? What aspects of the thoughts would you like to bring to your relationship? How will you do it?

resuming sex. (If you have questions about the medical risks of sex, you and your partner should discuss them with your doctor.)

If your efforts to renew your interest in sex are not as successful as you had hoped, think about getting sexual counseling. Psychologists and social workers who have experience working with people who have had cancer can talk with women and their partners about how treatment affects emotional and sexual responses. Licensed marriage and family counselors, licensed professional counselors, and licensed sex therapists with experience working with these issues can also help. A professional might be able to help you and your partner talk about topics that can be hard for you to discuss on your own. He or she can also suggest sexual techniques and answer questions.

Intimacy After Breast Surgery

The most common sexual side effect from breast surgery is feeling less attractive. In our culture, breasts are often viewed as an integral part of beauty and womanhood. A woman who has had her breast removed may feel less secure about whether a partner will accept her and still find her sexually appealing.

The breasts and nipples are also sources of sexual pleasure for many women and their partners. Touching the breasts is a common part of foreplay. Some women can reach orgasm just from having their breasts stroked. For many others, stroking the breasts adds to sexual excitement. Surgery for breast cancer can interfere with the pleasurable feelings of having the breasts touched. Women who have breast changes due to cancer sometimes miss the pleasure they felt from the stroking of the breast area during sex. After mastectomy, some women still enjoy being stroked around the area of the healed scar, but others dislike being touched there and might not enjoy being touched on the remaining breast and nipple, either. It might be pleasurable or exciting for your partner to stroke your whole body, including kissing your neck or touching your inner thighs or genital area. You might find new ways to replace the pleasure you used to feel.

If you had a segmental mastectomy or lumpectomy followed by radiation therapy, your breast might be scarred or might be different in shape, feel, or size. Some women have areas of numbness or decreased sensation near the surgical scar.

Some women who have had a mastectomy feel self-conscious being the partner "on top" during sex, because that position makes it obvious that the breast is missing or different. Some women who have had mastectomies wear a short nightgown or camisole—or even just a bra—with their prosthesis inside during sex. Other women find the breast prosthesis awkward or feel that it gets in the way. A woman who prefers not to wear a prosthesis might enjoy being touched around the site of the mastectomy and might feel no need to hide the scar. Talk to your partner about your comfort level and preferences so that you have the same expectations.

Intimacy and Breast Reconstruction

Breast reconstruction can boost feelings of wholeness and attractiveness. Some women find that breast reconstruction helps them enjoy sex more, even if it does not fully restore sensation. In a reconstructed breast, the feelings of pleasure from touching the breast and nipple can be decreased or even absent. This is because the nerves that supply feeling to the nipple run deep through the breast tissue and are sometimes cut during surgery. Sensation with a preserved or rebuilt nipple might also be weaker, although some feeling can return over time.

Dating After Breast Cancer

If you do not have a sexual partner, you have different concerns from women who are in relationships. You are probably wondering, for example, how and when you should tell someone you are dating about your history of breast cancer. You might also worry about how future lovers will react when they find out you've had cancer.

Some of the effects of cancer and its treatment are public, such as the loss of hair or skin changes. Others cannot be seen by a casual observer—there's no way to know that a woman on the street has had a mastectomy. The things that are not as noticeable on the outside can be just as painful, though, because the people who do see them are the ones whose acceptance and support matter most.

Sometimes the most private scar left by cancer is the damage done to your view of yourself. You might wonder how active you can be and even how long you will live. Maybe you hoped to marry or remarry before your diagnosis, but now you are wary of involving a partner in such an uncertain future.

Concerns about having children can also affect new relationships. You might not be able to have children because of cancer treatment. Or you might still be able to have children but are afraid that cancer will cut short the time you will have to see children grow up.

Talking About Your Cancer

Women who have had cancer often avoid talking about their illness when they are dating. At a time when closeness is so important, it can seem risky to draw his or her attention to your problems. After you have completed treatment, it can be tempting to try to forget that it ever happened.

Sometimes, you can ignore your history of cancer. But if a relationship becomes serious, silence is not the best plan. Before you decide to make a big commitment like marriage, you and your partner should talk about your cancer. This is especially true if your life expectancy or fertility has been affected by treatment. Otherwise, cancer could become the "skeleton in the closet," a secret that will limit your ability to confide in your partner. A truly loving partner needs to accept you and your health situation.

When to Talk About Your Cancer

If you have had a lumpectomy or mastectomy, when should you tell a new romantic interest about it? Telling the person during the first few minutes of meeting is probably too soon, but if you wait until you are about to get into bed together to reveal that you have had surgery on your breast, you risk a shocked reaction at an intimate moment. It is probably best to tell the other person about your cancer when you feel a sense of trust and friendship—a feeling that he or she likes you as a total person.

Ideally, a couple should discuss cancer when a relationship begins to become serious. Try having a talk when you and your partner are relaxed and in an intimate mood.

You can then ask your partner questions that leave room for different answers, such as, "I really like where our relationship is going, and I need you to know I had a mastectomy for breast cancer several years ago. How do you think that might affect our relationship?" You can also express your own feelings: "I had breast cancer ___ years ago. I guess I haven't wanted to bring it up because I'm afraid you'd rather be with someone who hasn't had it. It also scares me to remember that time in my life, but I need you to know about it. What are your thoughts or feelings about my having had cancer?"

You can even rehearse how to tell a dating partner about your experience with cancer. What message do you want to give? Try some different ways of saying it, and ask a friend for feedback. Did you come across the way you wanted to? Ask your friend to take the role of a new partner who rejects you because you have had cancer. Have your friend tell you what you dread hearing the most, and practice your response. Can you express your feelings in a dignified and satisfying way?

The Possibility of Rejection

The reality is that some potential lovers might reject you because of your cancer treatment. Of course, almost everyone gets rejected at some time. People without cancer reject each other because of looks, beliefs, personality, or their own issues. The tragedy, however, is that some single women with cancer limit themselves by not even trying to date. Instead of focusing on their good points, they convince themselves that no partner would accept them because of breast cancer and the effects of treatment. Although you will avoid being rejected if you stay at home, you'll also miss the chance to build happy, healthy relationships.

Improving Your Social Life

Try working on areas of your social life other than dating and sex. Build up your network of close friends, casual friends, and family. Make the effort to call, plan visits, or share activities. Get involved in a hobby, special interest group, or adult education course to broaden your social circle while enjoying yourself. Check out volunteer and support groups that are geared toward people who have faced cancer.

If you need to, remind yourself of what you have to offer another person by making a list of your good qualities. Whenever you catch yourself using cancer as an excuse not to meet new people or date, refer to your list of assets. See the sidebar on the next page for some questions to get you started. You might also want to explore individual or group

Why I Am Desirable

This exercise can help you remember that you have many wonderful and attractive qualities. It is for you to look at—**no one else**! Write enough glowing praise for yourself that looking at this list raises your self-esteem a notch if you need it. Start by answering the questions below, but don't stop there. Jot down your own questions and answers, too. Be specific about your good qualities, and don't be modest.

- What do I like about my looks?
- What are the best aspects of my personality?
- What are my special talents and skills?
- What dreams can I share with someone else?
- What can I give to a romantic partner?
- What makes me a good partner?

counseling with a professional counselor. Getting objective feedback about your strengths from others will help you maintain a more positive view of yourself.

If you feel shy about meeting new people, practice how to handle it. Talk to yourself in the mirror, or ask a close friend or family member to play the part with you. Think of meeting people and trying new things as part of a learning process rather than something you must do well on your first try.

Use the exercises in this chapter to boost your self-esteem and remind yourself of all you have to offer. Above all, be patient with yourself. You are a valuable and attractive woman and, with time, intimacy can once again be a satisfying and worthwhile part of your life.

CHAPTER 22

The Possibility of Facing Cancer Again

Once you have had breast cancer, the possibility always exists that you will have to face it again. When cancer comes back after treatment, it is called recurrence. Cancer can also occur in the other breast. This is usually a new cancer and is often referred to as a second primary breast cancer. Although most women stay cancer-free, even the thought of dealing with cancer again is scary. For some women, it can be hard to talk or even think about. For others, it can occupy their thoughts, making it hard to think about anything else. Either way, optimism, hope, and effective coping strategies can help you work through this difficult issue.

Because of the possibility of recurrence or a new cancer, it might be more accurate to think of cancer as a chronic lifelong disease that needs to be monitored and cared for throughout your life, rather than a one-time illness that can be cured by a short period of treatment.

What Is Recurrence and Why Does It Happen?

Recurrent cancer is cancer that comes back after treatment. Sometimes, no matter what type of treatment is used, a few cancer cells survive and eventually grow into new tumors. The cancer does not necessarily come back where it started. It can recur in other parts of your body, such as the lungs, liver, brain, nearby lymph nodes, and bones. If the cancer recurs after treatment, it is still considered breast cancer, no matter where in the body it is found. This is because the cancer cells themselves are still breast cancer cells, they have just moved to another part of the body. The cancer's primary site—the place it began—determines what kind of cancer it is.

Types of Recurrence

A recurrence is categorized according to its location in the body. Local recurrence is cancer that has returned in or near the place it was originally—such as in your mastectomy scar, on your chest wall, or in the breast tissue that remained after breast-conserving surgery (in the breast that originally had the cancer). Some of these can actually be new cancers (a second primary cancer), but there is often no way to tell for sure. Regional recurrence is when cancer is present in the tissue surrounding the breast but not in other parts of the body. Rarely, the cancer can recur in nearby lymph nodes, which is also considered regional recurrence. Distant recurrence is when the original cancer has spread to distant organs or tissue (such as the brain or liver). This is also known as metastatic disease. Sometimes, a local recurrence is found first, followed months or years later by the discovery of metastatic disease.

Cancer Recurrence Versus a Second Primary Cancer

Women who have had breast cancer are also at risk of a second breast cancer. A second cancer can develop in the breast that was originally treated as long as any breast tissue remains, even if it is only a few cells. Since even a mastectomy can leave a few breast cells behind, cancer can still develop after a mastectomy—in the remaining tissue, in the scar, or in the skin. Breast cancer can also develop in the opposite breast. Although a second breast cancer is different from recurrence, it can be difficult to tell them apart if it occurs in the same breast as the first cancer. Anyone who has had breast cancer is at increased risk for a new cancer developing in the other breast. Some estimates put the average risk at 5 percent over the first ten years after diagnosis and 10 percent over the first twenty years. The risk is known to be higher in women who carry gene mutations linked to breast cancer risk (such as the BRCA genes). Treatments such as chemotherapy and hormone therapy can lower the risk of both recurrence and a new breast cancer developing.

> **Questions to Ask Your Medical Team About Recurrence**
>
> - **Am I at high risk** for recurrence?
> - **Is there anything I can do** to decrease my chance of recurrence?
> - **How will I be monitored** for possible recurrence?

Tips for Coping with Fear of Cancer Recurrence

Consider the following tips for dealing with fear of recurrence:

- **Be informed.** Learn what you can do for your health now, and find out what services are available to you. This can give you a greater sense of control.
- **Express your feelings.** Expressing strong feelings can help you let go of them. You can talk to a friend, family member, or counselor. If you prefer not to discuss your cancer with others, try writing down your feelings.
- **Work toward having a positive attitude,** which can help you feel better about life now. Use your energy to focus on wellness and what you can do in the present moment to be as healthy as possible.
- **Find ways to help yourself relax.** Some women find meditation, yoga, deep breathing, or hypnosis to be helpful. Listen to soothing music. Treat yourself to a massage. Go for a long, quiet walk. Do whatever makes you feel restful and peaceful.
- **Be as active as you can.** Getting out of the house and focusing on doing something can divert your attention from cancer and the worries it brings. Exercise is a known way to reduce stress.
- **Participate in a support group.** Sharing your feelings with others who are in the same situation will help you feel less alone.
- **Control what you can.** Putting your life in order may make you feel less fearful. Being involved in your health care, keeping your appointments, and making positive changes in your lifestyle can also help you feel more in control.

Fear Is Normal

Once you have been treated for cancer, it is normal to be concerned that everyday aches and pains could be signs that the cancer has returned. Try to remember that everyone has aches and pains occasionally. If the pain increases or does not go away, contact your doctor. Do not hesitate to tell your doctors or other health care providers about any symptoms or side effects that concern you. Most of the time, such symptoms turn out not to be related to cancer, but it is still important to let your doctor know about them. For many women, the breast cancer does not come back. With each successful visit to your doctor, you will probably feel more reassured about your health. Your sense of vulnerability will diminish with time.

Another way to manage anxiety about possible recurrence is to follow through with your checkups after you have completed treatment. For some women, follow-up visits to the doctor help them feel confident that their body is being monitored for potential recurrence. These visits can allow you to get on with your life without focusing too much on the possibility of recurrence. However, for some, follow-up care can be stressful. The risk of recurrence can make you feel vulnerable and add a level of fearfulness to follow-up care.

If you have frequent anxious thoughts about recurrence that interfere with or prevent you from moving on with your life, or if your fears keep you from getting follow-up care, you may want to talk with a mental health professional. The coping mechanisms you have used throughout your cancer experience will also be helpful in dealing with your concerns about recurrence.

The Importance of Follow-Up Care

Although most recurrences happen within the first few years of the initial diagnosis, breast cancer can also recur years later, though this is less common. It is also important to realize that a second primary cancer can appear at any time. This makes follow-up care essential for women who have undergone treatment for breast cancer. Depending on the stage of your breast cancer and its treatment, routine follow-up will vary. After treatment ends, it is especially important to be alert to changes in your body and to report any unusual symptoms to your doctor.

One part of follow-up care is understanding your role in the early detection of cancer recurrence. For women who have had breast cancer treatment, mammography is one of the best tools for monitoring for recurrence or a new breast cancer. Because you are at risk for both of these, you need a mammogram at least yearly.

All mammography facilities are required to send the results to you within thirty days and to contact you within five working days if there is a problem with the mammogram. Some medical centers read mammograms on the spot. If you would like to get your results quickly, you might want to seek out such a facility.

Because mammography cannot detect all breast cancers, the American Cancer Society also recommends breast awareness and clinical breast examinations (CBE) by a doctor or other health care professional. Breast awareness means knowing how your breasts normally look and feel and being alert to any changes in your breasts. Mammography, CBEs, breast awareness, and other diagnostic tests for follow-up care were discussed in more detail in chapter 19.

Reducing Your Risk

The risk of recurrence depends on several factors that you cannot change, such as the stage and grade of the original cancer and certain tumor characteristics, such as the presence of hormone receptors or HER2 positivity. The effects of other factors, such as the risk factors for getting breast cancer in the first place, are unclear. How these risk factors affect the chance of recurrence or a new primary breast cancer is not clear.

As you have already learned, several factors associated with increased risk of breast cancer—age and family history, for example—cannot be changed. But you can change other factors that contribute to breast cancer risk—such as eating right, exercising, and reducing alcohol consumption.

Lifestyle Factors

Body weight: Studies have shown that women with breast cancer who are obese have worse survival, with an increased risk of death from breast cancer and other causes. The reason for this is not entirely clear, but the levels of certain hormones, such as insulin, adiponestin, leptin, and estrogen, may play a role. Although it has not yet been shown that losing weight after a breast cancer diagnosis helps prevent cancer recurrence or cancer-related death, this is being examined in a study going on now, called the Exercise and Nutrition to Enhance Recovery and Good Health for You (ENERGY) study. The ENERGY study is designed to examine the effect of diet and exercise as a weight management tool in overweight breast cancer survivors. Still, it is known that achieving a healthy weight has a number of health benefits, such as improving glucose tolerance, preventing cardiovascular disease, and lowering the risk of certain cancers.

Weight gain: Studies of women with breast cancer have linked weight gain after diagnosis with worse outcomes, even in women who do not become obese. Given this link, it makes sense for breast cancer survivors to try to prevent weight gain by eating a healthy diet and staying physically active.

Diet: A few studies have looked at the effects of specific diets on the risk of breast cancer recurrence, but the results have been unclear. One large study seemed to find a link between a low-fat diet and a lower risk of a new breast cancer, but another study did not. The reason behind these different findings is unclear: it could be due to the diet's effect on body weight or to differences in how strictly the women stuck to the diet. In the study that showed a benefit, women on the diet lost weight; in the other study, the diet had little effect on weight. Breast cancer risk also seemed to be lower in those who followed the diet more strictly. Still, even if following a healthy diet has not been proven to prevent cancer, it can help you feel better and keep your heart healthy.

Some people have expressed concerns about the effect of soy on breast cancer risk or outcomes. Soy foods are rich in isoflavones, a type of phytoestrogen. Phytoestrogens are plant-derived compounds that can act like estrogen or anti-estrogens in the body. Soy isoflavones can cause breast cancer cells to grow in test tubes and laboratory animals, leading some people to question whether they could lead to worse outcomes among women who have breast cancer. Studies looking at this, however, have shown no increased risk of recurrence or death in women who eat a lot of soy. In some women, a high soy intake may have even had a slight protective effect. In these studies, the use of soy isoflavone supplements was uncommon, so their safety in the breast cancer survivor is still not clear.

Alcohol: Alcohol intake is clearly linked to an increased risk of a primary breast cancer, but its effect on breast cancer recurrence is unclear. Some studies have linked alcohol consumption with worse outcomes, whereas others have not. Still, until there is a definitive answer, the best course of action is to drink alcohol sparingly, if at all.

Physical activity: Studies have shown that breast cancer survivors who are physically active have better outcomes than those who are not. Physically active women have better survival overall and are less likely to die of breast cancer. They also have better quality of life, less fatigue, and better physical function. Exercise can also lower your risk of high blood pressure, heart disease, diabetes, and some other types of cancer.

Adjuvant Therapy

Adjuvant therapy is treatment that is given after surgery has removed all visible cancer. Even when the surgeon has removed all the cancer that can be seen, a few cancer cells might remain. These cells can grow, multiply, and spread, leading to a recurrence. The goal of adjuvant therapy is to kill the remaining cancer cells, so that they never get the chance to grow, spread, or cause more tumors. This lowers the risk of recurrence.

Adjuvant therapy may include chemotherapy, targeted therapy, radiation therapy, and hormone therapy. Adjuvant chemotherapy for breast cancer generally starts soon after surgery and usually continues for three to six months. In early breast cancer, adjuvant chemotherapy has been shown to lower the risk of recurrence and help women live longer. In women with HER2-positive tumors, the drug trastuzumab (Herceptin) is given along with adjuvant chemotherapy. It is then continued for a total of one year. Using trastuzumab in this way has been shown to lower the risk of recurrence.

Adjuvant radiation therapy (to the underarm lymph nodes and/or to the remaining breast) also starts in the first few months after surgery and can continue for up to two months. Adjuvant radiation to the remaining breast is usually a part of breast-conserving therapy. Breast radiation after partial mastectomy has been shown to lower the risk of recurrence or a new cancer developing in the treated breast.

Adjuvant therapy with hormonal agents—drugs such as aromatase inhibitors, luteinizing hormone releasing hormone (LHRH) analogs, and tamoxifen—has been used for many years to reduce the risk of recurrence in early breast cancer. Many clinical trials have shown conclusively that continuing treatment with these drugs for at least five years reduces a woman's risk of recurrent breast cancer by almost 50 percent. This treatment also lowers the risk of a new cancer developing in the opposite breast. But not all women complete this treatment as recommended. These drugs have side effects, and many women say that they feel better when they do not take them. Five years can feel like a long time to take a drug when you have no signs of cancer and otherwise feel fine, but try to think of it as an investment in your future. Taking the medicine for the full five years gives you the best chance of not facing breast cancer again.

Neoadjuvant Chemotherapy

Neoadjuvant chemotherapy, which is giving chemotherapy before surgery to try to shrink the cancer, lowers the risk of distant recurrence. It seems to be as effective in lowering risk as giving the same chemotherapy after surgery (as adjuvant treatment).

Surgery

Some women who carry genes that put them at very high risk of breast cancer, such as those with BRCA mutations, choose to have surgery to lower their risk of a new (second) cancer. Often, this means removing the opposite healthy breast when cancer is diagnosed in one breast. This is a drastic option, but it can be a reasonable choice for women at very high risk for breast cancer.

Women with BRCA mutations who are premenopausal at the time of their breast cancer diagnosis also can choose to have their ovaries removed. Removing the ovaries lowers the estrogen available to promote the growth of cancer while also helping to prevent ovarian cancer (which can be common in women with BRCA mutations). Although this has not been proven to lower the risk of recurrence, it can decrease the chance of a new breast cancer forming.

Pregnancy

Because many breast cancers are sensitive to estrogen, there has been concern that high hormone levels during pregnancy could increase the chance of recurrence in women who have had breast cancer. Studies have shown, however, that pregnancy does not increase the risk of recurrence after successful treatment of breast cancer.

Doctors often counsel women to wait at least two years after their treatment is complete before becoming pregnant. The two-year waiting period is not a hard and fast rule. It is used because most recurrences of breast cancer happen during that time. Your risks, however, might be different. If you are thinking about becoming pregnant, you should discuss your risk of breast cancer recurrence with your doctors.

Menopausal Hormone Therapy

The known link between estrogen levels and breast cancer growth has discouraged many women and their doctors from choosing or recommending treatment with estrogen (sometimes called hormone replacement therapy [HRT] or just hormone therapy [HT]) to help relieve menopausal symptoms. Many women experience menopausal symptoms after treatment for breast cancer. This can occur naturally, such as when postmenopausal women stop taking HRT, or it can occur because of treatment, such as when pre-menopausal women undergo chemotherapy or removal of the ovaries. Drugs such as tamoxifen and aromatase inhibitors also can cause menopausal symptoms, such as hot flashes.

In the past, doctors have offered HRT (with estrogen, either alone or combined with a progestin) after breast cancer treatment to women with severe symptoms because early studies had shown no harm. But a well-designed study (the HABITS study) found that breast cancer survivors who were taking HRT were much more likely to have a new or recurrent breast cancer develop than women who were not taking the drugs. Most doctors now believe that it is unwise to prescribe HRT for women previously treated for breast cancer. Women with symptoms of menopause should talk with their doctor about their specific symptoms and the possible ways to treat them.

Other Cancers

Another serious concern for women treated for breast cancer is the possibility of being diagnosed with another type of cancer. For example, some women also are at increased risk for cancers of the ovary, uterus, lung, colon, rectum, thyroid, and connective tissue (sarcoma). The risk of melanoma and leukemia is also increased, but these are rare. Some of these cancers are linked to certain treatments. Most often, however, the second cancer is related to a common cancer-causing factor, such as a genetic factor or other risk factor. For example, breast and ovarian cancer have a common genetic link, as do breast and thyroid cancer. Being overweight or obese also is linked to higher risk for breast and colorectal cancer.

Radiation therapy for breast cancer is linked to an increased risk of lung cancer, especially in people who smoke. Radiation therapy to the breast also increases the risk of sarcomas of blood vessels (angiosarcomas), connective tissue, and bone (osteosarcomas). These cancers are rare and are most often seen in the remaining breast area, chest wall, and arm on the side that was treated with radiation therapy.

Treatment with some chemotherapy drugs is linked with an increased risk of leukemia, although this is rare. Tamoxifen treatment is linked to endometrial cancer. These conditions are rare and can develop years after the treatment. For many new cancer treatments, their long-term effects on the risk for a second cancer are not yet known. Still, it is important to note that second cancers related to treatment are rare. The small risk that these cancers will develop must be weighed against the benefits of treating your breast cancer now.

Dealing with a Recurrence or Second Cancer Diagnosis

Finding out that the cancer has returned or that a second cancer has developed can be extremely upsetting. It is normal to grieve—the thought of going through treatment again can make you feel depressed, hopeless, and afraid. You might feel betrayed by your body and your doctors: Didn't you feel better? Didn't they say you were doing fine? Doubts might start to creep in about the effectiveness of any treatment. If it didn't work the first time, why should it work this time? You might even blame yourself—did I do something to bring this on? Is there something I could have done to prevent it?

There is no way to know for certain why the cancer came back. Nobody can point to a single factor and say, "that's to blame." Although it won't be easy, you can face the challenges ahead. You've probably resolved some of the practical issues of dealing with breast cancer, and you know what to expect from a medical team and from treatment. Trying to maintain a positive attitude can help keep you on a constructive path.

Depending on how much time has passed since your initial diagnosis, you may want to reeducate yourself about treatment options. Significant advances in medical knowledge may offer you new or better treatment options.

To deal with some of the complex emotions you are going through, you might try such activities as relaxation, yoga, or imagery to help reduce stress and anxiety. It will also be important to reestablish your support system so that you do not have to deal with your new cancer diagnosis and treatment alone.

The Importance of Emotional Support

Enlisting support from family and friends might be more important now than ever before. The reassurance and support of close friends and loved ones is a strong foundation for handling a recurrence or second cancer. Joining a support group may also be extremely helpful not only for yourself but also for your family members, who are trying to cope with your situation, too.

Some people who have been in remission for a long time find it difficult to ask for help when they are dealing with cancer again because they are afraid of becoming a burden to their families. Don't let this fear stop you from being open and honest with your family about your feelings and your needs. Your family's support can make all the difference in your ability to maintain a positive outlook.

Things to Remember If Facing Recurrence

- **Take part in your medical care.** Ask questions, take notes, stay informed, and make informed decisions about your care.
- **Seek support.** Don't do it all yourself. Ask for help from your family, friends, and other supporters to help you get through this difficult time. Talk to others and share your feelings.
- **Take it easy on yourself.** You'll have good days and bad days. Allow yourself the time to work through your emotions and find constructive ways to deal with them.
- **Focus on healthy behaviors.** Before, during, and after treatment, it is important to eat a nutritious diet to keep up your strength and recover and heal as quickly as possible.
- **Stay active, both physically and mentally.** Try to be physically active on a regular basis if you're able. Keep your mind active, as well. Use complementary methods to ease stress and pain.

Treatment for Local Recurrence or a Second Cancer

Treatment for a local recurrence often involves surgery, which may be followed by radiation therapy, chemotherapy, hormone therapy, and/or targeted therapy.

In women who had a lumpectomy with radiation for the first cancer, a second cancer in the same breast is most often treated with mastectomy. Another lumpectomy is generally not an option because radiation can be given to an area only once. For women who have had lumpectomy and accelerated partial breast irradiation, it might be possible to save the breast if the cancer comes back at the lumpectomy site and there are no medical reasons not to use whole breast irradiation.

In women who have had mastectomy, a local recurrence may present as a tumor nodule in the mastectomy scar or on the chest wall. This can be treated by removing it surgically, often followed by radiation therapy to the chest wall (if radiation was not given before). Local recurrence might be treated with chemotherapy or hormone therapy to see whether the cancer will shrink before surgery. Your doctor may also recommend treatment after surgery, such as chemotherapy and/or hormone therapy.

A second primary cancer in the opposite breast is most often treated like any other breast cancer. You'll have the same surgical options, but the choices for treatment after surgery might be a little different, depending on how long ago you were treated for the first cancer. If you are still taking hormone therapy after the first cancer, for example, the new cancer might be resistant to that drug, and a different drug might be needed. Your prognosis and your treatment options will depend on your current state of health, your previous breast cancer treatment, and the size and location of the cancer.

Questions to Ask Your Medical Team If You Have a Recurrence

- **What type of recurrence** do I have?
- **How will my recurrence** be treated?
- **Since my first cancer diagnosis,** have any new treatments been introduced that could benefit me?
- **Is treatment for my recurrence covered** by my insurance company?
- **Will I have the same medical team** this time as I did the first time?
- **How long** will my treatment last?
- **If I have one recurrence,** does that mean I have a higher chance of future recurrences?
- **Are there any support groups** you can recommend to help me deal with my recurrence?

Treatment of Lymph Node Recurrence

Rarely, breast cancer recurs in the lymph nodes under the arm. This is most often treated with surgery to remove the lymph nodes. Further treatment depends on how long it has been since the original diagnosis and what treatments have been given previously. If the woman is on hormone therapy, the drug may be changed. If the woman has been off treatment for some time, chemotherapy and/or additional hormone therapy may be an option.

Advanced and Metastatic Cancer

Advanced (metastatic) cancer is cancer that has spread from its primary site to other parts of the body. Metastatic cancer is not generally thought to be curable. The main goal of treatment for metastatic disease is to help you feel better and live longer.

Breast cancer often spreads to the bone, but metastasis to the liver and lung is not uncommon. As the cancer progresses, metastasis to the brain may occur, but the cancer can spread anywhere, including the skin, eyes, or bone marrow. Sometimes metastatic disease is found by imaging tests before it causes symptoms. As the areas of metastasis grow larger, symptoms can occur. These symptoms depend on what areas are involved and can include bone pain, cough, shortness of breath, loss of appetite, weight loss, and neurological symptoms, such as pain, weakness, or headaches.

Metastatic breast cancer is often treated with systemic treatments such as chemotherapy, targeted therapy, and/or hormone therapy. These treatments can be very useful for cancer that has spread, because they affect cancer cells throughout the body. Radiation therapy might also be used, particularly to treat cancer in bones or when the cancer has spread to the brain. Other treatments might be needed, depending on problems caused by the cancer.

There is no right or wrong way to handle this stage of illness, and your choices about treatment will be personal and based on your needs, wishes, and abilities. It is important to know that even those who are not cured of cancer may go on living for months or even years, even though there may be changes in their lives. And though it can be hard to do, many families adjust to this kind of treatment schedule. Today, women treated for metastatic breast cancer are living longer and leading fuller lives.

American Cancer Society Recommendations for Early Breast Cancer Detection in Women Without Breast Symptoms

Women age forty and older should have a mammogram every year and should continue to do so for as long as they are in good health.

- Current evidence supporting mammograms is even stronger than in the past. In particular, evidence has confirmed that mammograms offer substantial benefit for women in their forties. Women can feel confident about the benefits associated with regular mammograms for finding cancer early. However, mammograms also have limitations and can miss some cancers. Mammograms with abnormal results also can lead to follow-up testing, sometimes including biopsies, which eventually show that no cancer is present.
- Women should be told about the benefits and limitations linked with yearly mammograms. Mammograms can miss some cancers. But despite their limitations, mammograms remain a very effective and valuable tool for decreasing suffering and death from breast cancer.
- Mammograms should be continued regardless of a woman's age, as long as she does not have serious, chronic health problems such as congestive heart failure, end-stage renal disease, chronic obstructive pulmonary disease, or moderate to severe dementia. Age alone should not be a reason to stop having regular mammograms. Women with serious health problems or short life expectancies should discuss with their doctors whether to continue having mammograms.

Women in their twenties and thirties should have a clinical breast examination (CBE) as part of a periodic health examination by a health professional, preferably every three years. Starting at age forty, women should have a CBE by a health professional every year.

- Clinical breast examination is done along with mammograms and gives women an opportunity to talk with their doctor or nurse about changes in their breasts, early detection testing, and factors in the woman's history that might make her more likely to have breast cancer.

- There may be some benefit in having the CBE shortly before the woman's regularly scheduled mammogram. The examination should include instructions on how women can become more familiar with their own breasts. Women should also be given information about the benefits and limitations of CBE and breast self-examination (BSE). The risk of breast cancer is very low for women in their twenties and gradually increases with age. Women should be told to promptly report any new breast symptoms to a health professional.

Breast self-examination is an option for women starting in their twenties. Women should be told about the benefits and limitations of breast self-examination. Women should immediately report any breast changes to their health professional.

- Beginning in their twenties, women should be told about the benefits and limitations of breast self-examination. Research has shown that breast self-examination plays a smaller role in finding breast cancer than finding a breast lump by chance or simply being aware of what is normal for each woman. Some women feel very comfortable doing regular self-examinations (usually monthly after their period), which involve a systematic step-by-step approach to examining the look and feel of one's breasts. Other women are more comfortable simply feeling their breasts in a less systematic approach, such as while showering or getting dressed or by doing occasional thorough examinations. Women should know how their breasts normally look and feel and report any new breast changes to a health professional as soon as they are found. Finding a breast change does not necessarily mean there is a cancer.

- Sometimes, women are so concerned about "doing it right" that they become stressed over the technique. Doing BSE regularly is one way for women to know how their breasts normally look and feel and to notice any changes. The goal, with or without BSE, is to immediately report any breast changes to a doctor or nurse.

- Women who choose to use a step-by-step approach to breast self-examination should have their technique reviewed during their physical examination by a health professional. It is okay for women to choose not to do BSE or not to do it on a regular schedule such as once every month. However, by doing the examination regularly, you get to know how your breasts normally look and feel and you can more readily find any changes. If a change occurs, such as development of a lump or swelling, skin irritation or dimpling, nipple pain or retraction (turning inward), redness or scaliness of the nipple or breast skin, or a discharge other than breast milk (such as staining of your sheets or bra), you should see your health care professional as soon as possible for evaluation. Remember that most of the time, however, these breast changes are not cancer.

Women at high risk (greater than 20 percent lifetime risk) should get an MRI and a mammogram every year. Women at moderately increased risk (15 to 20 percent lifetime risk) should talk with their doctors about the benefits and limitations of adding MRI screening to their yearly mammogram. Yearly MRI screening is not recommended for women whose lifetime risk of breast cancer is less than 15 percent.

- Women at high risk include those who meet one of the following criteria:
    - Have a known *BRCA1* or *BRCA2* gene mutation
    - Have a first-degree relative (parent, brother, sister, or child) with a *BRCA1* or *BRCA2* gene mutation, and have not had genetic testing themselves
    - Have a lifetime risk of breast cancer of 20 to 25 percent or greater, according to risk assessment tools that are based mainly on family history (see below)
    - Had radiation therapy to the chest when they were between the ages of ten and thirty years
    - Have Li-Fraumeni syndrome, Cowden syndrome, or Bannayan-Riley-Ruvalcaba syndrome, or a first-degree relative with one of these syndromes
- Women at moderately increased risk include those who meet one of these characteristics:
    - Have a lifetime risk of breast cancer of 15 to 20 percent, according to risk assessment tools that are based mainly on family history
    - Have a personal history of breast cancer, ductal carcinoma in situ (DCIS), lobular carcinoma in situ (LCIS), atypical ductal hyperplasia (ADH), or atypical lobular hyperplasia (ALH)
    - Have extremely dense breasts or unevenly dense breasts when viewed by mammograms

If MRI is used, it should be in addition to, not instead of, a screening mammogram. This is because although an MRI is a more sensitive test (it's more likely to detect cancer than a mammogram), it may still miss some cancers that a mammogram would detect.

For most women at high risk, screening with MRI and mammograms should begin at the age of thirty and continue for as long as a woman is in good health. But because the evidence is limited about the best age at which to start screening, this decision should be based on shared decision-making between patients and their health care providers, taking into account personal circumstances and preferences.

Several risk assessment tools, with names such as the Gail model, the Claus model, and the Tyrer-Cuzick model, are available to help health professionals estimate a woman's breast cancer risk. These tools give approximate, rather than precise, estimates of breast cancer risk based on different combinations of risk factors and different data sets. As a result, they may give different risk estimates for the same woman. For example, the Gail model bases its risk estimates on certain personal risk factors, such as current age, age at menarche (first menstrual period) and history of prior breast biopsies, along with any history of breast cancer in first-degree relatives. The Claus model estimates risk based on family history of breast cancer in both first and second-degree relatives. These two models could easily give different estimates using the same data. Results from any of the risk assessment tools should be discussed by a woman and her doctor when being used to decide whether to start MRI screening.

Women who get a screening MRI should do so at a facility that can do an MRI-guided breast biopsy at the same time, if needed. Otherwise, the woman will have to undergo a second MRI at another facility when she has the biopsy.

There is no evidence that MRI is an effective screening tool for women at average risk. Whereas MRI is more sensitive than mammography, it also has a higher false-positive rate (it is more likely to find something that turns out not to be cancer). This can lead to unneeded biopsies and other tests in many of the women screened, which can lead to worry and anxiety.

The American Cancer Society believes that the use of mammograms, MRI (in women at high risk), clinical breast examinations, and finding and reporting breast changes early, according to the recommendations outlined above, offer women the best chance to reduce their risk of dying of breast cancer. This multifaceted approach is clearly better than any one test alone.

Without question, a physical examination of the breast without a mammogram would miss the opportunity to detect many breast cancers that are too small for a woman or her doctor to feel but can be seen on mammograms. Mammograms are a sensitive screening method; however, a small percentage of breast cancers do not show up on mammograms but can be felt by a woman or her doctors. For women at high risk of breast cancer, such as those with BRCA gene mutations or a strong family history, both MRI and mammogram are recommended.

APPENDIX B

Women's Health and Cancer Rights Act

Federal law requires most group insurance plans that cover mastectomies to also cover breast reconstruction.

The Women's Health and Cancer Rights Act (WHCRA) helps protect many women with breast cancer who choose to have their breast reconstructed after mastectomy. The Act was signed into law on October 21, 1998. The US Departments of Labor and Health and Human Services oversee this law.

The WHCRA applies to the following health plans:
- group health plans for plan years starting on or after October 1, 1998
- group health plans, health insurance companies, and health maintenance organizations (HMOs), as long as the plan covers medical and surgical costs for mastectomy

Under the WHCRA, mastectomy benefits must cover the following procedures, devices, and/or issues:
- reconstruction of the breast that was removed by mastectomy
- surgery and reconstruction of the other breast to make the breasts look symmetrical or balanced after mastectomy
- any external breast prostheses (breast forms that fit into your bra) that are needed before or during the reconstruction
- any physical complications at all stages of mastectomy, including lymphedema

Mastectomy-related benefits may have a yearly deductible, which is the amount you must pay before any claims are paid. After you pay the deductible amount, the plan might also require you to pay coinsurance for mastectomy claims. Coinsurance is when the health plan pays less than the full cost of a claim and you must pay the difference. For instance, the company might cover 80 percent of your expenses after you pay the deductible, leaving you to pay the other 20 percent. This 20 percent also can be called a copayment or copay. But any deductible or coinsurance a plan requires for mastectomy-related claims must be like those it uses for other conditions it covers. So, for example, if a plan paid 80 percent of hospital and surgery fees for an appendectomy, but only 70 percent of hospital and surgery fees for breast reconstruction, it would violate the WHCRA.

Questions and Answers About the WHCRA

Does the WHCRA allow insurers to remove individuals from their plans so that they do not have to pay breast reconstruction benefits?

No. The WHCRA does not allow insurance plans and insurance companies to remove individuals from the plan or keep them from enrolling or renewing their coverage under the plan to avoid WHCRA requirements.

Does the WHCRA allow insurance plans to give doctors incentives to discourage women from having breast reconstruction after mastectomy?

No. The WHCRA does not allow insurance plans and insurance issuers to penalize doctors or cause them to provide care in ways that do not support the WHCRA. It also forbids insurance plans from rewarding doctors who discourage their patients from exploring possibilities for breast reconstruction.

Does my insurance provider have to tell me that I'm covered for breast reconstruction under the WHRCA?

Yes. The law requires insurance providers to notify you of this coverage when you enroll in their plan and every year after that.

What if my state has laws requiring that insurers cover breast reconstruction?

Several states have their own laws requiring that health plans that cover mastectomies also provide coverage for reconstructive surgery afterward. These state laws apply only to health plans that an employer buys from a commercial insurance company. If an employer is self-insured, state laws do not apply, but federal laws do. Federal laws like the WHCRA are enforced by the US Department of Labor.

A self-insured (or self-funded) plan is one in which the employer, rather than a commercial insurance company, pays for the insured person's health expenses. Some employers that self-insure will hire a commercial insurance company to write the checks and do other paperwork, even though the money for the payments still comes from the employer. So, unless you ask, it can be hard to tell whether you are in a self-insured or a commercial insurance plan.

If you are not sure about your plan's status, ask your employer's benefits manager. If you are in a commercial plan, you can contact your state's insurance department to find out whether your state provides extra protection that applies to your coverage. The WHCRA applies to self-insured plans that are not covered by state law and sets a minimum standard to be sure these services are available for all women in every state. This includes states with weak or no laws covering breast reconstruction.

I have received a breast cancer diagnosis and plan to have a mastectomy. How will the Women's Health and Cancer Rights Act affect my benefits?

Under the Act, group health plans, insurance companies, and HMOs that offer coverage for mastectomy must also cover reconstructive surgery after mastectomy. This includes reconstruction of the breast removed by mastectomy, reconstruction of the other breast (to give a more balanced look), breast prostheses, and treatment of physical complications at all stages of mastectomy, including lymphedema (swelling that sometimes happens after breast cancer treatment).

The WHCRA sets a floor (minimum requirement) so that women can have breast reconstruction after mastectomy, even if they live in states that don't force insurance companies to offer this coverage.

Does the WHCRA require that all group plans, insurance companies, and HMOs provide reconstructive surgery benefits?

In most cases, yes, as long as the insurance plan also covers medical and surgical benefits for mastectomy. But certain church plans and government plans may not be required to pay for reconstructive surgery. If you are insured under a health plan sponsored by a church or local government, check with your plan administrator to determine your coverage.

Under the WHCRA, can insurance providers impose deductibles or coinsurance requirements for reconstructive surgery in connection with mastectomy?

Yes. But the deductibles and coinsurance must be comparable to those required for other benefits under the plan or coverage. The company cannot make you pay a higher deductible or copay for breast reconstruction than you would pay for other types of surgery.

My state requires coverage for breast reconstruction the same as the coverage required by the WHCRA. My state also requires minimum hospital stays for mastectomy. If I have mastectomy *and* breast reconstruction, am I also entitled to the minimum hospital stay?

It depends. If you have coverage through a commercial insurance plan offered by your employer, you'd be entitled to the minimum hospital stay required by the state law. If you have coverage through your employer but your coverage isn't provided by a commercial insurance company or HMO (that is, your employer "self-insures" your coverage), then state law doesn't apply. In that case, even though the federal Women's Health and Cancer Rights Act would still apply, that Act does not require minimum hospital stays. To find out whether your group health plan is insured or self-insured (self-funded), contact your plan administrator. If you have coverage under a private health insurance policy (not through your employer), check with your state insurance commissioner's office to find out whether state law applies.

Are health plans required to give me notice of the WHCRA benefits?

Yes. Both health plans and health insurance issuers must give you notice of the WHCRA benefits. They must do this when you enroll and every year after that. The annual notice might be sent separately or it might be included in almost any written communication from the plan or insurer, such as newsletters, annual reports, policy renewal letters, or enrollment notices. Enrollment notices might include a phone number or website that you can use to get more information about coverage.

Does the WHCRA affect the amount that my health plan will pay my doctors?

No. the WHCRA doesn't prevent a plan or health insurance issuer from bargaining with doctors about payment amounts and types of payments. However, the law does forbid insurance plans and issuers from penalizing doctors or from providing incentives for doctors to provide care that is not consistent with WHCRA.

Do the WHCRA requirements apply to Medicare or Medicaid?

No. The law does not apply to Medicare and Medicaid.

Where can I get more information about my rights under the WHCRA?

If you have more questions or concerns, you can contact—

- the US Department of Labor, which has WHCRA information on its website (www.dol.gov/ebsa/Publications/whcra.html), or you can call them toll-free at 866-487-2365
- your health plan administrator (a number should be listed on your insurance card)
- your state insurance commissioner's office (The number should be listed in your local phone book in the state government section, or you can find it at the National Association of Insurance Commissioners' website [www.naic.org]. If you cannot find the number elsewhere, call 826-783-8300.)

See the resource guide starting on page 443 for other sources of help.

Benign Breast Conditions and Their Link to Breast Cancer Risk

Nonproliferative lesions that require biopsy for diagnosis:

- **Hyperplasia**, also known as epithelial hyperplasia or proliferative breast disease, is an overgrowth of cells lining the ducts or lobules. Hyperplasia is usually diagnosed with a core needle biopsy or a surgical biopsy. Breast cancer risk is different, according to the type. Based on the pattern of the cells, as viewed under a microscope, they may be classified as usual hyperplasia or atypical hyperplasia. Mild hyperplasia of the usual type does not increase the risk of breast cancer. See page 438 under "Proliferative lesions without atypia" for other types.

- **Adenosis** of the breast is a benign condition in which the breast lobules are enlarged and contain more glands than usual. Lobes are at the root of a woman's milk-producing system. Each lobe contains many smaller parts called lobules, which hold the bulbs that produce breast milk. Adenosis occurs when the lobules contain more bulbs than usual and become enlarged. Sometimes, the enlarged bulbs can be felt by breast self-examination, but often they cannot be felt. Calcifications can be seen in adenosis and may also show up in cancerous tumors. These cannot be distinguished by a mammogram; therefore, a biopsy must be taken and tested for a clear diagnosis. Other names for adenosis of the breast include mammary adenosis, aggregate adenosis, tumoral adenosis, or adenosis tumor. See information on sclerosing adenosis on page 439.

- **Duct ectasia** (also known as mammary duct ectasia) is common in women over fifty. It occurs when a breast duct widens and the walls thicken. This condition can cause the duct to become blocked and can lead to fluid buildup. Often, there are no symptoms with duct ectasia, and it is found on biopsy. Less often, duct ectasia may cause a sticky green or black discharge. The nipple may be pulled inward, and the breast tissue around it may be tender and red. Sometimes, scar tissue around the abnormal duct causes a hard lump that can be confused with cancer.

Duct ectasia may improve without treatment; warm compresses and antibiotics are sometimes helpful. If the symptoms do not go away, the abnormal duct can be removed through an incision (cut) at the edge of the areola (the darker colored area around the nipple). Duct ectasia does not increase breast cancer risk.

- **Fibrosis** is the overgrowth of tissue in the breast that forms small breast lumps. In **periductal fibrosis,** the tissue overgrowth is around the ducts of the mammary gland. This condition is more common in women going through menopause.

- **Benign phyllodes tumors** are similar to fibroadenomas and tend to occur in women ages thirty to fifty. These tumors contain both glandular and stromal tissue. They are rare, with both benign and malignant phyllodes tumors making up less than 1 percent of all breast tumors in women. A lump may be felt, but it is usually painless. Benign phyllodes tumors are removed with surgery. While they do not increase the risk of breast cancer, they can recur.

- **Single papillomas.** An intraductal papilloma is a tiny wart-like growth in breast tissue that sometimes punctures a duct. Papillomas are benign and are composed of fibrous tissue and blood vessels. An intraductal papilloma grows inside the milk ducts of the breast and can cause nipple discharge. If it is near a nipple, it may feel like a small lump. Multiple papillomas usually occur deeper inside the breast and cannot be felt (see more about multiple papillomas on page 439). Papillomas that produce symptoms—either a mass or discharge from the nipple—and papillomas that are found through core needle biopsy should be surgically removed. With these types of papillomas, there is a 5 to 40 percent chance that the papilloma will contain ductal carcinoma in situ or atypical ductal hyperplasia.

- **Fat necrosis** is a benign condition that consists of firm scar tissue, typically resulting from damage to fatty breast tissue. It can result from sports injuries, accidents, or even seat belt burn. It may also occur after any type of breast surgery, including biopsy and breast reconstruction. Once fatty tissue has been injured or has died, it can turn into scar tissue or collect as liquid within a cyst. Fat necrosis may cause breast pain, but it does not lead to the development of breast cancer.

- **Squamous cell metaplasia** is a very rare development in the breast. It indicates a change in cell differentiation, meaning the genetic instructions to certain types of cells are not normal. Squamous cells usually form in the most superficial layer of the epithelial linings of organs, such as the ducts of the breast. Although squamous cell metaplasia is a benign condition, it can be a cause for concern. It may be an early sign of squamous cell carcinoma of the breast, or it may be secondary to other breast cancers. Squamous cell carcinoma is rare, accounting for less than 1 percent of all breast cancers.
- **Apocrine metaplasia** is a nonproliferative breast lesion, usually associated with fibrocystic disease of the breast. (The term "proliferative" means that cells are growing in an unpredictable way, and such growth would usually be associated with carcinoma.) With apocrine metaplasia, the cell growth is limited and predictable and usually associated with some type of stress to the breast, such as formation of a cyst. Apocrine metaplasia is a benign condition that does not increase the risk of breast cancer. It is sometimes described as a "benign epithelial alteration" of breast tissue, which just means that the epithelial cells are undergoing a change. There are no clear distinctions for this condition on mammography, and it may appear as a mass or a lesion on the mammogram. Therefore, it should be followed up with a confirming ultrasound or a small biopsy.
- **Epithelial-related calcifications**. Calcifications are mineral deposits that are found in both noncancerous and cancerous lesions of the breast. They appear as white spots or flecks on a mammogram and are usually so small they can't be felt. Although breast calcifications are usually benign, there are certain patterns of calcifications with irregular shapes that could indicate breast cancer. Therefore, when certain patterns of calcifications are seen on a mammogram, a biopsy is usually done as follow-up. Unless there are other changes in the breast ducts or lobules that appear suspicious, microcalcifications and calcifications are not significant findings.
- Other benign tumors:
  - A **lipoma** is a growth of fat cells just below the surface of the skin. It is the most common type of noncancerous growth in soft tissue. Lipomas tend to be small and are not always felt, but mostly seen on breast mammography. Lipomas are not always easy to diagnose and may not be distinguishable

from cancerous tumors when observed through mammography or ultrasound. Therefore, excisional biopsy is required for a clear diagnosis.

- A breast **hamartoma** is a solid, benign mass made up of both connective and glandular tissues. It forms in the soft tissue of the breast and is frequently diagnosed in young women. This type of breast lesion requires regular monitoring, but no treatment. If it changes in shape or gets larger, a biopsy may be performed. Hamartomas rarely lead to the development of breast cancer.
- **Hemangiomas** are benign tumors of the blood vessels, which rarely occur in the breast. A hemangioma is usually diagnosed by physical examination. Even though these growths are benign, they have been found in mastectomy specimens and in autopsy findings of women who died of breast cancer. However, it is not widely accepted that hemangiomas are related to breast cancer or increase breast cancer risk.
- **Neurofibromas** are tumors of the peripheral nervous system. Breast neurofibromas are rare and tend to be associated with neurofibromatosis, a disorder that is genetically inherited and causes nerve tissues to grow into tumors.
- An **adenomyoepithelioma** is a benign tumor composed of myoepithelial cells. It rarely occurs in men and occurs, on average, in women aged sixty years. It usually forms as a mass and, though benign, is prone to recur.

Proliferative lesions without atypia:

- **Usual ductal hyperplasia** without atypia is an overgrowth of cells lining the ducts in which the cells still look close to normal. As mentioned above, mild hyperplasia is not a cause for concern. However, moderate or more extensive hyperplasia without atypia does increase the risk for breast cancer—one and one-half to two times that of a woman with no breast abnormalities.
- **Fibroadenomas** are benign tumors that are made up of glandular and stromal tissue. These noncancerous breast tumors are the most common breast lumps in young women, occurring most often in adolescent girls and women under the age of thirty. Fibroadenomas are not part of fibrocystic changes. A fibroadenoma can be felt as a lump and appears as a round or oval-shaped, smooth-edged mass. When a fibroadenoma contains cysts, sclerosing adenosis, epithelial calcifications, or papillary apocrine changes, it is considered a complex

fibroadenoma and is associated with an increased risk for breast cancer. Although some fibroadenomas will disappear without treatment, they can be bothersome and cause discomfort and even physical deformity. The best approach to confirm suspected fibroadenomas is through use of percutaneous core biopsy, with conservative follow-up. Rapid growth of a fibroadenoma, usually larger than three centimeters, is an indication for surgical excision.

- With **sclerosing adenosis**, the enlarged lobules in the breast have been distorted, or pulled out of shape, by fibrous tissue. Women with adenosis are at an increased risk for breast cancer. Those with sclerosing adenosis have about one and one-half to two times the risk of women with no breast changes. The risk is similar to that for women who have usual hyperplasia without atypia.

- **Multiple papillomas** (called papillomatosis), occur deeper within the breast than solitary papillomas. They present a different type of risk and require different management than solitary lesions and often appear in both breasts. To be considered "papillomatosis," some physicians believe there should be at least five clearly separate papillomas within a particular segment of breast tissue. Papillomatosis is a type of hyperplasia in which there are very small areas of cell growth within the ducts. Papillomatosis is also linked to a slightly increased risk for breast cancer. Ductograms are sometimes helpful in finding papillomas. If a papilloma is large enough to be felt, a needle biopsy can be done. On microscopic evaluation, doctors will look for atypical cellular features and, if many are present, the condition may be reclassified as "atypical ductal hyperplasia," requiring surgical excision.

- **Radial scar** is a condition that distorts the normal breast tissue, causing it to look like a scar when viewed under a microscope.

Proliferative lesions with atypia:

- In **atypical ductal hyperplasia (ADH)**, abnormal cells are found in the ducts.
- In **atypical lobular hyperplasia (ALH)**, abnormal cells are found in the lobules.

In ADH and ALH, there is excessive growth of cells in the ducts or lobules of the breast tissue, and the cells no longer resemble normal, healthy cells. The breast cells become abnormal in number, size, shape, growth pattern, and appearance. These conditions can only be diagnosed with a biopsy. They have a stronger effect on breast cancer risk—raising it three and a half to five times higher than normal. If a woman has either type of atypical hyperplasia, her doctor may recommend more frequent breast cancer screening and careful consideration of chemopreventive medications and other strategies to reduce breast cancer risk.

American Cancer Society Guidelines on Nutrition and Physical Activity for Cancer Prevention

Achieve and maintain a healthy weight throughout life.
- Be as lean as possible throughout life without being underweight.
- Avoid excess weight gain at all ages. For those who are currently overweight or obese, losing even a small amount of weight has health benefits and is a good place to start.
- Engage in regular physical activity and limit consumption of high-calorie foods and beverages as key strategies for maintaining a healthy weight.

Adopt a physically active lifestyle.
- Adults should engage in at least 150 minutes of moderate intensity or 75 minutes of vigorous intensity activity each week, or an equivalent combination, preferably spread throughout the week.
- Children and adolescents should engage in at least 1 hour of moderate or vigorous intensity activity each day, with vigorous intensity activity occurring at least three days each week.
- Limit sedentary behavior such as sitting, lying down, watching television, or other forms of screen-based entertainment.
- Doing some physical activity above usual activities, no matter what one's level of activity, can have many health benefits.

Consume a healthy diet, with an emphasis on plant foods.
- Choose foods and beverages in amounts that help achieve and maintain a healthy weight.
- Limit consumption of processed meat and red meat.
- Eat at least two and one-half cups of vegetables and fruits each day.
- Choose whole grains instead of refined grain products.

If you drink alcoholic beverages, limit consumption.

- Drink no more than one drink per day for women or two per day for men.

RESOURCE GUIDE

American Cancer Society Support Programs and Services

American Cancer Society

Toll-free number: 800-227-2345
Website: www.cancer.org

The American Cancer Society is the nationwide, community-based voluntary health organization dedicated to eliminating cancer as a major health problem by preventing cancer, saving lives, and diminishing suffering from cancer through research, education, advocacy, and service. Headquartered in Atlanta, Georgia, the Society has eleven Divisions, more than 900 local offices nationwide, and a presence in more than 5,100 communities.

The American Cancer Society provides educational materials, information, and patient services to help people with cancer and their loved ones understand cancer, manage their lives through treatment and recovery, and find the emotional support they need. A comprehensive resource for all your cancer-related questions, the Society can also put you in touch with community resources in your area.

And best of all, our help is free. For information about the programs and services listed below, visit www.cancer.org or call 800-227-2345.

American Cancer Society Cancer Action Network^{SM} (ACS CAN) is all about ensuring that fighting cancer is a top priority for our lawmakers. When constituents demand that legislators make fighting cancer a priority, they make a difference. All ACS CAN members are notified of cancer-related issues pending in government agencies. They are also notified when critical cancer issues are heading for a vote or are in danger of being ignored by our lawmakers. Visit www.acscan.org for more information.

American Cancer Society Cancer Survivors Network® comprises a community of cancer survivors, families, and friends. All have been touched by cancer and want to share their experiences, strength, and hope. Only those who have been there can truly understand.

The website is completely noncommercial and provides a private, secure way to find and communicate with others to share similar interests and experiences. Members control access to personal information. Visit www.acscsn.org to learn more.

Look Good…Feel Better® is a free, community-based program that teaches beauty techniques to female cancer patients to help them manage the appearance-related side effects of cancer treatment. The program is open to all women with cancer who are undergoing chemotherapy, radiation, or other forms of treatment. The thousands of volunteer beauty professionals who support Look Good…Feel Better are trained and certified by the Personal Care Products Council Foundation, the American Cancer Society, and the Professional Beauty Association | National Cosmetology Association at local, statewide, and national workshops. Visit http://lookgoodfeelbetter.org/ for more information.

The **American Cancer Society Patient Navigator Program** helps patients, families, and caregivers navigate the many systems needed during the cancer journey. Trained patient navigators at cancer treatment centers link those dealing with cancer to needed programs and resources. The "navigator" is a friendly, experienced, and approachable staff person who helps patients have a better experience while they are receiving care.

Reach To Recovery® helps people (female and male) cope with their breast cancer experience. This experience begins when someone is faced with the possibility of a breast cancer diagnosis and continues throughout the entire period that breast cancer remains a personal concern. Reach To Recovery volunteers offer understanding, support, and hope because they themselves have survived breast cancer and gone on to live normal, productive lives.

Road To Recovery® provides transportation to and from treatment for people who have cancer who do not have a ride or are unable to drive themselves. Volunteer drivers donate their time and the use of their cars so that patients can receive the life-saving treatments they need.

Hope Lodge® offers cancer patients and their families a free, temporary place to stay when their best hope for effective treatment may be in another city. Having to travel away from home to get care can place an extra emotional and financial burden on patients and caregivers during an already challenging time. Currently, there are thirty-one Hope

Lodge locations throughout the United States. Accommodations and eligibility requirements may vary by location, and room availability is first come, first served.

Relay For Life®, the American Cancer Society's signature event, is an overnight experience designed to bring together those who have been touched by cancer. At Relay, people from within the community gather to celebrate survivors, remember those lost to cancer, and to fight back against this disease. Relay participants help raise money and awareness to support the American Cancer Society in its life-saving mission to eliminate cancer as a major health issue. For more information, visit www.relayforlife.org.

"tlc" Tender Loving Care

The *"tlc"* magalog is the American Cancer Society's catalog and magazine for women. It offers helpful articles and a line of products made for women with cancer. Products include wigs, hairpieces, hats, turbans, breast forms, mastectomy bras, and swimwear. The *"tlc"* mission is to make these hard-to-find products affordable and readily available in the privacy of your own home. All proceeds from product sales go back into the American Cancer Society's programs and services for patients and survivors. To order products or catalogs, call 800-850-9445 or visit *"tlc"* at www.tlcdirect.org.

ADDITIONAL ORGANIZATIONS AND WEBSITES*

The following organizations can provide additional information and resources:

Breast Cancer Resources

Breastcancer.org
Website: www.breastcancer.org

Breastcancer.org is a nonprofit organization dedicated to providing the most reliable, complete, and up-to-date information about breast cancer and breast health, in addition to hosting an active and supportive online community.

Dr. Susan Love Research Foundation
Toll-free number: 866-569-0388
Telephone: 310-828-0060
Website: www.dslrf.org

The Dr. Susan Love Research Foundation is a nonprofit organization that works to eradicate breast cancer and improve the quality of women's health through innovative research, education, and advocacy.

National Breast Cancer Coalition
Toll-free number: 800-622-2838
Telephone: 202-296-7477
Website: www.stopbreastcancer.org

The National Breast Cancer Coalition (NBCC) strives to improve access to quality breast cancer care for all women—particularly the underserved and uninsured—from screening through diagnosis and treatment, through legislation and changes in systems of delivery of health care.

*Inclusion on this list does not imply endorsement by the American Cancer Society.

National Breast Cancer Foundation, Inc.

Website: www.nationalbreastcancer.org

The National Breast Cancer Foundation's mission is to save lives through early detection and to provide mammograms for those in need. Its mission includes increasing awareness through education, providing diagnostic breast care services for those in need, and providing nurturing support services.

National Lymphedema Network

Toll-free number: 800-541-3259

Telephone: 415-908-3681

Website: www.lymphnet.org

The National Lymphedema Network (NLN) is a nonprofit organization providing education and guidance to lymphedema patients, health care professionals, and the public by disseminating information on the prevention and management of lymphedema.

National Women's Health Information Center

Toll-free number: 800-994-9662

Website: http://womenshealth.gov

This website has a searchable database of information on various women's health issues, including breast cancer. Documents accessible through this site include information from the National Cancer Institute, the Centers for Disease Control and Prevention, and several other government agencies, as well as online links to medical dictionaries and journals.

Self-help for Women with Breast or Ovarian Cancer (SHARE)

Toll-free number: 866-891-2392

Telephone: 212-719-0364

Website: www.sharecancersupport.org

SHARE is a self-help organization that serves women who have been affected by breast cancer or ovarian cancer. Hotline volunteers are breast or ovarian cancer survivors. SHARE provides information, emotional support, printed materials, and referrals to national organizations.

Sisters Network® Inc.
Toll-free number: 866-781-1808
Telephone: 713-781-0255
Website: www.sistersnetworkinc.org

Sisters Network Inc. is a national African American breast cancer survivorship organization. This nonprofit organization is committed to increasing local and national attention on the devastating impact that breast cancer has in the African American community.

Susan G. Komen for the Cure®
Toll-free number: 877-GO-KOMEN (877-465-6636)
Website: ww5.komen.org

Susan G. Komen for the Cure is a large, national nonprofit organization that is working to end breast cancer in the United States and throughout the world. This organization invests in research, community health outreach, advocacy, and programs in more than fifty countries.

WomenStories
Toll-free number: 800-775-5790
Telephone: 716-881-7868
Website: www.womenstories.org

WomenStories, a nonprofit organization, benefits those who have been diagnosed with breast cancer and need the information and comfort that only other breast cancer survivors can provide.

Young Survival Coalition
Toll-free number: 877-972-1011
Telephone: 646-257-3000
Website: www.youngsurvival.org

Young Survival Coalition (YSC) is a global organization dedicated to the critical issues unique to young women (aged forty and younger) with breast cancer. This organization offers resources, connections, and outreach so women feel supported, empowered, and hopeful.

Breast Prostheses and Accessories

The following list includes a few of the prostheses and accessory manufacturers in the United States. These products sold by the following suppliers have not been tested or screened. The companies listed here are not necessarily endorsed by the American Cancer Society. To locate additional resources in your area, contact the American Cancer Society at 800-227-2345 or visit www.cancer.org.

Airway Mastectomy Products
Toll-free number: 800-888-0458
Telephone: 513-271-4594
Website: www.airwaymast.com

Bosom Buddy
Toll-free number: 800-262-2789
Website: www.bosombuddy.com

Freeman Manufacturing Company
Toll-free number: 800-253-2091
Website: www.freemanmfg.com

Gallery Mystique
E-mail: getinfo@gallerymystique.com
Website: www.gallerymystique.com

Jodee, Inc.
Toll-free number: 800-821-2767
Website: www.jodee.com

Ladies First, Inc.
Toll-free number: 800-497-8285
Website: www.ladiesfirst.com

Leading Lady Company

Toll-free number: 800-321-4804 or 800-832-3112 (in Ohio)

Website: www.leadinglady.com

Trulife

Toll-free number: 800-788-2267

Website: www.trulife.com

General Cancer Resources

American Society of Clinical Oncology

Toll-free number: 888-282-2552

Telephone: 571-483-1300

Website: www.asco.org, www.cancer.net (information for people with cancer)

The American Society of Clinical Oncology (ASCO) is an international medical society representing about ten thousand cancer specialists. The website includes patient guides, a glossary of cancer terms, an ASCO member oncologist locator, news and information about different cancers and drug treatments, information about cancer legislation, summaries of government reports, and links to related sites. The ASCO-sponsored Cancer-Net website provides information on types of cancer, coping, and patient support organizations.

Association of Community Cancer Centers

Telephone: 301-984-9496

Website: www.accc-cancer.org

The Association of Community Cancer Centers (ACCC) was founded to give oncology practitioners in the community a voice in the national oncology forum. ACCC includes more than seven hundred medical centers, hospitals, and cancer programs. The website features a searchable database of cancer centers listed by state, Internet resources for cancer survivors, and other useful information.

Cancer Research Institute

Toll-free number: 800-992-2623

Telephone: 212-688-7515

Website: www.cancerresearch.org

The Cancer Research Institute (CRI) is dedicated to the support and coordination of laboratory and clinical efforts that will lead to the immunological treatment, control, and prevention of cancer. The organization provides public information on cancer immunology and cancer treatment, helps locate immunotherapy clinical trials, and offers informational booklets on cancer.

National Cancer Institute

Toll-free number: 800-4-CANCER (800-422-6237)

TTY (Text Telephone): 800-332-8615

Website: www.cancer.gov

The National Cancer Institute (NCI) is a government agency that provides information on cancer research, diagnosis, and treatment to patients and health care providers. NCI also offers information about FDA-certified mammography facilities in local areas through its toll-free number. Callers can request free publications and have the opportunity to speak directly with a cancer specialist.

Cancer Information Service

Toll-free number: 800-4-CANCER (800-422-6237)

Live Help online chat: https://livehelp.cancer.gov

The NCI's Cancer Information Service (CIS) is a federally funded cancer education program that was established in 1975 as an essential part of the NCI's mission and information efforts. Accurate, up-to-date, and reliable information on cancer is provided through the toll-free number and through an online chat program. Help is available in both English and Spanish.

CancerTrials
Website: www.cancer.gov/clinicaltrials

Maintained by the NCI, this website offers information about ongoing cancer clinical trials and explanations of what a trial is and what is involved. Users can search for clinical trials by city, state, and type of cancer from a database of more than eight thousand trials in progress.

National Coalition for Cancer Survivorship
Toll-free number: 877-NCCS-YES (877-622-7937)
Telephone: 301-650-9127
Website: www.canceradvocacy.org

The National Coalition for Cancer Survivorship (NCCS) is a network of independent organizations working in the area of cancer survivorship and support. The website offers links to online cancer resources, support groups, survivorship programs, the Cancer Survival Toolbox™, and the NCCS newsletter.

National Comprehensive Cancer Network® (NCCN®)
Telephone: 215-690-0300
Website: www.nccn.org

The National Comprehensive Cancer Network® (NCCN®), a nonprofit alliance of the world's leading cancer centers, is dedicated to improving the quality and effectiveness of care provided to patients with cancer. The NCCN, made up of experts from many of the nation's leading cancer centers, develops cancer treatment guidelines for doctors to use when treating patients.

National Library of Medicine (includes MEDLINE)
Toll-free number: 888-FIND-NLM (888-346-3656)
Telephone: 301-594-5983
Website: www.nlm.nih.gov

The National Library of Medicine (NLM) collects, organizes, and makes available biomedical science information to investigators, educators, and health care professionals and carries out programs designed to strengthen medical library services in the United States.

HSR Project
Website: http://wwwcf.nlm.nih.gov/hsr_project/home_proj.cfm

Formerly the NLM Gateway, this site offers information about ongoing health services research and public health projects.

MEDLINEplus
Website: http://medlineplus.gov

MEDLINEplus is a database for consumer health information, including dictionaries; articles and journals from other organizations; textbooks; newsletters; and health news online for reading; and links to organizations that provide consumer information and clearinghouses that send health literature.

PubMed
Website: www.ncbi.nlm.nih.gov/PubMed

Also part of the National Library of Medicine, this database provides access to literature references in MEDLINE and other databases, with links to online journals. The website is searchable by key word.

University of Colorado Cancer Center Fund
Telephone: 303-724-7823
Website: www.cucancercenterfund.org

Through the counseling line of this nonprofit research center, people can request free publications and receive answers to questions about cancer. The website contains information about ongoing research and specific types of cancer.

US Department of Health and Human Services

Toll-free number: 877-696-6775

Website: www.hhs.gov

Website (Health Care Information): www.healthcare.gov

Centers for Disease Control and Prevention

Toll-free number: 800-CDC-INFO (800-232-4636)

TTY: 888-232-6348

Website: www.cdc.gov

The Centers for Disease Control and Prevention (CDC) is an agency of the US Department of Health and Human Services. Information about health topics can be found on the website with downloadable publications and links to related sources. The toll-free number can be used to locate free or low-cost mammography and Pap test centers in local areas.

National Health Information Center

Websites: www.health.gov/nhic/

The National Health Information Center (NHIC) is a health information referral service. NHIC connects health professionals and consumers who have health questions to the organizations that are best able to provide answers.

US Food and Drug Administration

Toll-free number: 888-INFO-FDA (888-463-6332)

Website: www.fda.gov

The US Food and Drug Administration (FDA) is responsible for regulating drugs, tobacco products, biological medical products, blood products, medical devices, and radiation-emitting devices, along with other products. The website has extensive information about all the products the FDA regulates.

Support for Patients and Families

CancerCare®
Toll-free number: 800-813-HOPE (800-813-4673)
Website: www.cancercare.org

CancerCare is a nonprofit social service agency that provides counseling and guidance to help cancer patients and their families and friends cope with the impact of cancer. CancerCare offers support groups; teleconferences for patients, friends, and family members; workshops, seminars, and clinics; and a newsletter and other publications.

CancerConnection
Telephone: 413-586-1642
Website: www.cancer-connection.org

CancerConnection is a community-based, nonprofit organization. Founded in 2000, it offers a haven where people living with cancer, their families, and their caregivers can learn how to cope with their changed lives and bodies and emotional turmoil by sharing strategies and resources.

Cancer Hope Network
Toll-free number: 800-552-4366
Telephone: 908-879-4039
Website: www.cancerhopenetwork.org

Cancer Hope Network is a nonprofit organization that provides free and confidential one-on-one support to cancer patients and their families. It matches cancer patients or family members with trained volunteers who have undergone and recovered from a similar cancer experience.

Cancer Support Community
Toll-free number: 888-793-9355
Telephone: 202-659-9709
Website: http://cancersupportcommunity.org/

In June 2011, Gilda's Club Worldwide and The Wellness Community officially merged to become the Cancer Support Community (CSC). CSC provides emotional and social support through a network of local affiliates and satellite locations.

CaringBridge.org
Telephone: 651-789-2300
Website: www.caringbridge.org

CaringBridge is a nonprofit organization that provides free websites to connect family and friends with someone experiencing a significant health challenge.

Hope for Two...The Pregnant with Cancer Network
Toll-free number: 800-743-4471
Website: www.pregnantwithcancer.org

Hope for Two...The Pregnant with Cancer Network is an international nonprofit organization that offers free support for women diagnosed with cancer while pregnant. It connects women who are currently pregnant with cancer with other women who have experienced a similar cancer diagnosis.

The Mautner Project
Telephone: 202-797-3570
Website: www.mautnerproject.org

This organization provides services and support to lesbians with cancer and their families and caregivers. The organization provides education and information about cancer to the lesbian community; education about the special concerns of lesbians with cancer and their loved ones to the health-providing community; and advocacy on lesbian health and cancer issues in national and local arenas.

National Association of Hospital Hospitality Houses, Inc.
Toll-free number: 800-542-9730
Website: www.nahhh.org

The National Association of Hospital Hospitality Houses, Inc. (NAHHH) provides information about hospital hospitality facilities, including Ronald McDonald Houses. These facilities provide lodging and other supportive services in a home-like environment, primarily for relatives of patients who are getting medical treatment outside their own community.

Patient Advocate Foundation
Toll-free number: 800-532-5274
Website: www.patientadvocate.org

Patient Advocate Foundation (PAF) is a national nonprofit organization that provides professional case management services to Americans with chronic, life-threatening, and debilitating illnesses. PAF case managers, assisted by doctors and health care attorneys, serve as liaisons between patients and their insurers, employers, and/or creditors to resolve insurance, job retention, and/or debt crisis matters as they relate to their diagnoses.

Stupid Cancer (formerly called The I'm Too Young for This Cancer Foundation)
Toll-free number: 877-735-4673
Website: www.stupidcancer.org

Stupid Cancer is the nation's largest support community for young adults with cancer. This nonprofit organization empowers young adults affected by cancer by building community, improving quality of life, and providing meaningful survivorship through age-appropriate support, programs, and services.

Well Spouse Foundation
Toll-free number: 800-838-0879
Website: www.wellspouse.org

The Well Spouse Foundation is a national organization that provides support to partners of the chronically ill and/or disabled. They offer letter-writing support groups, a bimonthly newsletter, annual conferences, and weekend meetings. They also make referrals to local support groups throughout the country.

Resources for Children and Adolescents

Cancercare for Kids

Toll-free number: 800-813-HOPE (800-813-4673)
Website: www.cancercareforkids.org

Cancercare for Kids is an online support program for teens with a parent, sibling, or other family member who has cancer. The toll-free number is also for anyone who has cancer or has a loved one with cancer.

Cancer Really Sucks

Website: www.cancerreallysucks.org

Cancer Really Sucks is an Internet-only resource designed for teens by teens who have loved ones facing cancer.

CLIMB®

Telephone: 303-322-1202
Website: www.childrenstreehousefdn.org

CLIMB® (Children's Lives Include Moments of Bravery) is a support group program for children of adult cancer patients. CLIMB is a program that helps children find the courage to deal with cancer in their families.

KidsCope

Website: www.kidscope.org

KidsCope is an Internet-only resource for children and families. Its mission is to help children and families understand the effects of cancer or chemotherapy on a loved one, to provide suggestions for coping, and to develop innovative programs and materials that communicate a message of hope.

Kids Konnected

Toll-free number: 800-899-2866

Telephone: 949-582-5443

Website: www.kidskonnected.org

Kids Konnected is a national, nonprofit organization that provides friendship, under-standing, education, and support for kids and teens who have a parent with cancer or have lost a parent with cancer. It provides answers to questions about cancer, support for children with a parent affected by cancer, an information packet with books and infor-mation specific to the needs of each child, referrals to local groups with monthly meetings, a quarterly newsletter for children, summer camps, socials, and grief workshops.

Caregiving and Hospice Resources

American College of Physicians

Toll-free number: 800-523-1546

Telephone: 215-351-2400

Website: www.acponline.org

This organization provides a free book called the *American College of Physicians Home Care Guide for Advanced Cancer* to help caregivers deal with the complex issues of caring for someone with cancer.

Caregiving.com

Toll-free number: 800-394-5334

Telephone: 773-343-6341

Website: www.caregiving.com

This grassroots organization provides practical information on being a caregiver, man-aging the stresses of caregiving, and solutions for caregiving situations.

Family Caregiver Alliance

Toll-free number: 800-445-8106

Telephone: 415-434-3388

Website: www.caregiver.org

The Family Caregiver Alliance (FCA) offers programs at the national, state, and local level to support and sustain caregivers. The website contains fact sheets, online support groups, newsletters, and links to other resources.

Hospice Net
Website: www.hospicenet.org

Hospice Net is an independent nonprofit organization that works exclusively through the Internet. The website includes information for patients and caregivers about hospice care, information about grief and loss, and a hospice locator service.

National Alliance for Caregiving
Website: www.caregiving.org

The National Alliance for Caregiving is a nonprofit coalition of national organizations focusing on issues of family caregiving. The Alliance was created to conduct research, do policy analysis, develop national programs, increase public awareness of family caregiving issues, work to strengthen state and local caregiving coalitions, and represent the US caregiving community internationally.

National Family Caregivers Association
Toll-free number: 800-896-3650
Telephone: 301-942-6430
Website: www.nfcacares.org

The National Family Caregivers Association (NFCA) educates, supports, empowers, and speaks up for the more than fifty million Americans who care for loved ones with a chronic illness or disability or the frailties of old age. It provides information, education, public awareness, and advocacy.

National Hospice & Palliative Care Organization
Toll-free number: 800-646-6460
Telephone: 703-837-1500
Website: www.nhpco.org

The National Hospice and Palliative Care Organization (NHPCO) is the largest non-profit membership organization representing hospice and palliative care programs and professionals in the United States. The organization is committed to improving end-of-life care and expanding access to hospice care, with the goal of profoundly enhancing quality of life for dying people and their loved ones.

Benefits, Employment, Legal, and Financial Resources

Americans with Disability Act (ADA)
Toll-free number: 800-514-0301
TTY: 800-514-0383
Website: www.ada.gov

This service employs specialists who can answer questions about the Americans with Disabilities Act (ADA) and provide information about the programs and services available through state and local governments. The website has a list of free booklets and publications you can order or read online. Many of these publications are available in languages other than English.

Cancer and Careers
Website: www.cancerandcareers.org

This organization is a resource for working people with cancer and their employers. The website offers news, articles, charts, checklists, tips, and also provides a link to an online community of experts, patients, and survivors.

Cancer Legal Resource Center
Toll-free number: 866-THE-CLRC (866-843-2572)
Website: www.disabilityrightslegalcenter.org/cancer-legal-resource-center

The Cancer Legal Resource Center (CLRC) is a national, joint program of the Disability Rights Legal Center and Loyola Law School Los Angeles. The CLRC provides free information and resources on cancer-related legal issues to cancer survivors, caregivers, health care professionals, employers, and others coping with cancer.

Eldercare Locator
Toll-free number: 800-677-1116
Website: www.eldercare.gov

The Eldercare Locator, a public service of the Administration on Aging, US Department of Health and Human Services, is a nationwide service that connects older Americans and their caregivers with information on senior services.

Federal Citizen Information Center
Toll-free number: 800-FED-INFO (800) 333-4636
TTY: 800-326-2996
Website: http://gsa.gov/portal/content/101085

The Federal Citizen Information Center (FCIC), in the Office of Citizen Services and Innovative Technologies, provides US government information and services directly to the public. It currently offers a variety of information channels, including websites, web chat, telephone, print, social media and e-mail.

Financial Planning Association
Toll-free number: 800-322-4237
Website: www.fpanet.org

The Financial Planning Association (FPA®) offers free information on personal finance and answers to general questions about financial planning, makes referrals to FPA members who are Certified Financial Planners™, and sets up free financial planning services to qualified people and families in need.

Insurance Information Institute
Telephone: 212-346-5500
National Consumer Help Line: 800-942-4242
Website: www.iii.org/services

For more than fifty years, the Insurance Information Institute (III) has provided information, analysis, and referrals to improve public understanding of insurance issues.

Internal Revenue Service
Toll-free number: 800-829-1040
Website: www.irs.gov

The Internal Revenue Service (IRS) is the agency with the Department of the Treasury that is responsible for collecting taxes and the interpretation and enforcement of the Internal Revenue Code.

Medicare Rights Center (for those with Medicare)
Toll-free number: 800-333-4114
Website: www.medicarerights.org

The Medicare Rights Center can help you understand your rights and benefits, navigate the Medicare system, and get quality medical care. They can also help you apply for programs that can reduce prescription drugs and medical care expenses, and guide you through the appeals process if drugs you need are denied through your Medicare prescription drug plan.

National Association of Insurance Commissioners
Telephone: 816-783-8300
Website: www.naic.org

The National Association of Insurance Commissioners (NAIC) is the US insurance industry standard-setting and regulatory support organization. For state insurance department phone numbers, visit http://www.naic.org/state_web_map.htm.

National Endowment for Financial Education
Telephone: 303-741-6333
Website: www.nefe.org

The National Endowment for Financial Education (NEFE) provides financial education and practical information to people at all financial stages. They provide numerous programs for consumers, including the NEFE High School Financial Planning Program® (HSFPP). All NEFE resources are available at no cost.

National Foundation for Credit Counseling
Toll-free number: 800-388-2227
Telephone: 202-677-4300
Website: www.nfcc.org

The National Foundation for Credit Counseling (NFCC) is the nation's largest financial counseling organization. The NFCC Member Agency Network includes more than seven hundred community-based offices that provide financial counseling and education to consumers in person, over the phone, or online.

Needy Meds
Toll-free number: 800-503-6897
Website: www.needymeds.org

NeedyMeds is a resource offering information on thousands of programs that may be able to offer assistance to people in need. NeedyMeds strives to provide accurate and current information, but the specific organizations providing services should be contacted directly for questions. NeedyMeds does offer a free drug discount card that may help obtain a substantially lower price on your medications.

Pharmaceutical Research and Manufacturers Association of America
Telephone: 202-835-3400
Website: www.phrma.org

The Pharmaceutical Research and Manufacturers of America (PhRMA) represents the country's leading pharmaceutical research and biotechnology companies.

Partnership for Prescription Assistance
Toll-free number: 888-4PPA-NOW (888-477-2669)
Website: www.pparx.org

The Partnership for Prescription Assistance helps qualifying patients without prescription drug coverage get the medicines they need through the program that is right for them.

Social Security Administration
Toll-free number: 800-772-1213
TTY: 800-325-0778
Website: www.socialsecurity.gov

The Social Security Administration (SSA) has general information, qualification criteria, and information about how to apply for program benefits (such as Social Security Disability Income and Supplemental Security Income if you cannot work). The SSA also makes referrals to local SSA and Medicare/Medicaid offices.

US Department of Agriculture
Telephone: 202-720-2791
Website: www.usda.gov

Women, Infants, and Children (WIC) Program
Website: www.fns.usda.gov/wic

The Special Supplemental Nutrition Program for Women, Infants, and Children (WIC) provides federal grants to states for supplemental foods, health care referrals, and nutrition education for low-income pregnant, breastfeeding, and non-breast-feeding postpartum women, and to infants and children up to age five who are found to be at nutritional risk.

Supplemental Nutrition Assistance Program (formerly called Food Stamps Program)
Toll-free number: 800-221-5689
Website: www.fns.usda.gov/snap

Supplemental Nutrition Assistance Program (SNAP) offers nutrition assistance to millions of eligible, low-income individuals and families and provides economic benefits to communities.

US Department of Health and Human Services
Toll-free number: 877-696-6775
Website: www.hhs.gov

Hill-Burton Program
Toll-free number: 800-638-0742
Website: http://www.hhs.gov/ocr/civilrights/understanding/Hill-Burton

The Hill-Burton Act authorizes funding for hospitals and other medical facilities so they can offer free or low-cost services to people who cannot pay. Eligibility for Hill-Burton is based on family size and income. Patients can apply for Hill-Burton assistance at any time, before or after they receive care.

Medicaid
Toll-free number: 877-267-2323
TTY: 866-226-1819
Website: www.medicaid.gov

This office of the US Department of Health and Human Services can provide information about Medicaid coverage and eligibility. Your state social service or human service agency can best answer your questions about your benefits and eligibility. To locate contact information for your state, visit www.cms.gov/apps/contacts.

Medicare
Toll-free number: (800-MEDICARE) 800-633-4227
TTY: 877-486-2048
Website: www.medicare.gov

This office of the US Department of Health and Human Services provides literature, answers questions, and gives referrals to state Medicare offices and local HMOs with Medicare contracts.

Office of Family Assistance

Toll-free number: 877-696-6775

Telephone: 202-401-9275

Website: www.acf.hhs.gov/programs/ofa/help

This office provides contact information by state or territory for family assistance, including Temporary Assistance for Needy Families (TANF) in your state.

US Department of Labor

Toll-free number: 866-4-USA-DOL (866-487-2365)

Website: www.dol.gov

This department of the US government is responsible for occupational safety, wage and hour standards, unemployment insurance benefits, re-employment services, and some economic statistics.

Employee Benefits Security Administration

Toll-free number: 866-444-3272

Website: www.dol.gov/ebsa

The Employee Benefits Security Administration (EBSA) has information on employee benefit laws, including COBRA, FMLA, and HIPAA requirements for employer-based health coverage and self-insured health plans. This website also has information on recent changes in health care laws. Information for military reservists who must leave their private employers for active duty can be found at www.dol.gov/elaws/vets/userra/mainmenu.asp.

Job Accommodation Network

Toll-free number: 800-526-7234

TTY: 877-781-9403

Website: www.askjan.org

The Job Accommodation Network is a free consulting service of the US Department of Labor that gives information on the Americans with Disability Act (ADA), your rights, how to talk to an employer, and how to ask for accommodations. A list of available publications can be found online at http://askjan.org/media/index.htm.

Wage and Hour Division

Toll-free number: (866-4-USWAGE) 866-487-9243
TTY: 877-889-5627
Website: http://www.dol.gov/whd/fmla/

The Wage and Hour Division can provide more information about the Family and Medical Leave Act (FMLA), including school employee rules, how it impacts state law, employer policy variations, changes for military families, and more. A direct link for citizens/employees can be found at http://www.dol.gov/dol/topic/benefits-leave/fmla.htm.

US Department of Veterans Affairs

Toll-free number: 800-827-1000
Website: www.va.gov

The Department of Veterans Affairs can provide information on veterans' medical benefits and the qualifications necessary to receive them. Call 877-222-8387 or visit www.va.gov/healtheligibility to find out whether you are eligible for veterans' benefits.

US Equal Employment Opportunity Commission

Toll-free number: 800-669-4000
TTY: 800-669-6820
Website: www.eeoc.gov

The US Equal Employment Opportunity Commission (EEOC) has information on all federal equal employment regulations, practices, and policies; how to file charges of workplace discrimination; and how to find EEOC in your area. Their publication *Questions and Answers About Cancer in the Workplace and the Americans with Disability Act (ADA)* can be found at www.eeoc.gov/facts/cancer.html.

Other Professional Organizations

American Academy of Physical Medicine and Rehabilitation (for locating physiatrists)
Toll-free number: 847-737-6000
Website: www.aapmr.org

The American Academy of Physical Medicine and Rehabilitation is the national medical society representing more than 7,500 physicians who are specialists in the field of physical medicine and rehabilitation. The website has information about the specialty of physical medicine and rehabilitation. They provide a searchable database (www.aapmr.org/patients/findphysician) to help you locate physiatrists in your area.

American Association for Marriage and Family Therapy
Telephone: 703-838-9808
Website: www.aamft.org

The American Association for Marriage and Family Therapy (AAMFT) is the professional association for the field of marriage and family therapy. AAMFT provides referrals to local marriage and family therapists. They also provide educational materials to help couples live with illness and other issues related to families and health.

American Counseling Association
Toll-free number: 800-347-6647
Website: www.counseling.org

The American Counseling Association (ACA) is a nonprofit professional and educational organization dedicated to the growth and enhancement of the counseling profession. ACA provides information to consumers for how to locate a professional counselor through the National Board of Certified Counselors (www.nbcc.org/counselorfind) and other sources.

American Physical Therapy Association
Toll-free number: 800-999-APTA (800-999-2782)
Website: www.apta.org

The American Physical Therapy Association (APTA) is a national professional organization representing more than seventy-two thousand members. The organization represents and promotes the profession of physical therapy and strives to further the profession's role in the prevention, diagnosis, and treatment of movement dysfunctions and the enhancement of the physical health and functional abilities of members of the public.

American Psychiatric Association

Toll-free number: 888-35-PSYCH (888-357-7924)
Website: www.psych.org

The American Psychiatric Association provides information on mental health and referrals. It represents more than thirty-six thousand psychiatric physicians from the United States and around the world.

American Psychological Association

Toll-free number: 800-374-2721
Telephone: 202-336-5500
Website: www.apa.org

The American Psychological Association (APA) is a scientific and professional organization that represents psychology in the United States. The APA offers referrals to psychologists in local areas (http://locator.apa.org). They also provide information on family issues, parenting, and health.

American Society of Plastic Surgeons

Telephone: 847-228-9900
Website: www.plasticsurgery.org

The American Society of Plastic Surgeons (ASPS) is the largest plastic surgery specialty organization in the world. ASPS is composed of more than seven thousand physician members and represents more than 94 percent of all board-certified plastic surgeons in the United States who perform cosmetic and reconstructive surgery.

Association of Oncology Social Work
Telephone: 215-599-6093
Website: www.aosw.org

The Association of Oncology Social Work (AOSW) and its members work to increase awareness about the social, emotional, educational, and spiritual needs of cancer patients. This is accomplished through research, writing, workshops and lectures, and collaborations with other patient advocacy groups, as well as national and international oncology organizations whose primary focus is access to quality care for cancer patients.

National Association of Social Workers
Toll-free number: 800-742-4089
Telephone: 202-408-8600
Website: www.naswdc.org

The National Association of Social Workers (NASW) is the largest membership organization of professional social workers in the world. The NASW Register of Clinical Social Workers, available on the website under "Find a Social Worker," is a resource the public can use to identify social workers who are qualified by education, experience, and credentials to provide mental health services.

REFERENCES

Chapter 1: What Is Cancer?

Abeloff MD, Wolff AC, Weber BL, et al. Cancer of the breast. In: Abeloff MD, Armitage JO, Lichter AS, et al, eds. *Clinical Oncology*. 4th ed. Philadelphia, PA: Elsevier; 2008: 1875–1943.

American Cancer Society. *Cancer Facts and Figures 2012*. Atlanta, GA: American Cancer Society; 2012.

Burstein HJ, Harris JR, Morrow M. Malignant tumors of the breast. In: DeVita VT, Lawrence TS, Rosenberg SA, eds. *DeVita, Hellman, and Rosenberg's Cancer: Principles and Practice of Oncology*. 8th ed. Philadelphia, PA: Lippincott Williams & Wilkins; 2008: 1606–1654.

Dillon DA, Guidi AJ, Schnitt SJ. Pathology of invasive breast cancer. In: Harris JR, Lippman ME, Morrow M, Osborne CK, eds. *Diseases of the Breast*. 4th ed. Philadelphia, PA: Lippincott Williams & Wilkins; 2010: 374–407.

Howlader N, Noone AM, Krapcho M, Neyman N, Aminou R, Waldron W, Altekruse SF, Kosary CL, Ruhl J, Tatalovich Z, Cho H, Mariotto A, Eisner MP, Lewis DR, Chen HS, Feuer EJ, Cronin KA, Edwards BK (eds). *SEER Cancer Statistics Review, 1975–2008*, National Cancer Institute. Bethesda, MD, http://seer.cancer.gov/csr/1975_2008/, based on November 2010 SEER data submission, posted to the SEER website, 2011.

Santen RJ, Mansel R. Benign breast disorders. *N Engl J Med*. 2005;353(3):275–285.

Schnitt SJ, Collins LC. Pathology of benign breast disorders. In: Harris JR, Lippman ME, Morrow M, Osborne CK, eds. *Diseases of the Breast*. 4th ed. Philadelphia, PA: Lippincott Williams & Wilkins; 2010: 69–85.

Simpson PT, Reis-Filho JS, Lakhani SR. Lobular carcinoma in situ: biology and pathology. In: Harris JR, Lippman ME, Morrow M, Osborne CK, eds. *Diseases of the Breast*. 4th ed. Philadelphia, PA: Lippincott Williams & Wilkins. 2010: 333–340.

Chapter 2: Who Gets Breast Cancer?

Abeloff MD, Wolff AC, Weber BL, et al. Cancer of the breast. In: Abeloff MD, Armitage JO, Lichter AS, et al, eds. *Clinical Oncology*. 4th ed. Philadelphia, PA: Elsevier; 2008: 1875–1943.

American Cancer Society. *Cancer Facts and Figures 2012*. Atlanta, GA: American Cancer Society; 2012.

Anderson GL, Clebowski RT, Aragaki AK, Kuller LH, Manson JE, Gass M, Bluhm E, Connelly S, Hubbell FA, Lane D, Martin L, Ockene J, Rohan T, Schenken R, Wactawski-Wende J. Conjugated equine oestrogen and breast cancer incidence and mortality in postmenopausal women with hysterectomy: extended follow-up of the Women's Health Initiative randomised placebo-controlled trial. *Lancet Oncol*. 2012;13(5):476–486. Epub 2012 Mar 7.

Anderson GL, Limacher M, Assaf AR, Bassford T, Beresford SA, Black H, Bonds D, Brunner R, Brzyski R, Caan B, Chlebowski R, Curb D, Gass M, Hays J, Heiss G, Hendrix S, Howard BV, Hsia J, Hubbell A, Jackson R, Johnson KC, Judd H, Kotchen JM, Kuller L, LaCroix AZ, Lane D, Langer RD, Lasser N, Lewis CE, Manson J, Margolis K, Ockene J, O'Sullivan MJ, Phillips L, Prentice RL, Ritenbaugh C, Robbins J, Rossouw JE, Sarto G, Stefanick ML, Van Horn L, Wactawski-Wende J, Wallace R, Wassertheil-Smoller S; Women's Health Initiative Steering Committee. Effects of conjugated equine estrogen in postmenopausal women with hysterectomy: the Women's Health Initiative randomized controlled trial. *JAMA*. 2004;291(14):1701–1712.

Antiperspirants/deodorants and breast cancer. National Cancer Institute website. http://www.cancer.gov/cancertopics/factsheet/Risk/AP-Deo. Accessed February 16, 2012.

Beral V; Million Women Study Collaborators. Breast cancer and hormone-replacement therapy in the Million Women Study. *Lancet*. 2003;362(9382):419–427.
  Erratum in:
  Lancet. 2003;362(9390):1160.

Bio-identicals: sorting myths from facts. US Food and Drug Administration website. http://www.fda.gov/forconsumers/consumerupdates/ucm049311.htm. Accessed February 14, 2012.

Burstein HJ, Harris JR, Morrow M. Malignant tumors of the breast. In: DeVita VT, Lawrence TS, Rosenberg SA, eds. *DeVita, Hellman, and Rosenberg's Cancer: Principles and Practice of Oncology.* 8th ed. Philadelphia, PA: Lippincott Williams & Wilkins; 2008: 1606–1654.

California Environmental Protection Agency. Proposed identification of environmental tobacco smoke as a toxic air contaminant, part B: health effects of exposure to environmental tobacco smoke. www.oehha.ca.gov/air/environmental_tobacco/pdf/app3partb2005.pdf. Published June 24, 2005. Accessed November 7, 2011.

Chen LC, Weiss NS, Newcomb P, Barlow W, White E. Hormone replacement therapy in relation to breast cancer. *JAMA.* 2002;287(6):734–741.

Chen WY, Rosner B, Hankinson SE, Colditz GA, Willett WC. Moderate alcohol consumption during adult life, drinking patterns, and breast cancer risk. *JAMA.* 2011;306(17):1884–1890.

Chen X, Lu W, Zheng W, Gu K, Chen Z, Zheng Y, Shu XO. Obesity and weight change in relation to breast cancer survival. *Breast Cancer Res Treat.* 2010;122(3):823–833. Epub 2010 Jan 8.

Claus EB, Risch N, Thompson WD. Autosomal dominant inheritance of early-onset breast cancer. Implications for risk prediction. *Cancer.* 1994;73(3):643–651.

Collaborative Group on Hormonal Factors in Breast Cancer. Breast cancer and breastfeeding: collaborative reanalysis of individual data from 47 epidemiological studies in 30 countries, including 50,302 women with breast cancer and 96,973 women without the disease. *Lancet.* 2002;360(9328):187–195.

Collaborative Group on Hormonal Factors in Breast Cancer. Familial breast cancer: collaborative reanalysis of individual data from 52 epidemiological studies including 58,209 women with breast cancer and 101,986 women without the disease. *Lancet.* 2001;358(9291):1389–1399.

Darbre PD, Aljarrah A, Miller WR, Coldham NG, Sauer MJ, Pope GS. Concentrations of parabens in human breast tumours. *J Appl Toxicol.* 2004;24(1):5–13.

Gail MH, Brinton LA, Byar DP, Corle DK, Green SB, Schairer C, Mulvihill JJ. Projecting individualized probabilities of developing breast cancer for white females who are being examined annually. *J Natl Cancer Inst.* 1989;81(24):1879–1886.

Genetics of breast and ovarian cancer (PDQ®). National Cancer Institute website. http://www.cancer.gov/cancertopics/pdq/genetics/breast-and-ovarian/HealthProfessional. Accessed February 14, 2012.

Giusti RM, Iwamoto K, Hatch EE. Diethylstilbestrol revisited: a review of the long-term health effects. *Ann Intern Med.* 1995;122(10):778–788.

Heiss G, Wallace R, Anderson GL, Aragaki A, Beresford SA, Brzyski R, Chlebowski RT, Gass M, LaCroix A, Manson JE, Prentice RL, Rossouw J, Stefanick ML; WHI Investigators. Health risks and benefits 3 years after stopping randomized treatment with estrogen and progestin. *JAMA.* 2008;299(9):1036–1045.

Hoover RN, Hyer M, Pfeiffer RM, Adam E, Bond B, Cheville AL, Colton T, Hartge P, Hatch EE, Herbst AL, Karlan BY, Kaufman R, Noller KL, Palmer JR, Robboy SJ, Saal RC, Strohsnitter W, Titus-Ernstoff L, Troisi R. Adverse health outcomes in women exposed in utero to diethylstilbestrol. *N Engl J Med.* 2011;365(14):1304–1314.

Howlader N, Noone AM, Krapcho M, Neyman N, Aminou R, Waldron W, Altekruse SF, Kosary CL, Ruhl J, Tatalovich Z, Cho H, Mariotto A, Eisner MP, Lewis DR, Chen HS, Feuer EJ, Cronin KA, Edwards BK (eds). *SEER Cancer Statistics Review, 1975–2008*, National Cancer Institute. Bethesda, MD, http://seer.cancer.gov/csr/1975_2008/, based on November 2010 SEER data submission, posted to the SEER website, 2011.

Kabat GC, Cross AJ, Park Y, Schatzkin A, Hollenbeck AR, Rohan TE, Sinha R. Meat intake and meat preparation in relation to risk of postmenopausal breast cancer in the NIH-AARP diet and health study. *Int J Cancer.* 2009;124(10):2430–2435.

Kabat GC, Kim M, Adams-Campbell LL, Caan BJ, Chlebowski RT, Neuhouser ML, Shikany JM, Rohan TE; WHI Investigators. Longitudinal study of serum carotenoid, retinol, and tocopherol concentrations in relation to breast cancer risk among postmenopausal women. *Am J Clin Nutr.* 2009;90(1):162–169. Epub 2009 May 27.

Kushi LH, Doyle C, McCullough M, Rock CL, Demark-Wahnefried W, Bandera EV, Gapstur S, Patel AV, Andrews K, Gansler T; American Cancer Society 2010 Nutrition and Physical Activity Guidelines Advisory Committee. American Cancer Society guidelines on nutrition and physical activity for cancer prevention: reducing the risk of cancer with healthy food choices and physical activity. *CA Cancer J Clin.* 2012;62(1):30–67.

Li CI, Beaber EF, Chen Tang MT, Porter PL, Daling JR, Malone KE. Effect of depo-medroxyprogesterone acetate on breast cancer risk among women 20 to 44 years of age. *Cancer Res.* 2012 Apr 15;72(8):2028-2035. Epub 2012 Feb 27.

McTiernan A, Kooperberg C, White E, Wilcox S, Coates R, Adams-Campbell LL, Woods N, Ockene J; Women's Health Initiative Cohort Study. Recreational physical activity and the risk of breast cancer in postmenopausal women: the Women's Health Initiative Cohort Study. *JAMA.* 2003;290(10):1331–1336.

Mirick DK, Davis S, Thomas DB. Antiperspirant use and the risk of breast cancer. *J Natl Cancer Inst.* 2002;94(20):1578–1580.

National Toxicology Program. Bisphenol A (BPA). National Institute of Environmental Health Sciences website. http://www.niehs.nih.gov/health/assets/docs_a_e/bisphenol_a_bpa_508.pdf. Accessed February 16, 2012.

Norat T, Chan D, Lau R, Vieira R. The associations between food, nutrition and physical activity and the risk of breast cancer. WCRF/AICR *Systematic Literature Review Continuous Update Project Report.* World Cancer Research Fund/American Institute for Cancer Research website. http://www.dietandcancerreport.org/cancer_resource_center/downloads/cu/cu_breast_cancer_report_2008.pdf. Issued November 7, 2008. Accessed February 16, 2012.

Olsson HL, Ingvar C, Bladström A. Hormone replacement therapy containing progestins and given continuously increases breast carcinoma risk in Sweden. *Cancer.* 2003;97(6):1387–1392.

Online Mendelian Inheritance in Man, OMIM®. McKusick-Nathans Institute of Genetic Medicine, Johns Hopkins University (Baltimore, MD). http://omim.org/. Accessed February 14, 2012.

Reproductive history and breast cancer risk. National Cancer Institute website. http://www.cancer.gov/cancertopics/factsheet/Risk/reproductive-history. Accessed August 1, 2012.

Rossouw JE, Anderson GL, Prentice RL, LaCroix AZ, Kooperberg C, Stefanick ML, Jackson RD, Beresford SA, Howard BV, Johnson KC, Kotchen JM, Ockene J; Writing Group for the Women's Health Initiative Investigators. Risks and benefits of estrogen plus progestin in healthy postmenopausal women: principal results from the Women's Health Initiative Randomized Controlled Trial. *JAMA.* 2002;288(3):321–333.

Santen RJ, Mansel R. Benign breast disorders. *N Engl J Med.* 2005;353(3):275–285.

Saslow D, Boetes C, Burke W, Harms S, Leach MO, Lehman CD, Morris E, Pisano E, Schnall M, Sener S, Smith RA, Warner E, Yaffe M, Andrews KS, Russell CA; American Cancer Society Breast Cancer Advisory Group. American Cancer Society guidelines for breast screening with MRI as an adjunct to mammography. *CA Cancer J Clin.* 2007;57(2):75–89.
    Erratum in:
    CA Cancer J Clin. 2007;57(3):185

Schnitt SJ, Collins LC. Pathology of benign breast disorders. In: Harris JR, Lippman ME, Morrow M, Osborne CK, eds. *Diseases of the Breast.* 4th ed. Philadelphia, PA: Lippincott Williams & Wilkins; 2010: 69–85.

Simpson PT, Reis-Filho JS, Lakhani SR. Lobular Carcinoma in situ: biology and pathology. In: Harris JR, Lippman ME, Morrow M, Osborne CK, eds. *Diseases of the Breast.* 4th ed. Philadelphia, PA: Lippincott Williams & Wilkins. 2010: 333–340.

Skegg DC, Noonan EA, Paul C, Spears GF, Meirik O, Thomas DB. Depot medroxyprogesterone acetate and breast cancer. A pooled analysis of the World Health Organization and New Zealand studies. *JAMA.* 1995;273(10):799–804.

Smith-Warner SA, Spiegelman D, Yaun SS, van den Brandt PA, Folsom AR, Goldbohm RA, Graham S, Holmberg L, Howe GR, Marshall JR, Miller AB, Potter JD, Speizer FE, Willett WC, Wolk A, Hunter DJ. Alcohol and breast cancer in women: a pooled analysis of cohort studies. *JAMA.* 1998;279(7):535–540.

Thompson D, Easton DF; The Breast Cancer Linkage Consortium. Cancer incidence in BRCA1 mutation carriers. *J Natl Cancer Inst.* 2002;94(18):1358–1365.

Tyrer J, Duffy SW, Cuzick J: A breast cancer prediction model incorporating familial and personal risk factors. *Stat Med.* 2004;23(7):1111–1130.
> Erratum in:
> *Stat Med.* 2005;24(1):156.

US Department of Health and Human Services. The health consequences of involuntary exposure to tobacco smoke: a report of the surgeon general. 2006. http://www.surgeongeneral.gov/library/secondhand smoke/. Issued June 27, 2006. Accessed November 3, 2011.

US Preventive Services Task Force. Genetic risk assessment and BRCA mutation testing for breast and ovarian cancer susceptibility: recommendation statement. *Ann Intern Med.* 2005;143(5):355–361.
> Erratum in
> *Ann Intern Med.* 2005;143(7):547.

Chapter 3: Your Breast Cancer Workup

Arpino G, Generali D, Sapino A, Lucia del M, Frassoldati A, de Laurentis M, Paolo P, Mustacchi G, Cazzaniga M, De Placido S, Conte P, Cappelletti M, Zanoni V, Antonelli A, Martinotti M, Puglisi F, Berruti A, Bottini A, Dogliotti L. Gene expression profiling in breast cancer: a clinical perspective. *Breast.* 2013;22(2):109–120.

Breast cancer treatment. (PDQ®). National Cancer Institute website. http://www.cancer.gov/cancertopics/pdq/treatment/breast/healthprofessional. Accessed March 4, 2013.

Brenton JD, Carey LA, Ahmed AA, Caldas C. Molecular classification and molecular forecasting of breast cancer: Ready for clinical application? *J Clin Oncol.* 2005;23(29):7350–7360. Epub 2005 Sep 6.

Fenton JJ, Abraham L, Taplin SH, Geller BM, Carney PA, D'Orsi C, Elmore JG, Barlow WE; Breast Cancer Surveillance Consortium. Effectiveness of computer-aided detection in community mammography practice. *J Natl Cancer Inst.* 2011;103(15):1152–1161. Epub 2011 Jul 27.

Fenton JJ, Taplin SH, Carney PA, Abraham L, Sickles EA, D'Orsi C, Berns EA, Cutter G, Hendrick RE, Barlow WE,

Elmore JG. Influence of computer-aided detection on performance of screening mammography. *N Engl J Med.* 2007;356(14):1399–1409.

MRI of the breast. Radiological Society of North America, Inc. website. http://www.radiologyinfo.org/en/info.cfm?pg=breastmr. Reviewed April 24, 2012. Accessed September 11, 2012.

Pisano ED, Gatsonis C, Hendrick E, Yaffe M, Baum JK, Acharyya S, Conant EF, Fajardo LL, Bassett L, D'Orsi C, Jong R, Rebner M; Digital Mammographic Imaging Screening Trial (DMIST) Investagators Group. Diagnostic performance of digital versus film mammography for breast-cancer screening. *N Eng J Med.* 2005;353(17):1773–1783. Epub 2005 Sep 16.
> Erratum in:
> *N Eng J Med.* 2006;355(17):1840.

Ross JS, Hatzis C, Symmans F, Pusztai L, Hortobágyi GN. Commercialized multigene predictors of clinical outcome for breast cancer. *Oncologist.* 2008;13(5):477–493.
> Erratum in
> *Oncologist.* 2008;13(8). doi 10. 1634/theoncologist.2007-0248.

Sala M, Comas M, Macià F, Martinez J, Casamitjana M, Castells X. Implementation of digital mammography in a population-based breast cancer screening program: effect of screening round on recall rate and cancer detection. *Radiology.* 2009;252(1):31–39. Epub 2009 May 6.

Smith RA, D'Orsi C, Newell MS. Screening for breast cancer. In: Harris JR, Lippman ME, Morrow M, Osborne CK, eds. *Diseases of the Breast.* 4th ed. Philadelphia, PA: Lippincott Williams & Wilkins; 2010:87–115.

Yang WT, Le-Petross HT, Macapinlac H, Carkaci S, Gonzalez-Angulo AM, Dawood S, Resetkova E, Hortobagyi GN, Cristofanilli M. Inflammatory breast cancer: PET/CT, MRI, mammography, and sonography findings. *Breast Cancer Res Treat.* 2008;109(3):417–426. Epub 2007 Jul 26.

Chapter 4: Understanding Your Diagnosis

American Joint Committee on Cancer. Breast. In: *AJCC Cancer Staging Manual.* 7th ed. New York: Springer; 2010: 347–369.

Chapter 5: Coping with Your Diagnosis and Moving Forward

Ali SA, Gupta S, Sehgal R, Vogel V. Survival outcomes in pregnancy associated breast cancer: a retrospective case control study. *Breast J.* 2012;18(2):139–144.

Cardonick E, Dougherty R, Grana G, Gilmandyar D, Ghaffar S, Usmani A. Breast cancer during pregnancy: maternal and fetal outcomes. *Cancer J.* 2010;16(1):76-82.

Christ GH, Christ AE. Current approaches to helping children cope with a parent's terminal illness. *CA Cancer J Clin.* 2006;56(4):197–212.

Harpham WS. *When a Parent Has Cancer: A Guide to Caring for Your Children.* New York: HarperCollins, 2004.

Pirl WF. Evidence report on the occurrence, assessment, and treatment of depression in cancer patients. *JNCI Monographs.* 2004;(32):32–39. doi: 10.1093/jncimonographs/lgh026.

Thastum M, Johansen MB, Gubba L, Olesen LB, Romer G. Coping, social relations, and communication: a qualitative exploratory study of children of parents with cancer. *Clin Child Psychol Psychiatry.* 2008;13(1):123–138.

Thastum M, Watson M, Kienbacher C, Piha J, Steck B, Zachariae R, Baldus C, Romer G. Prevalence and predictors of emotional and behavioural functioning of children where a parent has cancer: a multinational study. *Cancer.* 2009;115(17):4030–4039.

Walton JR, Prasad MR. Obstetric and neonatal outcomes of cancer treated during pregnancy. *Clin Obstet Gynecol.* 2011;54(4):567-573.

Watson M, St James-Roberts I, Ashley S, Tilney C, Brougham B, Edwards L, Baldus C, Romer G. Factors associated with emotional and behavioural problems among school age children of breast cancer patients. *Br J Cancer.* 2006;94(1):43–50.

When someone in your family has cancer. National Cancer Institute website. http://www.cancer.gov/cancertopics/when-someone-in-your-family-archived/page1. Accessed May 19, 2010. Content no longer available.

Chapter 6: Making the Medical System Work for You

Facts about hospital accreditation. The Joint Commission website. http://www.jointcommission.org/facts_about_hospital_accreditation/. Accessed December 14, 2012.

How to find a doctor or treatment facility if you have cancer. National Cancer Institute website. http://www.cancer.gov/cancertopics/factsheet/Therapy/doctor-facility. Reviewed June 29, 2009. Accessed December 14, 2012.

Chapter 7: Exploring Treatment Options

No references.

Chapter 8: Surgery

Ahmed AK, Hahn DE, Hage JJ, Bleiker EM, Woerdeman LA. Temporary banking of the nipple-areola complex in 97 skin-sparing mastectomies. *Plast Reconstr Surg.* 2011;127(2):531–539.

Chung AP, Sacchini V. Nipple-sparing mastectomy: where are we now? *Surg Oncol.* 2008;17(4):261–266. Epub 2008 May 5.
    Erratum in
    Surg Oncol. 2010;19(2):114

Crowe JP, Kim JA, Yetman R, Banbury J, Patrick RJ, Baynes D. Nipple-sparing mastectomy: technique and results of 54 procedures. *Arch Surg.* 2004;139(2):148–150.

Gärtner R, Jensen MB, Nielsen J, Ewertz M, Kroman N, Kehlet H. Prevalence of and factors associated with persistent pain following breast cancer surgery. *JAMA.* 2009;302(18):1985–1992.

Giuliano AE, Hunt KK, Ballman KV, Beitsch PD, Whitworth PW, Blumencranz PW, Leitch AM, Saha S, McCall LM, Morrow M. Axillary dissection vs no axillary dissection in women with invasive breast cancer and sentinel node metastasis. *JAMA.* 2011;305(6):569–575.

Graeser MK, Engel C, Rhiem K, Gadzicki D, Bick U, Kast K, Froster UG, Schlehe B, Bechtold A, Arnold N, Preisler-Adams S, Nestle-Kraemling C, Zaino M, Loeffler M, Kiechle M, Meindl A, Varga D, Schmutzler RK. Contralateral breast cancer risk in BRCA1 and BRCA2 mutation carriers. *J Clin Oncol.* 2009;27(35):5887–5892. doi: 10.1200/JCO.2008.19.9430. Epub 2009 Oct 26.

Harness JK, Vetter TS, Salibian AH. Areola and nipple-areola-sparing mastectomy for breast cancer treatment and risk reduction: report of an initial experience in a community hospital setting. *Ann Surg Oncol.* 2011;18(4):917–922. Epub 2010 Oct 7.

Jensen JA, Orringer JS, Giuliano AE. Nipple-sparing mastectomy in 99 patients with a mean follow-up of 5 years. *Ann Surg Oncol.* 2011;18(6):1665–1670. Epub 2010 Dec 21.

Lawenda BD, Mondry TE, Johnstone PA. Lymphedema: a primer on the identification and management of a chronic condition in oncologic treatment. *CA Cancer J Clin.* 2009;59(1):8–24.

Moskovitz AH, Anderson BO, Yeung RS, Byrd DR, Lawton TJ, Moe RE. Axillary web syndrome after axillary dissection. *Am J Surg.* 2001;181(5):434–439.

Nattinger AB. Variation in the choice of breast-conserving surgery or mastectomy: Patient or physician decision making? *J Clin Oncol.* 2005;23(24):5429–5431.

Petit JY, Veronesi U, Orecchia R, Luini A, Rey P, Intra M, Didier F, Martella S, Rietjens M, Garusi C, DeLorenzi F, Gatti G, Leon ME, Casadio C. Nipple-sparing mastectomy in association with intra operative radiotherapy (ELIOT): a new type of mastectomy for breast cancer treatment. *Breast Cancer Res Treat.* 2006;96(1):47–51. Epub 2005 Oct 27.

Petit JY, Veronesi U, Rey P, Rotmensz N, Botteri E, Rietjens M, Garusi C, De Lorenzi F, Martella S, Bosco R, Manconi A, Luini A, Galimberti V, Veronesi P, Ivaldi GB, Orecchia R. Nipple-sparing mastectomy: risk of nipple-areolar recurrences in a series of 579 cases. *Breast Cancer Res Treat.* 2009;114(1):97–101. Epub 2008 Mar 22.

Vadivelu N, Schreck M, Lopez J, Kodumudi G, Narayan D. Pain after mastectomy and breast reconstruction. *Am Surg.* 2008;74(4):285–296.

Vilholm OJ, Cold S, Rasmussen L, Sindrup SH. The postmastectomy pain syndrome: an epidemiological study on the prevalence of chronic pain after surgery for breast cancer. *Br J Cancer.* 2008;99(4):604–610.

Chapter 9: Other Treatments for Breast Cancer

Albert JM, Pan IW, Shih YC, Jiang J, Buchholz TA, Giordano SH, Smith BD. Effectiveness of radiation for prevention of mastectomy in older breast cancer patients treated with conservative surgery. *Cancer.* 2012;118(19):4642–4651. doi: 10.1002/cncr.27457.

Bachelot T, Bourgier C, Cropet C, Ray-Coquard I, Ferrero JM, Freyer G, Abadie-Lacourtoisie S, Eymard JC, Debled M, Späeth D, Legouffe E, Allouache D, El Kouri C, Pujade-Lauraine E. Randomized phase II trial of everolimus in combination with tamoxifen in patients with hormone receptor-positive, human epidermal growth factor receptor 2-negative metastatic breast cancer with prior exposure to aromatase inhibitors: a GINECO study. *J Clin Oncol.* 2012;30(22):2718–2724. Epub 2012 May 7.

Bamias A, Kastritis E, Bamia C. Moulopoulos LA, Melakopoulos I, Papadimitriou C, Terpos E, Dimopoulos MA. Osteonecrosis of the jaw in cancer after treatment with bisphosphonates: incidence and risk factors. *J Clin Oncol.* 2005;23(34):8580–8587.

Baselga J, Campone M, Piccart M, Burris HA 3rd, Rugo HS, Sahmoud T, Noguchi S, Gnant M, Prichard KI, Lebrun F, Beck JT, Ito Y, Yardley D, Deleu I, Perez A, Bachlot T, Vittori L, Xu Z, Mukhopadhyay P, Lebwohl D, Hortobagyi GN. Everolimus in postmenopausal hormone-receptor-positive advanced breast cancer. *N Engl J Med.* 2012;366(6):520–529. Epub 2011 Dec 7.

Baselga J, Cortés J, Kim SB, Im SA, Hegg R, Im YH, Roman L, Pedrini JL, Pienkowski T, Knott A, Clark E, Benyunes MC, Ross G, Swain SM; CLEOPATRA Study Group. Pertuzumab plus trastuzumab plus docetaxel for metastatic breast cancer. *N Engl J Med.* 2012;366(2):109–119. Epub 2011 Dec 7.

Baselga J, Semiglazov V, van Dam P, Manikhas A, Bellet M, Mayordomo J, Campone M, Kubista E, Griel R, Bianchi G, Steinseifer J, Molloy B, Tokaji E, Gardner H, Phillips P, Stumm M, Lane HA, Dixon JM, Jonat W, Rugo HS. Phase II randomized study of neoadjuvant everolimus plus letrozole compared with placebo plus letrozole in patients with estrogen receptor-positive breast cancer. *J Clin Oncol.* 2009;27(16):2630–2637. Epub 2009 Apr 20.

Benitez PR, Keisch ME, Vicini F, Stolier A, Scroggins T, Walker A, White J, Hedberg P, Hebert M, Arthur D, Zannis V, Quiet C, Streeter O, Silverstein M. Five-year results: the initial clinical trial of MammoSite balloon brachytherapy for partial breast irradiation in early-stage breast cancer. *Am J Surg.* 2007;194(4):456–462.

Blackwell KL, Burstein HJ, Storniolo AM, Rugo HS, Sledge G, Aktan G, Ellis C, Florance A, Vukelja S, Bischoff J, Baselga J, O'Shaughnessy J. Overall survival benefit with lapatinib in combination with trastuzumab for patients with human epidermal growth factor receptor 2-positive metastatic breast cancer: final results from the EGF104900 Study. *J Clin Oncol.* 2012;30(21): 2585–2592. doi: 10.1200/JCO.2011.35.6725. Epub 2012 Jun 11.

Blackwell KL, Burstein HJ, Storniolo AM, Rugo H, Sledge G, Koehler M, Ellis C, Casey M, Vukelja S, Bischoff J, Baselga J, O'Shaughnessy J. Randomized study of Lapatinib alone or in combination with trastuzumab in women with ErbB2-positive, trastuzumab-refractory metastatic breast cancer. *J Clin Oncol.* 2010;28(7): 1124–1130. Epub 2010 Feb 1.

Briot K, Tubiana-Hulin M, Bastit L, Kloos I, Roux C. Effect of a switch of aromatase inhibitors on musculoskeletal symptoms in postmenopausal women with hormone-receptor-positive breast cancer: the ATOLL (articular tolerance of letrozole) study. *Breast Cancer Res Treat.* 2010;120(1):127–134. Epub 2009 Dec 25.

Burstein HJ, Sun Y, Dirix LY, Jiang Z, Paridaens R, Tan AR, Awada A, Ranade A, Jiao S, Schwartz G, Abbas R, Powell C, Turnbull K, Vermette J, Zacharchuk C, Badwe R. Neratinib, an irreversible ErbB receptor tyrosine kinase inhibitor, in patients with advanced ErbB2-positive breast cancer. *J Clin Oncol.* 2010;28(8): 1301–1307. Epub 2010 Feb 8.

Chang G, Meadows ME, Orav EJ, Antin JH. Mental status changes after hematopoietic stem cell transplantation. *Cancer.* 2009;115(19):4625–4635. doi: 10.1002/cncr.24496.

Clarke M, Collins R, Darby S, Davies C, Elphinstone P, Evans E, Godwin J, Gray R, Hicks C, James S, MacKinnon E, McGale P, McHugh T, Peto R, Taylor C, Wang Y; Early Breast Cancer Trialists' Collaborative Group (EBCTCG). Effects of radiotherapy and of differences in the extent of surgery for early breast cancer on local recurrence and 15-year survival: an overview of the randomised trials. *Lancet.* 2005;366(9503):2087–2106.

Coleman RE, Marshall H, Cameron D, Dodwell D, Burkinshaw R, Keane M, Gil M, Houston SJ, Grieve RJ, Barrett-Lee PJ, Ritchie D, Pugh J, Gaunt C, Rea U,

Peterson J, Davies C, Hiley V, Gregory W, Bell R; AZURE Investigators. Breast cancer adjuvant therapy with zoledronic Acid. *N Engl J Med.* 2011;365(15):1396–1405. Epub 2011 Sep 25.

Coleman RE, Winter MC, Cameron D, Bell R, Dodwell D, Keane MM, Gil M, Ritchie D, Passos-Coelho JL, Wheatley D, Burkinshaw R, Marshall SJ, Thorpe H; AZURE (BIG01/04) Investigators. The effects of adding zoledronic acid to neoadjuvant chemotherapy on tumour response: exploratory evidence for direct anti-tumour activity in breast cancer. *Br J Cancer.* 2010;102(7):1099–1105. Epub 2010 Mar 16.

Corrao A. A comparison of APBI brachytherapy techniques: MammoSite, SAVI, Contura, and Axxent. Talk presented at: American Association of Medical Dosimetrists 2010 Annual Meeting; June 13-17, 2010. http://www.medicaldosimetry.org/meetings/2010 presentations/4-Corrao.pdf. Accessed March 1, 2013.

Davies C, Pan H, Godwin J, Gray R, Arriagada R, Raina V, Abraham M, Alencar VH, Badran A, Bonfill X, Bradbury J, Clarke M, Collins R, Davis SR, Delmestri A, Forbes JF, Haddad P, Hou MF, Inbar M, Khaled H, Kielanowska J, Kwan WH, Mathew BS, Mittra I, Müller B, Nicolucci A, Peralta O, Pernas F, Petruzelka L, Pienkowski T, Radhika R, Rajan B, Rubach MT, Tort S, Urrútia G, Valentini M, Wang Y, Peto R; for the Adjuvant Tamoxifen: Longer Against Shorter (ATLAS) Collaborative Group. Long-term effects of continuing adjuvant tamoxifen to 10 years versus stopping at 5 years after diagnosis of oestrogen receptor-positive breast cancer: ATLAS, a randomised trial. *Lancet.* 2013;381(9869):805-816.

Department of Health and Human Services, Food and Drug Administration. Proposal to withdraw approval for the breast cancer indication for AVASTIN (Bevacizumab), Decision of the commissioner. Docket No. FDA-2010-N-0621. Issued November 18, 2011. http://www.fda.gov/downloads/NewsEvents/Newsroom/UCM280546.pdf

Early Breast Cancer Trialists' Collaborative Group (EBCTCG), Darby S, McGale P, Correa C, Taylor C, Arriagada R, Clarke M, Cutter D, Davies C, Ewertz M, Godwin J, Gray R, Pierce L, Whelan T, Wang Y, Peto R. Effect of radiotherapy after breast-conserving surgery on 10-year recurrence and 15-year breast cancer death: meta-analysis of individual patient data for 10,801 women in 17 randomised trials. *Lancet.* 2011;378(9804):1707–1716. Epub 2011 Oct 19.

Early Breast Cancer Trialists' Collaborative Group (EBCTCG). Effects of chemotherapy and hormonal therapy for early breast cancer on recurrence and 15-year survival: an overview of the randomised trials. *Lancet.* 2005;365(9472):1687-1717.

FDA briefing document, oncology drug advisory committee meeting, BLA STN 125085/191 and 192, Avastin (bevacizumab). http://www.fda.gov/downloads/AdvisoryCommittees/CommitteesMeetingMaterials/Drugs/OncologicDrugsAdvisoryCommittee/UCM219224.pdf. Published July 20, 2010. Accessed April 2, 2013.

Fizazi K, Lipton A, Mariette X, Body JJ, Rahim Y, Gralow JR, Gao G, Wu L, Sohn W, Jun S. Randomized phase II trial of denosumab in patients with bone metastases from prostate cancer, breast cancer, or other neoplasms after intravenous bisphosphonates. *J Clin Oncol.* 2009;27(10):1564-1571. Epub 2009 Feb 23.

Gnant M, Mlineritsch B, Luschin-Ebengreuth G, Kainberger F, Kässmann H, Piswanger-Sölkner JC, Seifert M, Ploner F, Menzel C, Dubsky P, Fitzal F, Bjelic-Radisic V, Steger G, Greil R, Marth C, Kubista E, Samonigg H, Wohlmuth P, Mittlböck M, Jakesz R; Austrian Breast and Colorectal Cancer Study Group (ABCSG). Adjuvant endocrine therapy plus zoledronic acid in premenopausal women with early-stage breast cancer: 5-year follow-up of the ABCSG-12 bone-mineral density substudy. *Lancet Oncol.* 2008(9):840-849. Epub 2008 Aug 19.

Goss PE, Smith IE, O'Shaughnessy J, Ejlertsen B, Kaufmann M, Boyle F, Buzdar AU, Fumoleau P, Gradishar W, Martin M, Moy B, Piccart-Gebhart M, Pritchard KI, Lindquist D, Chavarri-Guerra Y, Aktan G, Rappold E, Williams LS, Finkelstein DM; TEACH investigators. Adjuvant lapatinib for women with early-stage HER2-positive breast cancer: a randomised, controlled, phase 3 trial. *Lancet Oncol.* 2013;14(1):88-96. doi: 10.1016/S1470-2045(12)70508-9. Epub 2012 Dec 10.

Gray RG, Rea D, Handley K, Bowden SJ, Perry P, Earl HM, Poole CJ, Bates T, Chetiyawardana S, Fernando IN, Grieve R, Nicoll J, Rayter Z, Robinson A, Salman A, Yarnold J, Bathers S, Marshall A, Lee M; on behalf of aTTom Collaborative Group. Long-term effects of continuing adjuvant tamoxifen to 10 years versus stopping at 5 years in 6,953 women with early breast cancer. *J Clin Oncol* (Meeting Abstracts). 2013;31 (18-Suppl 5).

Khan AJ, Dale RG, Arthur DW, Haffty BG, Todor DA, Vicini FA. Ultrashort courses of adjuvant breast radiotherapy: wave of the future or a fool's errand? *Cancer.* 2012;118(8):1962-1970. doi: 10.1002/cncr.26457.

Lawenda BD, Mondry TE, Johnstone PA. Lymphedema: a primer on the identification and management of a chronic condition in oncologic treatment. *CA Cancer J Clin.* 2009;59(1):8-24.

Learn about breast conservation therapy. Cianna Medical website. http://www.ciannamedical.com/for_women/therapy.htm. Accessed March 1, 2013.

Miller K, Wang M, Gralow J, Dickler M, Cobleigh M, Perez EA, Shenkier T, Cella D, Davidson NE. Paclitaxel plus bevacizumab versus paclitaxel alone for metastatic breast cancer. *N Engl J Med.* 2007;357(26):2666-2676.

Pavlakis N, Schmidt R, Stockler M. Bisphosphonates for breast cancer. *Cochrane Database Syst Rev.* 2005;(3): CD003474.

Sauter G, Lee J, Bartlett JM, Slamon DJ, Press MF. Guidelines for human epidermal growth factor receptor 2 testing: biologic and methodologic considerations. *J Clin Oncol.* 2009 Mar 10;27(8):1323-33. Epub 2009 Feb 9.

Schagen SB, Muller MJ, Boogerd W, Rosenbrand RM, van Rhijn D, Rodenhuis S, van Dam FS. Late effects of adjuvant chemotherapy on cognitive function: a follow-up study in breast cancer patients. *Ann Oncol.* 2002;13(9):1387-1397.

Smith BD, Arthur DW, Buchholz TA, Haffty BG, Hahn CA, Hardenbergh PH, Julian TB, Marks LB, Todor DA, Vicini FA, Whelan, TJ, White J, Wo JY, Harris JR. Accelerated partial breast irradiation consensus statement from the American Society for Radiation Oncology (ASTRO). *Int J Radiat Oncol Bio Phys.* 2009;74(4):987-1001.

Stopeck AT, Lipton A, Body JJ, Steger GG, Tonkin K, de Boer RH, Lichinitser M, Fujiwara Y, Yardley DA, Viniegra M, Fan M, Jiang Q, Dansey R, Jun S, Braun A. Denosumab compared with zoledronic acid for the treatment of bone metastases in patients with advanced breast cancer: a randomized, double-blind study. *J Clin Oncol.* 2010;28(35):5132-5139. Epub 2010 Nov 8.

Syrjala KL, Artherholt SB, Kurland BF, Langer SL, Roth-Roemer S, Elrod JB, Dikmen S. Prospective neurocognitive function over 5 years after allogeneic hematopoietic cell transplantation for cancer survivors compared with matched controls at 5 years. *J Clin Oncol.* 2011;29(17):2397–2404. doi: 10.1200/JCO.2010.33.9119. Epub 2011 May 2.

van de Velde CJ, Rea D, Seynaeve C, Putter H, Hasenburg A, Vannetzel JM, Paridaens R, Markopoulos C, Hozumi Y, Hille ET, Kieback DG, Asmar L, Smeets J, Nortier JW, Hadji P, Bartlett JM, Jones SE. Adjuvant tamoxifen and exemestane in early breast cancer (TEAM): a randomised phase 3 trial. *Lancet.* 2011;377(9762):321-31. doi: 10.1016/S0140-6736(10)62312-4.

Verma S, Miles D, Gianni L, Krop IE, Welslau M, Baselga J, Pegram M, Oh DY, Diéras V, Guardino E, Fang L, Lu MW, Olsen S, Blackwell K; EMILIA Study Group. Trastuzumab emtansine for HER2-positive advanced breast cancer. *N Engl J Med.* 2012;367(19):1783-1791. doi: 10.1056/NEJMoa1209124. Epub 2012 Oct 1.

Vogel VG, Costantino JP, Wickerham DL, Cronin WM, Cecchini RS, Atkins JN, Bevers TB, Fehrenbacher L, Pajon ER Jr, Wade JL 3rd, Robidoux A, Margolese RG, James J, Lippman SM, Runowicz CD, Ganz PA, Reis SE, McCaskill-Stevens W, Ford LG, Jordan VC, Wolmark N; National Surgical Adjuvant Breast and Bowel Project (NSABP). Effects of tamoxifen vs raloxifene on the risk of developing invasive breast cancer and other disease outcomes: the NSABP Study of Tamoxifen and Raloxifene (STAR) P-2 trial. *JAMA.* 2006;295(23):2727–2741. Epub 2006 Jun 5.
> Erratum in
> *JAMA.* 2006;296(24):2926.
> *JAMA.* 2007;298(9):973.

Vogel VG, Costantino JP, Wickerham DL, Cronin WM, Cecchini RS, Atkins JN, Bevers TB, Fehrenbacher L, Pajon ER, Wade JL 3rd, Robidoux A, Margolese RG, James J, Runowicz CD, Ganz PA, Reis SE, McCaskill-Stevens W, Ford LG, Jordan VC, Wolmark N; National Surgical Adjuvant Breast and Bowel Project. Update of the National Surgical Adjuvant Breast and Bowel Project Study of Tamoxifen and Raloxifene (STAR) P-2 Trial: preventing breast cancer. *Cancer Prev Res* (Phila). 2010;3(6):696–706. Epub 2010 Apr 19.

Whelan T, MacKenzie R, Julian J, Levine M, Shelley W, Grimard L, Lada B, Lukka H, Perera F, Fyles A, Laukkanen E, Gulavita S, Benk V, Szechtman B. Randomized trial of breast irradiation schedules after lumpectomy for women with lymph node-negative breast cancer. *J Natl Cancer Inst.* 2002;94(15):1143–1150.

Whelan TJ, Pignol JP, Levine MN, Julian JA, MacKenzie R, Parpia S, Shelley W, Grimard L, Bowen J, Lukka H, Perera F, Fyles A, Schneider K, Gulavita S, Freeman C. Long-term results of hypofractionated radiation therapy for breast cancer. *N Engl J Med.* 2010;362(6):513–520.

Chapter 10: Treatment Options Based on Your Situation

Abdel-Hady el-S, Hemida RA, Gamal A, El-Zafarany M, Toson E, El-Bayoumi MA. Cancer during pregnancy: perinatal outcome after in utero exposure to chemotherapy. *Arch Gynecol Obstet.* 2012;286(2):283–286. doi: 1007/s00404-012-2287-5.

Abeloff MD, Wolff AC, Weber BL, et al. Cancer of the breast, unusual problems encountered in breast cancer: breast cancer and pregnancy. In: Abeloff MD, Armitage JO, Niederhuber JE, Kastan MB, McKenna WG, eds. *Clinical Oncology.* 4th ed. Philadelphia, PA: Elsevier; 2008:1933.

Ali SA, Gupta S, Sehgal R, Vogel V. Survival outcomes in pregnancy associated breast cancer: a retrospective case control study. *Breast J.* 2012;18(2):139–144.

American Joint Committee on Cancer. *AJCC Cancer Staging Manual.* 7th ed. New York: Springer; 2010.

Ayyappan AP, Kulkarni S, Crystal P. Pregnancy-associated breast cancer: spectrum of imaging appearances. *Br J Radiol.* 2010;83(990):529–534.

Bartels RH, van der Linden YM, van der Graaf WT. Spinal extradural metastasis: review of current treatment options. *CA Cancer J Clin.* 2008;58(4):245–259.

Barthelmes L, Davidson LA, Gaffney C, Gateley CA. Pregnancy and breast cancer. *BMJ.* 2005;330(7504):1375–1378.

Belfiore G, Tedeschi E, Ronza FM, Belfiore MP, Della Volpe T, Zeppetella G, Rotondo A. Radiofrequency ablation of bone metastases induces long-lasting palliation in patients with untreatable cancer. *Singapore Med J.* 2008;49(7):565–570.

Berger A, Portenoy RK, Weissman DE, eds. *Principles and Practice of Supportive Oncology.* Philadelphia, PA: Lippincott-Raven; 1998.

Berger JC, Clericuzio CL. Pierre Robin sequence associated with first trimester fetal tamoxifen exposure.

Am J Med Genet A. 2008;146A(16):2141–2144. doi: 10.1002/ajmg.a.32432.

Breast cancer treatment and pregnancy (PDQ®). National Cancer Institute website. http://www.cancer.gov/cancertopics/pdq/treatment/breast-cancer-and-pregnancy/healthprofessional/allpages. Accessed August 1, 2012.

Burstein HJ, Harris JR, Morrow M. Malignant tumors of the breast. In DeVita VT Jr, Lawrence TS, Rosenberg SA, eds. *Cancer: Principles and Practice of Oncology*. 9th ed. Philadelphia, PA: Lippincott Williams & Wilkins; 2011: 1437–1438.

Cardonick E, Dougherty R, Grana G, Gilmandyar D, Ghaffar S, Usmani A. Breast cancer during pregnancy: maternal and fetal outcomes. *Cancer J*. 2010;16(1):76–82.

Chow E, Finkelstein JA, Sahgal A, Coleman RE. Metastatic cancer to the bone. In: DeVita VT, Lawrence TS, Rosenberg SA, eds. *DeVita, Hellman, and Rosenberg's Cancer: Principles & Practice of Oncology*. 9th ed. Philadelphia, PA: Lippincott Williams & Wilkins; 2011: 2192–2204.

Coleman RE. Clinical features of metastatic bone disease and risk of skeletal morbidity. *Clin Cancer Res*. 2006;12 (20 Pt 2):6243s–6249s.

Coleman RE, Guise TA, Lipton A, Roodman GD, Berebson JR, Body JJ, Boyce BF, Calvi LM, Hadji P, McCloskey EV, Saad F, Smith MR, Suva LJ, Taichman RS, Vessella RL, Weilbaecher KN. Advancing treatment for metastatic bone cancer: consensus recommendations from the Second Cambridge Conference. *Clin Cancer Res*. 2008;14(20):6387–6395. doi: 10.1158/1078-0432.CCR-08-1572.

Coleman RE, Holen I. Bone metastasis. In: Abeloff MD, Armitage JO, Niederhuber JE. Kastan MB, McKenna WG, eds. *Abeloff's Clinical Oncology*. 4th ed. Philadelphia, PA: Elsevier; 2008: 845–871.

Dawood S, Cristofanilli M. Inflammatory breast cancer: what progress have we made? *Oncology* (Williston Park). 2011;25(3):264–270, 273.

Dawood S, Cristofanilli M. What progress have we made in managing inflammatory breast cancer? *Oncology* (Williston Park). 2007;21(6):673–679; discussion 679–680, 686–687.

Dawood S, Merajver SD, Viens P, Vermeulen PB, Swain SM, Buchholz TA, Dirix LY, Levine PH, Lucci A, Krishnamurthy S, Robertson FM, Woodward WA, Yang WT, Ueno NT, Cristofanilli M. International expert panel on inflammatory breast cancer: consensus statement for standardized diagnosis and treatment. *Ann Oncol*. 2011;22(3):515–523. Epub 2010 Jul 5.

Donnelly EH, Smith JM, Farfán EB, Ozcan I. Prenatal radiation exposure: background material for counseling pregnant patients following exposure to radiation. *Disaster Med Public Health Prep*. 2011;5(1):62–68.

Early Breast Cancer Trialists' Collaborative Group (EBCTCG), Darby S, McGale P, Correa C, Taylor C, Arriagada R, Clarke M, Cutter D, Davies C, Ewertz M, Godwin J, Gray R, Pierce L, Whelan T, Wang Y, Peto R. Effect of radiotherapy after breast-conserving surgery on 10-year recurrence and 15-year breast cancer death: meta-analysis of individual patient data for 10,801 women in 17 randomised trials. *Lancet*. 2011;378(9804):1707–1716. Epub 2011 Oct 19.

Early Breast Cancer Trialists' Collaborative Group (EBCTCG). Effects of chemotherapy and hormonal therapy for early breast cancer on recurrence and 15-year survival: an overview of the randomised trials. *Lancet*. 2005;365(9472):1687–1717.

Early Breast Cancer Trialists' Collaborative Group (EBCTCG), Peto R, Davies C, Godwin J, Gray R, Pan HC, Clarke M, Cutter D, Darby S, McGale P, Taylor C, Wang YC, Bergh J, Di Leo A, Albain K, Swain S, Piccart M, Pritchard K. Comparisons between different olychemotherapy regimens for early breast cancer: meta-analyses of long-term outcome among 100,000 women in 123 randomised trials. *Lancet*. 2012;379(9814):432–444. Epub 2011 Dec 5.

Filippakis GM, Zografos G. Contraindications of sentinel lymph node biopsy: are there any really? *World J Surg Oncol*. 2007;5:10. doi: 10.1186/1477-7819-5-10.

Finlay IG, Mason MD, Shelley M. Radioisotopes for the palliation of metastatic bone cancer: a systematic review. *Lancet Oncol*. 2005;6(6):392–400.

Fizazi K, Lipton A, Mariette X, Body JJ, Rahim Y, Gralow JR, Gao G, Wu L, Sohn W, Jun S. Randomized phase II trial of denosumab in patients with bone metastases from prostate cancer, breast cancer, or other neoplasms after intravenous bisphosphonates. *J Clin Oncol*. 2009;27(10):1564–1571. Epub 2009 Feb 23.

Gambino A, Gorio A, Carrara L, Agoni L, Franzini R, Lupi GP, Maggino T, Romagnolo C, Sartori E, Pecorelli S. Cancer in pregnancy: maternal and fetal implications on decision-making. *Eur J Gynaecol Oncol.* 2011;32(1):40–45.

Giuliano AE, Hunt KK, Ballman KV, Beitsch PD, Whitworth PW, Blumencranz PW, Leitch AM, Saha S, McCall LM, Morrow M. Axillary dissection vs no axillary dissection in women with invasive breast cancer and sentinel node metastasis. *JAMA.* 2011;305(6):569–575.

Grigg A. Special issues in pregnancy, specific malignancies: breast cancer. In: Abeloff MD, Armitage JO, Niederhuber JE, Kastan MB, McKenna WG, eds. *Clinical Oncology.* 4th ed. Philadelphia, PA: Elsevier; 2008: 1054–1055.

Guidroz JA, Scott-Conner CEH, Weigel RJ. Management of pregnant women with breast cancer. *J Surg Oncol.* 2011;103(4):337–340. doi: 10.1002/jso.21673.

Hance KW, Anderson WF, Devesa SS, Young HA, Levine PH. Trends in inflammatory breast carcinoma incidence and survival: the Surveillance, Epidemiology, and End Results program at the National Cancer Institute. *J Natl Cancer Inst.* 2005;97(13):966–975. doi: 10.1093/jnci/dji172.

Hartsell WF, Scott CB, Bruner DW, Scarantino CW, Ivker RA, Roach M 3rd, Suh JH, Demas WF, Movsas B, Petersen IA, Konski AA, Cleeland CS, Janjan NA, DeSilvio M. Randomized trial of short- versus long-course radiotherapy for palliation of painful bone metastases. *J Natl Cancer Inst.* 2005;97(11):798–804.

Hennessy BT, Gonzalez-Angulo AM, Hortobagyi GN, Cristofanilli M, Wan Kau S, Broglio K, Fornage B, Singletary SE, Sahin A, Buzdar AU, Valero V. Disease-free and overall survival after pathologic complete disease remission of cytologically proven inflammatory breast carcinoma axillary lymph node metastases after primary systemic chemotherapy. *Cancer.* 2006;106(5):1000–1006.

Howlader N, Noone AM, Krapcho M, Neyman N, Aminou R, Waldron W, Altekruse SF, Kosary CL, Ruhl J, Tatalovich Z, Cho H, Mariotto A, Eisner MP, Lewis DR, Chen HS, Feuer EJ, Cronin KA (eds). *SEER Cancer Statistics Review, 1975–2009* (Vintage 2009 Populations), National Cancer Institute. Bethesda, MD, http://seer.cancer.gov/csr/1975_2009_pops09/, based on November 2011 SEER data submission, posted to the SEER website, April 2012.

Kaufman B, Trudeau M, Awada A, Blackwell K, Bachelot T, Salazar V, DeSilvio M, Westlund R, Zaks T, Spector N, Johnston S. Lapatinib monotherapy in patients with HER2-overexpressing relapsed or refractory inflammatory breast cancer: final results and survival of the expanded HER2+ cohort in EGF103009, a phase II study. *Lancet Oncol.* 2009;10:581–588. Epub 2009 Apr 27.

Kenan S, Mechanick JI. Skeletal complications. In: Kufe DW, Bast RC, Hait WN, et al. (eds.) *Cancer Medicine.* 7th ed. Lewiston, NY: BC Decker; 2006: 2085–2094.

Liotta LA, Kohn EC. Invasion and metastasis. In: Kufe DW, Pollock RE, Weichselbaum RR, Bast RC, Gansler TS, Holland JF, Frei E, eds. *Cancer Medicine 6.* Hamilton, Ontario: BC Decker; 2003: 151–160.

Lipton A, Steger GG, Figueroa J, Alvarado C, Solal-Celigny, Jaques Body J, de Boer R, Berardi R, Gascon P, Tonkin KS, Coleman RE, Paterson AHG, Gao GM, Kinsey AC, Peterson MC, Jun S. Extended efficacy and safety of denosumab in breast cancer patients with bone metastases not receiving prior bisphosphonate therapy. *Clin Cancer Res.* 2008;14(20):6690–6696.

Litton JK, Theriault RL. Breast cancer and pregnancy: current concepts in diagnosis and treatment. *Oncologist.* 2010;15(12):1238–1247.

Loibl S, von Minckwitz G, Gwyn K, Ellis P, Blohmer JU, Schlegelberger B, Keller M, Harder S, Theriault RL, Crivellari D, Klingebiel T, Louwen F, Kaufmann M. Breast carcinoma during pregnancy, international recommendations from an expert meeting. *Cancer.* 2006;106(2):237–246.

Molckovsky A, Madarnas Y. Breast cancer in pregnancy: a literature review. *Breast Cancer Res Treat.* 2008;108(3):333–338.

Murphy CG, Mallam D, Stein S, Patil S, Howard J, Sklarin N, Hudis CA, Gemignani ML, Seidman AD. Current or recent pregnancy is associated with adverse pathologic features but not impaired survival in early breast cancer. *Cancer.* 2012;118(13):3254–3259. doi: 10.1002/cncr.26654.

Coping with advanced cancer. National Cancer Institute website. NIH Pub No 12-0856 http://www.cancer.gov/cancertopics/advancedcancer/page1. Updated January 2012. Accessed May 16, 2012.

National Comprehensive Cancer Network. NCCN clinical guidelines in oncology™. Breast cancer, V.2.2013. http://www.nccn.org/professionals/physician_gls/pdf/breast.pdf. Accessed July 31, 2012.

Panades M, Olivotto IA, Speers CH, Shenkier T, Olivotto TA, Weir L, Allan SJ, Truong PT. Evolving treatment strategies for inflammatory breast cancer: a population based survival analysis. *J Clin Oncol.* 2005;23(9):1941–1950.

Ries LAG, Eisner MP. Cancer of the female breast. In: Ries LAG, Young JL, Keel GE, Eisner MP, Lin YD, Horner M-J, eds. SEER Survival Monograph: Cancer Survival Among Adults: U.S. SEER Program, 1988-2001, Patient and Tumor Characteristics. National Cancer Institute, SEER Program, NIH Pub. No. 07-6215, Bethesda, MD, 2007. http://seer.cancer.gov/publications/survival/. Accessed July 22, 2008.

Rosen LS, Gordon D, Kaminski M, Howell A, Belch A, Mackey J, Apffelstaedt J, Hussein MA, Coleman RE, Reitsma D, Chen BL, Seaman JJ. Long-term efficacy and safety of zoledronic acid compared with pamidronate disodium in the treatment of skeletal complications in patients with advanced multiple myeloma or breast carcinoma: a randomized, double-blind, multicenter, comparative trial. *Cancer.* 2003;98(8):1735–1744.

Sinclair S, Swain SM. Primary systemic chemotherapy for inflammatory breast cancer. *Cancer.* 2010;116(11 Suppl):2821–2828.

Stopeck AT, Lipton A, Body JJ, Steger GG, Tonkin K, de Boer RH, Lichinitser M, Fujiwara Y, Yardley DA, Viniegra M, Fan M, Jiang Q, Dansey R, Jun S, Braun A. Denosumab compared with zoledronic acid for the treatment of bone metastases in patients with advanced breast cancer: a randomized, double-blind study. *J Clin Oncol.* 2010;28(35):5132–5139. Epub 2010 Nov 8.

Sukumvanich P. Review of current treatment options for pregnancy-associated breast cancer. *Clin Obstet Gynecol.* 2011;54(1):164–172.

Viswanathan S, Ramaswamy B. Pregnancy-associated breast cancer. *Clin Obstet Gynecol.* 2011;54(4):546–555. doi: 10.1097/GRF.0b013e318236e436.

Yang WT, Dryden MJ, Gwyn K, Whitman GJ, Theriault R. Imaging of breast cancer diagnosed and treated with chemotherapy during pregnancy. *Radiology.* 2006;239(1):52–60.

Chapter 11: Clinical Trials

Bennett CL, Adams JR, Knox KS, Kelahan AM, Silver SM, Bailes JS. Clinical trials: are they a good buy? *J Clin Oncol.* 2001;19(23):4330–4339.

Getz K, Borfitz D. *Informed Consent: The Consumer's Guide to the Risks and Benefits of Volunteering for Clinical Trials.* Boston, MA: CenterWatch; 2002.

Learning about clinical trials. National Cancer Institute website. http://www.cancer.gov/clinicaltrials. Accessed September 26, 2012.

New approaches to cancer drug development and clinical trials: questions and answers. National Cancer Institute website. http://www.cancer.gov/newscenter/pressreleases/PhaseZeroNExTQandA/print?page=&keyword=. Accessed September 20, 2012.

Should I enter a clinical trial? A patient reference guide for adults with a serious or life-threatening illness. ECRI Institute website. http://www.ecri.org/Documents/Clinical_Trials_Patient_Reference_Guide.pdf. Published February 2002. Accessed September 21, 2012.

Streiner DL, Norman GR. Drug trial phases. *Community Oncology.* 2009;6(1):36–40.

Stryker JE, Wray RJ, Emmons KM, Winer E, Demetri G. Understanding the decisions of cancer clinical trial participants to enter research studies: factors associated with informed consent, patient satisfaction, and decisional regret. *Patient Educ Couns.* 2006;63(1–2):104–109.

US Department of Health and Human Services. Medicare and clinical research studies [pamphlet]. Centers for Medicare and Medicaid Services website. http://www.medicare.gov/Publications/Pubs/pdf/02226.pdf. Published March 2010. Accessed September 20, 2012.

Chapter 12: Complementary and Alternative Therapies

Astin JA, Shapiro SL, Eisenberg DM, Forys KL. Mind-body medicine: state of the science, implications for practice. *J Am Board Fam Pract.* 2003;16(2):131–147.

Bass SS, Cox CE, Salud CJ, Lyman GH, McCann C, Dupont E, Berman C, Reintgen DS. The effects of postinjection massage on the sensitivity of lymphatic mapping in breast cancer. *J Am Coll Surg.* 2001;192(1):9–16.

Bower JE, Woolery A, Sternlieb B, Garet D. Yoga for cancer patients and survivors. *Cancer Control.* 2005;12(3):165–171.

Bradt J, Dileo C, Grocke D, Magill L. Music interventions for improving psychological and physical outcomes in cancer patients. *Cochrane Database Syst Rev.* 2011;(8): CD006911.

Breitbart W. Spirituality and meaning in supportive care: spirituality- and meaning-centered group psychotherapy interventions in advanced cancer. *Support Care Cancer.* 2002;10(4):272–280. Epub 2001 Aug 28.

Buckle J. Use of aromatherapy as a complementary treatment for chronic pain. *Altern Ther Health Med.* 1999;5(5):42–51.

Burish TG, Jenkins RA. Effectiveness of biofeedback and relaxation training in reducing the side effects of cancer chemotherapy. *Health Psychol.* 1992;11(1):17–23.

Cassileth B. *The Alternative Medicine Handbook: The Complete Reference Guide to Alternative and Complementary Therapies.* New York: W.W. Norton; 1998.

Cassileth B, Vickers AJ. Massage therapy for symptom control: outcome study at a major cancer center. *J Pain Symptom Manage.* 2004;28(3):244–249.

Cawthorn A. A review of the literature surrounding the research into aromatherapy. *Complement Ther Nurs Midwifery.* 1995;1(4):118–120.

Cepeda MS, Carr DB, Lau J, Alvarez H. Music for pain relief. *Cochrane Database Syst Rev.* 2006;(2):CD004843.

Cerrato PL. Aromatherapy: is it for real? *RN.* 1998;61: 51–52.

Clark M, Isaacks-Downton G, Wells N, Redlin-Frazier S, Eck C, Hepworth JT, Chakravarthy B. Use of preferred music to reduce emotional distress and symptom activity during radiation therapy. *J Music Ther.* 2006;43(3):247–265.

Consumer information on dietary supplements. US Food and Drug Administration website. http://www.fda.gov/ Food/DietarySupplements/ConsumerInformation/defaul t.htm. Updated October 9, 2012. Accessed December 10, 2012.

Deng G, Cassileth BR. Integrative oncology: complementary therapies for pain, anxiety, and mood disturbance. *CA Cancer J Clin.* 2005;55(2):109–116.

Dietary supplements. US Food and Drug Administration website. http://www.fda.gov/food/dietarysupplements/ default.htm. Updated November 16, 2012. Accessed December 10, 2012.

Dincer F, Linde K. Sham interventions in randomized clinical trials of acupuncture—a review. *Complement Ther Med.* 2003;11(4):235–242.

Elkins G, Fisher W, Johnson A. Mind-body therapies in integrative oncology. *Curr Treat Options Oncol.* 2010;11(3–4):128–140.

Eller LS. Guided imagery interventions for symptom management. *Annu Rev Nurs Res.* 1999;17:57–84.

Ernst E, ed. *The Desktop Guide to Complementary and Alternative Medicine: An Evidence-Based Approach.* New York: Mosby; 2001.

Ernst G, Strzyz H, Hagmeister H. Incidence of adverse effects during acupuncture therapy-a multicentre survey. *Complement Ther Med.* 2003;11(2):93–97.

Ezzo JM, Richardson MA, Vickers A, Allen C, Dibble SL, Issell BF, Lao L, Pearl M, Ramirez G, Roscoe J, Shen J, Shivnan JC, Streitberger K, Treish I, Zhang G. Acupuncture-point stimulation for chemotherapy-induced nausea or vomiting. *Cochrane Database Syst Rev.* 2006;(2):CD002285.

Ezzone S, Baker C, Rosselet R, Terepka E. Music as an adjunct to antiemetic therapy. *Oncol Nurs Forum.* 1998;25(9):1551–1556.

Fellowes D, Barnes K, Wilkinson S. Aromatherapy and massage for symptom relief in patients with cancer. *Cochrane Database Syst Rev.* 2004;(2):CD002287

Finniss DG, Kaptchuk TJ, Miller F, Benedetti F. Biological, clinical, and ethical advances of placebo effects. *Lancet.* 2010;375(9715):686–695.

Flory N, Lang E. Practical hypnotic interventions during invasive cancer diagnosis and treatment. *Hematol Oncol Clin North Am.* 2008;22(4):709–725, ix.

Hernandez-Reif M, Ironson G, Field T, Hurley J, Katz G, Diego M, Weiss S, Fletcher MA, Schanberg S, Kuhn C, Burman I. Breast cancer patients have improved immune and neuroedocrine functions following massage therapy. *J Psychosom Res*. 2004;57(1):45–52.

Hilliard RE. The effects of music therapy on the quality and length of life of people diagnosed with terminal cancer. *J Music Ther*. 2003;40(2):113–137.

Huebscher R, Shuler P. Mind-body-spirit interventions. In Huebscher R, Shuler P, eds. *Natural, Alternative, and Complementary Health Care Practices*. St. Louis, MO: Mosby; 2003:762–787.

Integration of behavioral and relaxation approaches into the treatment of chronic pain and insomnia. NIH Technology Assessment Panel on Integration of Behavioral and Relaxation Approaches into the Treatment of Chronic Pain and Insomnia. *JAMA*. 1996;276(4):313–318.

An introduction to acupuncture. National Center for Complementary and Alternative Medicine website. http://nccam.nih.gov/health/acupuncture/. Accessed May 22, 2013.

Kaptchuk TJ, Friedlander E, Kelley JM, Sanchez MN, Kokkotou E, Singer JP, Kowalczykowski M, Miller FG, Kirsch I, Lembo AJ. Placebos without deception: a randomized controlled trial in irritable bowel syndrome. *PLoS One*. 2010;5(12):e15591.

Key TJ, Thorogood M, Appleby PN, Burr ML. Dietary habits and mortality in 11,000 vegetarians and health conscious people: results of a 17 year follow up. *BMJ*. 1996;313(7060):775–779.

Kolcaba K, Fox C. The effects of guided imagery on comfort of women with early stage breast cancer undergoing radiation therapy. *Oncol Nurs Forum*. 1999;26(1):67–72.

Krout RE. The effects of single-session music therapy interventions on the observed and self-reported levels of pain control, physical comfort, and relaxation of hospice patients. *Am J Hosp Palliat Care*. 2001;18(6):383–390.

Kushi LH, Doyle C, McCullough M, Rock CL, Demark-Wahnefried W, Bandera EV, Gapstur S, Patel AV, Andrews K, Gansler T; American Cancer Society 2010 Nutrition and Physical Activity Guidelines Advisory Committee. American Cancer Society guidelines on nutrition and physical activity for cancer prevention: reducing the risk of cancer with healthy food choices and physical activity. *CA Cancer J Clin*. 2012;62(1):30–67. doi: 10.3322/caac.20140.

Levitan AA. The use of hypnosis with cancer patients. *Psychiatr Med*. 1992;10(1):119–131.

Manipulation & body-based methods: massage & related bodywork. Complementary/Integrative Medicine Education Resources, The University of Texas M.D. Anderson Cancer Center website. http://www.mdanderson.org/education-and-research/resources-for-professionals/clinical-tools-and-resources/cimer/therapies/manipulative-and-body-based-methods/body-based-methods.html. Accessed May 22, 2013.

Masters KS, Spielmans GI, Goodson JT. Are there demonstrable effects of distant intercessory prayer? A meta-analytic review. *Ann Behav Med*. 2006;32(1):21–26.

Moadel AB, Shah C, Wylie-Rosett J, Harris MS, Patel SR, Hall CB, Sparano JA. Randomized controlled trial of yoga among a multiethnic sample of breast cancer patients: effects on quality of life. *J Clin Oncol*. 2007;25(28):4387–4395. Epub 2007 Sep 4.

Montgomery GH, Bovbjerg DH, Schnur JB, David D, Goldfarb A, Weltz CR, Schechter C, Graff-Zivin J, Tatrow K, Price DD, Silverstein JH. A randomized clinical trial of a brief hypnosis intervention to control side effects in breast surgery patients. *J Natl Cancer Inst*. 2007;99(17):1304–1312.

Mustian KM, Katula JA, Zhao H. A pilot study to assess the influence of tai chi chuan on functional capacity among breast cancer survivors. *J Support Oncol*. 2006;4(3):139–145.

Mytko JJ, Knight SJ. Body, mind and spirit: towards the integration of religiosity and spirituality in cancer quality of life research. *Psychooncology*. 1999;8(5):439–450.

NIH Technology Assessment Panel. Integration of behavioral and relaxation approaches into the treatment of chronic pain and insomnia. *JAMA*. 1996;276(4):313–318.

Pain control: a guide for people with cancer and their families. National Cancer Institute website. http://www.cancer.gov/cancertopics/paincontrol. Accessed June 12, 2008.

Prayer. Aetna InteliHealth website. http://www.intelihealth.com/IH/ihtIH/WSIHW000/8513/34968/360051.html. Accessed May 23, 2013.

Post-White J, Kinney ME, Savik KS, Gau JB, Wilcox C, Lerner I. Therapeutic massage and healing touch improve symptoms in cancer. *Integr Cancer Ther.* 2003;2(4):332–344.

Rao MR, Raghuram N, Nagendra HR, Gopinath KS, Srinath BS, Diwakar RB, Patil S, Bilimagga SR, Rao N, Varambally S. Anxiolytic effects of a yoga program in early breast cancer patients undergoing conventional treatment: a randomized controlled trial. *Complement Ther Med.* 2009;17(1):1–8. Epub 2008 Oct 14.

Roffe L, Schmidt K, Ernst E. A systematic review of guided imagery as an adjuvant cancer therapy. *Psychooncology.* 2005;14(8):607–617.

Sharp DM, Walker MB, Chaturvedi A, Upadhyay S, Hamid A, Walker AA, Bateman JS, Braid F, Ellwood K, Hebblewhite C, Hope T, Lines M, Walker LG. A randomised, controlled trial of the psychological effects of reflexology in early breast cancer. *Eur J Cancer.* 2010;46(2):312–322. Epub 2009 Nov 10.

Sherman KJ, Cherkin DC, Eisenberg DM, Erro J, Hrbek A, Deyo RA. The practice of acupuncture: who are the providers and what do they do? *Ann Fam Med.* 2005; 3(2):151–158.

Simonton CO, Simonton SM, Creighton JL. *Getting Well Again.* Los Angeles, CA: Tarcher Books; 1992.

Smith JE, Richardson J, Hoffman C, Pilkington K. Mindfulness-based stress reduction as supportive therapy in cancer care: systematic review. *J Adv Nurs.* 2005;52(3):315–327.
    Errtaum in:
    J Adv Nurs. 2006;53(5):618.

Smith MC, Kemp J, Hemphill, Vojir CP. Outcomes of therapeutic massage for hospitalized cancer patients. *J Nurs Scholarsh.* 2002;34(3):257–262.

Speca M, Carlson LE, Goodey E, Angen M. A randomized, wait-list controlled clinical trial: the effect of a mindfulness meditation-based stress reduction program on mood and symptoms of stress in cancer outpatients. *Psychosom Med.* 2000;62(5):613–622.

Spencer JW, Jacobs JJ. *Complementary/Alternative Medicine: An Evidence-Based Approach.* St. Louis, MO: Mosby; 1999.

Tai chi. Aetna InteliHealth website. http://www.intelihealth.com/IH/ihtIH?d=dmtContent&c=358867. Accessed May 23, 2013.

Vadiraja HS, Raghavendra RM, Nagarathna R, Nagendra HR, Rekha M, Vanitha N, Gopinath KS, Srinath BS, Vishweshwara MS, Madhavi YS, Ajaikumar BS, Ramesh BS, Nalini R, Kumar V. Effects of a yoga program on cortisol rhythm and mood states in early breast cancer patients undergoing adjuvant radiotherapy: a randomized controlled trial. *Integr Cancer Ther.* 2009;8(1):37–46. Epub 2009 Feb 3.
    Erratum in:
    Integr Cancer Ther. 2009;8(2):195.

Walker EM, Rodriguez AI, Kohn B, Ball RM, Pegg J, Pocock JR, Nunez R, Peterson E, Jakary S, Levine RA. Acupuncture versus venlafaxine for the management of vasomotor symptoms in patients with hormone receptor-positive breast cancer: a randomized controlled trial. *J Clin Oncol.* 2010;28(4):634–640. Epub 2009 Dec 28.

Walsh SM, Martin SC, Schmidt LA. Testing the efficacy of a creative-arts intervention with family caregivers of patients with cancer. *J Nurs Scholarsh.* 2004;36(3):214–219.

Weinrich SP, Weinrich MC. The effect of massage on pain in cancer patients. *Appl Nurs Res.* 1990;3(4):140–145.

Yoga. Aetna InteliHealth website. http://www.intelihealth.com/IH/ihtIH?d=dmtContent&c=358876. Accessed May 22, 2013.

Chapter 13: Coping with Symptoms and Side Effects

Asher A. Cognitive dysfunction among cancer survivors. *Am J Phys Med Rehabil.* 2011;90(5 Suppl 1):S16–S26. doi: 10.1097/PHM.0b013e31820be463.

Azim HA Jr, Bellettini G, Liptrott SJ, Armeni ME, Dell'Acqua V, Torti F, Di Nubila B, Galimberti V, Peccatori F. Breastfeeding in breast cancer survivors: pattern, behaviour and effect on breast cancer outcome. *Breast.* 2010;19(6):527–531.

Berger A, Portenoy RK, Weissman DE, eds. *Principles and Practice of Supportive Oncology.* Philadelphia, PA: Lippincott-Raven; 1998.

Boykoff N, Moieni M, Subramanian SK. Confronting chemobrain: an in-depth look at survivors' reports of impact on work, social networks, and health care response. *J Cancer Surviv*. 2009;3(4):223–232. doi: 10.1007/s11764-009-0098-x. Epub 2009 Sep 16.

Bruera E, Kim HN. Cancer pain. *JAMA*. 2003;290(18): 2476–2479.

CancerCare. Chemobrain Information Series: Cognitive Problems after Chemotherapy. http://www.cancercare.org/pdf/fact_sheets/fs_chemobrain_cognitive.pdf. Accessed May 16, 2012.

Cassileth BR, Keefe FJ. Integrative and behavioral approaches to the treatment of cancer-related neuropathic pain. *Oncologist*. 2010;15(2):19–23. doi: 10.1634/theoncologist.2009-S504.

Cobo A, Meseguer M, Remohí J, Pellicer A.Use of cryo-banked oocytes in an ovum donation programme: a prospective, randomized, controlled, clinical trial. *Hum Reprod*. 2010;25(9):2239–2246. doi: 10.1093/humrep/deq146. Epub 2010 Jun 30.

Davis MP. Recent development in therapeutics for breakthrough pain. *Expert Rev Neurother*. 2010;10(5): 757–773. doi: 10.1586/ern.10.41.

Díaz N, Menjón S, Rolfo C, García-Alonso P, Carulla J, Magro A, Miramón J, Rodríguez CA, de Castellar R, Gasquet JA. Patients' perception of cancer-related fatigue: results of a survey to assess the impact on their everyday life. *Clin Transl Oncol*. 2008;10(11):753–757.

Duijts SF, van Beurden M, Oldenburg HS, Hunter MS, Kieffer JM, Stuiver MM, Gerritsma MA, Menke-Pluymers MB, Plaisier PW, Rijna H, Lopes Cardozo AM, Timmers G, van der Meij S, van der Veen H, Bijker N, de Widt-Levert LM, Geenen MM, Heuff G, van Dulken EJ, Boven E, Aaronson NK. Efficacy of cognitive behavioral therapy and physical exercise in alleviating treatment-induced menopausal symptoms in patients with breast cancer: results of a randomized, controlled, multicenter trial. *J Clin Oncol*. 2012;30(33):4124–4133. doi: 10.1200/JCO.2012.41.8525.

Ernst E, Bergholdt S, Jørgensen JS, Andersen CY. The first woman to give birth to two children following transplantation of frozen/thawed ovarian tissue. *Hum Reprod*. 2010;25(5):1280–1281. doi: 10.1093/humrep/deq033. Epub 2010 Feb 19.

Escalante CP, Kallen MA, Valdres RU, Morrow PK, Manzullo EF. Outcomes of a cancer-related fatigue clinic in a comprehensive cancer center. *J Pain Symptom Manage*. 2010;39(4):691–701. doi: 10.1016/j.jpainsymman.2009.09.010. Epub 2010 Mar 11.

Ferguson RJ, Ahles TA, Saykin AJ, McDonald BC, Furstenberg CT, Cole BF, Mott LA. Cognitive-behavioral management of chemotherapy-related cognitive change. *Psychooncology*. 2007;16(8):772–777.

Foley KM, Abernathy A. Management of cancer pain. In: DeVita VT Jr, Lawrence TS, Rosenberg SA, eds. *Cancer: Principles and Practice of Oncology*. 8th ed. Philadelphia, PA: Lippincott Williams and Wilkins; 2008: 2757–2790.

Graham PH. Compression prophylaxis may increase the potential for flight-associated lymphoedema after breast cancer treatment. *Breast*. 2002;11(1):66–71.

Hayes SC, Johansson K, Stout NL, Prosnitz R, Armer JM, Gabram S, Schmitz KH. Upper-body morbidity after breast cancer: incidence and evidence for evaluation, prevention, and management within a prospective surveillance model of care. *Cancer*. 2012;118(8 Suppl):2237–2249. doi: 10.1002/cncr.27467.

Hede, K. Chemobrain is real but may need new name. *J Natl Cancer Inst*. 2008;100(3):162–163, 169. doi: 10.1093/jnci/djn007. Epub 2008 Jan 29.

Hickey M, Peate M, Saunders CM, Friedlander M. Breast cancer in young women and its impact on reproductive function. *Hum Reprod Update*. 2009;15(3):323–339.

Hurter B, Bush NJ. Cancer-related anemia: clinical review and management update. *Clin J Oncol Nurs*. 2007;11(3):349–359.

Jacobs A, Wegewitz U, Sommerfeld C, Grossklaus R, Lampen A. Efficacy of isoflavones in relieving vasomotor menopausal symptoms - a systematic review. *Mol Nutr Food Res*. 2009;53(9):1084–1097. doi: 10.1002/mnfr.200800552.

Katz A. *Breaking the Silence on Cancer and Sexuality: A Handbook for Healthcare Providers*. Pittsburg, PA; Oncology Nursing Society: 2007.

Lawenda BD, Mondry TE, Johnstone PA. Lymphedema: a primer on the identification and management of a chronic condition in oncologic treatment. *CA Cancer J Clin*. 2009;59(1):8–24.

Leach MJ, Moore V. Black cohosh (Cimicifuga spp.) for menopausal symptoms. *Cochrane Database Syst Rev.* 2012;9:CD007244. doi: 10.1002/14651858.CD007244. pub2.

Lee S, Song JY, Ku SY, Kim SH, Kim T. Fertility preservation in women with cancer. *Clin Exp Reprod Med.* 2012;39(2):46–51. doi: 10.5653/cerm.2012.39.2.46. Epub 2012 Jun 30.

Lethaby AE, Brown J, Marjoribanks J, Kronenberg F, Roberts H, Eden J. Phytoestrogens for vasomotor menopausal symptoms. *Cochrane Database Syst Rev.* 2007;(4):CD001395.

Mann E, Smith MJ, Hellier J, Balabanovic JA, Hamed H, Grunfeld EA, Hunter MS. Cognitive behavioural treatment for women who have menopausal symptoms after breast cancer treatment (MENOS 1): a randomised controlled trial. *Lancet Oncol.* 2012;13(3):309–318. Epub 2012 Feb 15.

Mayo Clinic. Chemobrain. http://www.mayoclinic.com/health/chemo-brain/DS01109. Accessed May 16, 2012.

Morris MC, Evans DA, Tangney CC, Bienias JL, Wilson RS. Associations of vegetable and fruit consumption with age-related cognitive change. *Neurology.* 2006;67: 1370–1376.

Fatigue PDQ® (Health Professional version). National Cancer Institute website. Updated August 29, 2012. http://www.cancer.gov/cancertopics/pdq/supportivecare/fatigue/HealthProfessional. Accessed November 26, 2012.

Nausea and Vomiting PDQ®. National Cancer Institute website. Updated September 28, 2012. http://www.cancer.gov/cancertopics/pdq/supportivecare/nausea/Patient. Accessed February 11, 2013.

Pain control: support for people with cancer. National Cancer Institute website. http://www.cancer.gov/cancertopics/paincontrol/page1. Accessed September 20, 2010.

The prevalence and types of sexual dysfunction in people with cancer. National Cancer Institute website. http://www.cancer.gov/cancertopics/pdq/supportivecare/sexuality/HealthProfessional Accessed November 20, 2012.

National Comprehensive Cancer Network. Adult Cancer Pain. *NCCN Practice Guidelines in Oncology*, V.1.2010. http://www.nccn.org/professionals/physician_gls/PDF/pain.pdf. Accessed September 20, 2010.

National Comprehensive Cancer Network. Antiemesis. *NCCN Clinical Practice Guidelines in Oncology*–v.1.2013. http://www.nccn.org/professionals/physician_gls/pdf/antiemesis.pdf. Accessed February 11, 2013.

National Comprehensive Cancer Network. Cancer- and Chemotherapy-Induced Anemia. *NCCN Clinical Practice Guidelines in Oncology*–V.1.2013. http://www.nccn.org/professionals/physician_gls/pdf/anemia.pdf. Accessed August 15, 2012.

National Comprehensive Cancer Network. Cancer-Related Fatigue. *NCCN Clinical Practice Guidelines in Oncology*–V.1.2013. http://www.nccn.org/professionals/physician_gls/pdf/fatigue.pdf. Accessed November 26, 2012.

National Lymphedema Network Advisory Committee. Position statement of the National Lymphedema Network, topic: exercise. National Lymphedema Network website. http://www.lymphnet.org/pdfDocs/nlnexercise.pdf. Updated May 2011. Accessed November 12, 2012.

National Lymphedema Network Advisory Committee. Position statement of the National Lymphedema Network, topic: lymphedema risk reduction practices. National Lymphedema Network website. http://www.lymphnet.org/pdfDocs/nlnriskreduction.pdf. Updated May 2012. Accessed November 12, 2012.

Paskett ED, Dean JA, Oliveri JM, Harrop JP. Cancer-related lymphedema risk factors, diagnosis, treatment, and impact: a review. *J Clin Oncol.* 2012;30(30):3726–3733. doi: 10.1200/JCO.2012.41.8574. Epub 2012 Sep 24.

Reid-Arndt SA, Cox CR. Stress, coping and cognitive deficits in women after surgery for breast cancer. *J Clin Psychol Med Settings.* 2012;19(2):127–137. doi: 10.1007/s10880-011-9274-z.

Reid-Arndt SA, Yee A, Perry MC, Hsieh C. Cognitive and psychological factors associated with early posttreatment functional outcomes in breast cancer survivors. *J Psychosoc Oncol.* 2009;27(4):415–434. doi: 10.1080/07347330903183117.

Rosenbaum EH. Anemia causes and treatment. Cancer Supportive Care website. Updated July 15, 2008. http://www.cancersupportivecare.com/anemiacause.html. Accessed August 15, 2012.

Schagen SB, Muller MJ, Boogerd W, Rosenbrand RM, van Rhijn D, Rodenhuis S, van Dam FS. Late effects of adjuvant chemotherapy on cognitive function: a follow-up study in breast cancer patients. *Ann Oncol.* 2002;13(9):1387–1397.

Schilder CM, Seynaeve C, Linn SC, Boogerd W, Beex LV, Gundy CM, Nortier JW, van de Velde CJ, van Dam FS, Schagen SB. Cognitive functioning of postmenopausal breast cancer patients before adjuvant systemic therapy, and its association with medical and psychological factors. *Crit Rev Oncol Hematol.* 2010;76(2):133–141. doi: 10.1016/j.critrevonc.2009. 11.001. Epub 2009 Dec 24.

Schwartzberg LS. Chemotherapy-induced nausea and vomiting: clinician and patient perspectives. *J Support Oncol.* 2007;5(2 Suppl 1):5–12.

Shilling V, Jenkins V. Self-reported cognitive problems in women receiving adjuvant therapy for breast cancer. *Eur J Oncol Nurs.* 2007;11(1):6–15. Epub 2006 Jul 17.

Silverman DH, Dy CJ, Castellon SA, Lai J, Pio BS, Abraham L, Waddell K, Petersen L, Phelps ME, Ganz PA. Altered frontocortical, cerebellar, and basal ganglia activity in adjuvant-treated breast cancer survivors 5-10 years after chemotherapy. *Breast Cancer Res Treat.* 2007;103(3):303–311. Epub 2006 Sep 29.

Smith RE, Tchekmedyian S. Practitioners' practical model for managing cancer-related anemia. *Oncology (Williston Park).* 2002;16(9 Suppl 10):55–63. http://www.cancernetwork.com/display/article/10165/67 853. Accessed September 2, 2010.

Stout NL, Pfalzer LA, Springer B, Levy E, McGarvey CL, Danoff JV, Gerber LH, Soballe PW. Breast cancer-related lymphedema: comparing direct costs of a prospective surveillance model and a traditional model of care. *Phys Ther.* 2012;92(1):152–163. doi: 10.2522/ptj.20100167.

Stout Gergich NL, Pfalzer LA, McGarvey C, Springer B, Gerber LH, Soballe P. Preoperative assessment enables the early diagnosis and successful treatment of lymphedema. *Cancer.* 2008;112(12):2809–2819. doi: 10.1002/cncr.23494.

Vardy J, Rourke S, Tannock IF. Evaluation of cognitive function associated with chemotherapy: a review of published studies and recommendations for future research. *J Clin Oncol.* 2007;25(17):2455–2463. Epub 2007 May 7.

Walker EM, Rodriguez AI, Kohn B, Ball RM, Pegg J, Pocock JR, Nunez R, Peterson E, Jakary S, Levine RA. Acupuncture versus venlafaxine for the management of vasomotor symptoms in patients with hormone receptor-positive breast cancer: a randomized controlled trial. *J Clin Oncol.* 2010;28(4):634–640. Epub 2009 Dec 28.

Wefel JS, Saleeba AK, Buzdar AU, Meyers CA. Acute and late onset cognitive dysfunction associated with chemotherapy in women with breast cancer. *Cancer.* 2010;116(14):3348–3356. doi: 10.1002/cncr.25098.

Wickham R. Evolving treatment paradigms for chemotherapy-induced nausea and vomiting. *Cancer Control.* 2012;19(2 Suppl):3–9.

Wiffen PJ, McQuay HJ. Oral morphine for cancer pain. *Cochrane Database Syst Rev.* 2007;(4):CD003868.

Wu HS, McSweeney M. Cancer-related fatigue: "It's so much more than just being tired." *Eur J Oncol Nurs.* 2007;11(2):117–125. Epub 2006 Jul 7.

Chapter 14: Staying Emotionally Healthy During Treatment

American Psychiatric Association. *Diagnostic and Statistical Manual of Mental Disorders* DSM-IV-TR (Text Revision). 4th ed. American Psychiatric Publishing, Inc.; Arlington, VA: 2000.

Jacobsen PB, Jim HS. Psychosocial interventions for anxiety and depression in adult cancer patients: achievements and challenges. *CA Cancer J Clin.* 2008;58:214–230. doi: 10.3322/CA.2008.0003. Epub 2008 Jun 16.

National Institute of Mental Health. Mental Health Topics. http://www.nimh.nih.gov. Accessed August 26, 2011.

Parker PA, Baile WF, de Moor C, Cohen L. Psychosocial and demographic predictors of quality of life in a large sample of cancer patients. *Psychooncology.* 2003;12:183–193.

Petticrew M, Bell R, Hunter D. Influence of psychological coping on survival and recurrence in people with cancer: systematic review. *BMJ.* 2002;325(7372):1066.

Pirl WF. Evidence report on the occurrence, assessment, and treatment of depression in cancer patients. JNCI Monographs. 2004(32):32–39. http://jncimono.oxfordjournals.org/cgi/content/abstract/2004/32/32. Accessed August 26, 2011.

Rodin G, Lloyd N, Katz M, Green E, Mackay JA, Wong RK; Supportive Care Guidelines Group of Cancer Care Ontario Program in Evidence-Based Care. The treatment of depression in cancer patients: a systematic review. *Support Care Cancer.* 2007;15(2):123–136. Epub 2006 Oct 21.

White CA, Macleod U. ABCs of psychological medicine: cancer. *BMJ.* 2002;325(7360):377–380.

Chapter 15: Breast Reconstruction and Prostheses

American Cancer Society. *Cancer Facts and Figures 2013.* Atlanta, GA: American Cancer Society; 2013.

Ananthakrishnan P, Lucas A. Options and considerations in the timing of breast reconstruction after mastectomy. *Cleve Clin J Med.* 2008;75 Suppl 1:S30–S33.

Andrades P, Fix RJ, Danilla S, Howell RE 3rd, Campbell WJ, De la Torre J, Vasconez LO. Ischemic complications in pedicle, free, and muscle sparing transverse rectus abdominal myocutaneous flaps for breast reconstruction. *Ann Plast Surg.* 2008;60(5):562–567.

Bishara MR, Ross C, Sur M. Primary anaplastic large cell lymphoma of the breast arising in reconstruction mammoplasty capsule of saline filled breast implant after radical mastectomy for breast cancer: an unusual case presentation. *Diagn Pathol.* 2009;4:11. doi: 10.1186/1746-1596-4-11.

Boehmler JH 4th, Butler CE, Ensor J, Kronowitz SJ. Outcomes of various techniques of abdominal fascia closure after TRAM flap breast reconstruction. *Plast Reconstr Surg.* 2009;123(3):773–781.

Breast reconstruction. American Society of Plastic Surgeons website. http://www.plasticsurgery.org/Patients_and_Consumers/Procedures/Reconstructive_Procedures/Breast_Reconstruction.html. Accessed February 6, 2012.

Djohan R, Gage E, Bernard S. Breast reconstruction options following mastectomy. *Cleve Clin J Med.* 2008;75 Suppl 1:S17–S23.

Farhadi J, Maksvytyte GK, Schaefer DJ, Pierer G, Scheufler O. Reconstruction of the nipple-areola complex: an update. *J Plast Reconstr Aesthet Surg.* 2006;59(1):40–53.

Gerber B, Krause A, Dieterich M, Kundt G, Reimer T. The oncological safety of skin sparing mastectomy with conservation of the nipple-areola complex and autologous reconstruction: an extended follow-up study. *Ann Surg.* 2009;249(3):461–468. doi: 10.1097/SLA.obo13e31819ao44f.

Guerra AB, Metzinger SE, Bidros RS, Gill PS, Dupin CL, Allen RJ. Breast reconstruction with gluteal artery perforator (GAPS) Flaps: a critical analysis of 142 cases. *Ann Plast Surg.* 2004;52(2):118–125.

Kim SM, Park JM. Mammographic and ultrasonographic features after autogenous myocutaneous flap reconstruction mammoplasty. *J Ultrasound Med.* 2004;23(2):275–282.

Kufe DW, Pollock RE, Weichselbaum RR, Bast RC, Gansler TS, Holland JF, Frei E, eds. *Cancer Medicine 6.* Hamilton, Ontario: BC Decker; 2003.

Li S, Lee AK. Silicone implant and primary breast ALK1-negative anaplastic large cell lymphoma, fact or fiction? *Int J Clin Exp Pathol.* 2009;3(1):117–127.

Namnoum JD. Expander/implant reconstruction with AlloDerm: recent experience. *Plast Reconstr Surg.* 2009;124(2):387–394.

Newman MI, Samson MC, Tamburrino JF, Swartz KA, Brunworth L. An investigation of the application of laser-assisted indocyanine green fluorescent dye angiography in pedicle transverse rectus abdominus myocutaneous breast reconstruction. *Can J Plast Surg.* 2011;19(1):e1–e5.

Newman MI, Swartz KA, Samson MC, Mahoney CB, Diab K. The true incidence of near-term postoperative complications in prosthetic breast reconstruction utilizing human acellular dermal matrices: a meta-analysis. *Aesthetic Plast Surg.* 2011;35(1):100–106. Epub 2010 Dec 24.

Nguyen MD, Chen C, Colakoğlu S, Morris DJ, Tobias AM, Lee BT. Infectious complications leading to explantation in implant-based breast reconstruction with alloderm. *Eplasty*. 2010;10:e48.

Resnick B, Belcher AE. Breast reconstruction. Options, answers, and support for patients making a difficult personal decision. *Am J Nurs*. 2002;102(4):26–33; quiz 34.

Spear SL, Parikh PM, Reisin E, Menon NG. Acellular dermis-assisted breast reconstruction. *Aesth Plast Surg*. 2008;32(3):418–425. doi: 10.1007/s00266-008-9128-8.

Taylor CW, Horgan K, Dodwell D. Oncological aspects of breast reconstruction. *Breast*. 2005;14(2):118–130.

US Food and Drug Administration. Breast implant surgery. http://www.fda.gov/MedicalDevices/ ProductsandMedicalProcedures/ImplantsandProsthetics/ BreastImplants/ucm064176.htm. Updated June 22, 2011. Accessed February 6, 2012.

US Food and Drug Administration. FDA update on the safety of silicone gel-filled breast implants. http://www. fda.gov/downloads/MedicalDevices/ProductsandMedical Procedures/ImplantsandProsthetics/BreastImplants/UCM 260090.pdf. Published June 2011. Accessed April 30, 2013.

US Food and Drug Administration. Guidance for industry and FDA staff—saline, silicone gel, and alternative breast implants. http://www.fda.gov/ MedicalDevices/DeviceRegulationandGuidance/ GuidanceDocuments/ucm071228.htm. Published November 17, 2006. Accessed February 6, 2012.

US Food and Drug Administration. Medical device safety communication: reports of anaplastic large cell lymphoma (ALCL) in women with breast implants. http://www.fda.gov/MedicalDevices/Safety/AlertsandNot ices/ucm240000.htm. Updated November 20, 2012. Accessed February 6, 2012.

Vadivelu N, Schreck M, Lopez J, Kodumudi G, Narayan D. Pain after mastectomy and breast reconstruction. *Am Surg*. 2008;74(4):285–296

Chapter 16: Employment and Workplace Issues

Fact sheet #28: The Family and Medical Leave Act of 1993. United States Department of Labor website. http://www.dol.gov/whd/regs/compliance/whdfs28.pdf. Accessed April 11, 2013.

The Family and Medical Leave Act of 1993 as amended. United States Department of Labor website. http://www.dol.gov/whd/fmla/fmlaAmended.htm. Accessed April 11, 2013.

The Family and Medical Leave Act, the Americans with Disabilities Act, and Title VII of the Civil Rights Act of 1964. US Equal Employment Opportunity Commission website. http://www.eeoc.gov/policy/docs/fmlaada.html. Accessed April 11, 2013.

Filing a charge of discrimination. US Equal Employment Opportunity Commission website. http://www.eeoc.gov/ employees/charge.cfm. Accessed April 10, 2013.

Leave benefits: family & medical leave. United States Department of Labor website. http://www.dol.gov/dol/ topic/benefits-leave/fmla.htm. Accessed April 11, 2013.

Office of Disability Employment Policy. Employment rights: Who has them and who enforces them. United States Department of Labor website. http://www.dol.gov/ odep/pubs/fact/rights.htm. Accessed April 11, 2013.

US Department of Justice. A guide to disability rights laws. Americans with Disabilities Act website. http://www.ada.gov/cguide.htm. Published July 2009. Updated April 9, 2012. Accessed April 8, 2013.

Chapter 17: Insurance and Your Rights

About Medicare health plans. Medicare.gov website. http://www.medicare.gov/sign-up-change-plans/ medicare-health-plans/medicare-health-plans.html. Accessed April 8, 2013.

CHAMPVA. United States Department of Veterans Affairs website. http://www.va.gov/hac/forbeneficiaries/ champva/champva.asp. Accessed April 8, 2013.

Hudson KL, Holohan MK, Collins FS. Keeping pace with the times–The Genetic Information Nondiscrimination Act of 2008. *N Eng J Med*. 2008;358(25):2661–2663.

National Cancer Institute. *Facing Forward: A Guide for Cancer Survivors*. (NIH Publication No. 94-2424. Revised July 1994).

Scam alerts: bogus health plans. Coalition Against Insurance Fraud website. http://www.insurancefraud.org/ bogus_health.htm. Accessed August 24, 2012. Content no longer available.

US Department of Agriculture, Food and Nutrition Service. How to get food help [pamphlet]. Publication No. FNS-416. http://www.fns.usda.gov/cga/publications/ConsumerBrochure.pdf. Published November 2010. Accessed April 8, 2013.

US Department of Health and Human Services. Children's health insurance program. Medicaid.gov website. http://www.medicaid.gov/Medicaid-CHIP-Program-Information/By-Topics/Childrens-Health-Insurance-Program-CHIP/Childrens-Health-Insurance-Program-CHIP.html. Accessed August 28, 2012.

US Department of Health and Human Services. Has your health insurer denied payment for a medical service? You have a right to appeal. Healthcare.gov website. http://www.healthcare.gov/news/factsheets/2012/06/appeals06152012a.html. Accessed August 27, 2012.

US Department of Health and Human Services. Health claim appeals: a guide to resolving health insurance disputes. America's Health Insurance Plans website. http://www.healthclaimappeals.org/home.html. Accessed December 2, 2010. Content no longer available.

Chapter 18: Finances and Cancer Treatment

National Endowment for Financial Education. How to find a financial professional sensitive to cancer issues: financial guidance for cancer survivors and their families. American Cancer Society website. http://www.cancer.org/acs/groups/content/@editorial/documents/document/acsq-020181.pdf. Accessed April 28, 2013.

National Endowment for Financial Education. In treatment: financial guidance for cancer survivors and their families. American Cancer Society website. http://www.cancer.org/acs/groups/content/@editorial/documents/document/acsq-020182.pdf. Accessed May 1, 2013.

Special Caregiver's Section: Supporting the Woman with Cancer

Given BA, Given CW, Kozachik S. Family support in advanced cancer. CA Cancer J Clin. 2001;51(4):213–231.

Glajchen M. The emerging role and needs of family caregivers in cancer care. J Supportive Oncol. 2004;2(2):145–155.

Mellon S, Northouse LL, Weiss LK. A population-based study of the quality of life of cancer survivors and their family caregivers. Cancer Nurs. 2006;29(2):120–131; quiz 132–133.

Nijboer C, Triemstra M, Tempelaar R, Mulder M, Sanderman R, van den Bos GA. Patterns of caregiver experiences among partners of cancer patients. Gerontologist. 2000;40(6):738–746.

Pellegrino R, Formica V, Portarena I, Mariotti S, Grenga I, Del Monte G, Roselli M. Caregiver distress in the early phases of cancer. Anticancer Res. 2010;30(11):4657–4663.

Rivera HR. Depression symptoms in cancer caregivers. Clin J Oncol Nurs. 2009;13(2):195–202.

Chapter 19: Taking Care of Yourself After Cancer: Health and Wellness

Carmichael AR. Obesity and prognosis of breast cancer. Obes Rev. 2006 Nov;7(4):333–340.

Doyle C, Kushi LH, Byers T, Courneya KS, Demark-Wahnefried W, Grant B, McTiernan A, Rock CL, Thompson C, Gansler T, Andrews KS; 2006 Nutrition, Physical Activity and Cancer Survivorship Advisory Committee; American Cancer Society. Nutrition and physical activity during and after cancer treatment: an American Cancer Society guide for informed choices. CA Cancer J Clin. 2006;56(6):323–353.

IARC strengthens its findings on several carcinogenic personal habits and household exposures [news release]. Lyon, France: World Health Organization International Agency for Research on Cancer; November 2, 2009. http://www.iarc.fr/en/media-centre/pr/2009/pdfs/pr196_E.pdf. Accessed May 1, 2013.

Ligibel J. Obesity and breast cancer. Oncology (Williston Park). 2011;25(11):994–1000.

McDonald S, Saslow D, Alciati MH. Performance and reporting of clinical breast examination: A review of the literature. CA Cancer J Clin. 2004;54:345–361.

Rock CL, Doyle C, Demark-Wahnefried W, Meyerhardt J, Courneya KS, Schwartz AL, Bandera EV, Hamilton KK, Grant B, McCullough M, Byers T, Gansler T. Nutrition and physical activity guidelines for cancer survivors. CA Cancer J Clin. 2012;62(4):243–274. doi: 10.3322/caac.21142.

Saunders KJ, Pilgrim CA, Pennypacker HS. Increased proficiency of search in breast self-examination. *Cancer.* 1986;58:2531–2537.

Chapter 20: Emotional Wellness After Treatment: Moving On

Björneklett HG, Lindemalm C, Rosenblad A, Ojutkangas ML, Letocha H, Strang P, Bergkvist L. A randomised controlled trial of support group intervention after breast cancer treatment: results on anxiety and depression. *Acta Oncol.* 2012;51(2):198–207. doi: 10.3109/0284186X. 2011.610352. Epub 2011 Sep 19.

Helgeson VS, Cohen S, Schulz R, Yasko J. Education and peer discussion group interventions and adjustment to breast cancer. *Arch Gen Psychiatry.* 1999;56:340–347.

Richardson JL, Shelton DR, Krailo M, Levine AM. The effect of compliance with treatment on survival among patients with hematologic malignancies. *J Clin Oncol.* 1990;8:356–364.

Spiegel D, Bloom JR, Kraemer HC, Gottheil E. Effect of psychosocial treatment on survival of patients with metastatic breast cancer. *Lancet.* 1989;2(8668):888–891.

Zabalegui A, Sanchez S, Sanchez PD, Juando C. Nursing and cancer support groups. *J Adv Nurs.* 2005;51:369–381.

Chapter 21: Intimacy After Cancer Treatment

Dorval M, Guay S, Mondor M, Mâsse B, Falardeau M, Robidoux A, Deschênes L, Maunsell E. Couples who get closer after breast cancer: frequency and predictors in a prospective investigation. *J Clin Oncol.* 2005;23(15): 3588–3596.

Chapter 22: The Possibility of Facing Cancer Again

Abrahamson PE, Gammon MD, Lund MJ, Flagg EW, Porter PL, Stevens J, Swanson CA, Brinton LA, Eley JW, Coates RJ. General and abdominal obesity and survival among young women with breast cancer. *Cancer Epidemiol Biomarkers Prev.* 2006;15(10):1871-1877.

Azim HA Jr, Santoro L, Pavlidis N, Gelber S, Kroman N, Azim H, Peccatori FA. Safety of pregnancy following breast cancer diagnosis: a meta-analysis of 14 studies. *Eur J Cancer.* 2011;47(1):74–83. Epub 2010 Oct 11.

Beasley JM, Kwan ML, Chen WY, Weltzien EK, Kroenke CH, Lu W, Nechuta SJ, Cadmus-Bertram L, Patterson RE, Sternfeld B, Shu XO, Pierce JP, Caan BJ. Meeting the physical activity guidelines and survival after breast cancer: findings from the after breast cancer pooling project. *Breast Cancer Res Treat.* 2012;131(2):637–643. doi: 10.1007/s10549-011-1770-1. Epub 2011 Sep 21.

Bradshaw PT, Ibrahim JG, Stevens J, Cleveland R, Abrahamson PE, Satia JA, Teitelbaum SL, Neugut AI, Gammon MD. Postdiagnosis change in bodyweight and survival after breast cancer diagnosis. *Epidemiology.* 2012;23(2):320–327.

Caan BJ, Kwan ML, Hartzell G, Castillo A, Slattery ML, Sternfeld B, Weltzien E. Pre-diagnosis body mass index, post-diagnosis weight change, and prognosis among women with early stage breast cancer. *Cancer Causes Control.* 2008;19(10):1319–1328. Epub 2008 Aug 28.

Caan BJ, Natarajan L, Parker B, Gold EB, Thomson C, Newman V, Rock CL, Pu M, Al-Delaimy W, Pierce JP. Soy food consumption and breast cancer prognosis. *Cancer Epidemiol Biomarkers Prev.* 2011;20(5):854–858. Epub 2011 Feb 25.

Chen X, Lu W, Zheng W, Gu K, Chen Z, Zheng Y, Shu XO. Obesity and weight change in relation to breast cancer survival. *Breast Cancer Res Treat.* 2010;122(3): 823–833. Epub 2010 Jan 8.

Chlebowski RT, Blackburn GL, Thomson CA, Nixon DW, Shapiro A, Hoy MK, Goodman MT, Giuliano AE, Karanja N, McAndrew P, Hudis C, Butler J, Merkel D, Kristal A, Caan B, Michaelson R, Vinciguerra V, Del Prete S, Winkler M, Hall R, Simon M, Winters BL, Elashoff RM. Dietary fat reduction and breast cancer outcome: interim efficacy results from the Women's Intervention Nutrition Study. *J Natl Cancer Inst.* 2006;98(24):1767–1776.

Clarke M, Collins R, Darby S, Davies C, Elphinstone P, Evans E, Godwin J, Gray R, Hicks C, James S, MacKinnon E, McGale P, McHugh T, Peto R, Taylor C, Wang Y; Early Breast Cancer Trialists' Collaborative Group (EBCTCG). Effects of radiotherapy and of differences in the extent of surgery for early breast cancer on local recurrence and 15-year survival: an overview of the randomised trials. *Lancet.* 2005;366(9503):2087–2106.

Cuzick J, Sestak I, Baum M, Buzdar A, Howell A, Dowsett M, Forbes JF; ATAC/LATTE investigators.

Effect of anastrozole and tamoxifen as adjuvant treatment for early-stage breast cancer: 10-year analysis of the ATAC trial. *Lancet Oncol.* 2010;11(12):1135–1141. Epub 2010 Nov 17.

Demicheli R, Bonadonna G, Hrushesky WJ, Retsky MW, Valagussa P. Menopausal status dependence of the timing of breast cancer recurrence after surgical removal of the primary tumour. *Breast Cancer Res.* 2004;6(6):R689–R696.

Dong JY, Qin LQ. Soy isoflavones consumption and risk of breast cancer incidence or recurrence: a meta-analysis of prospective studies. *Breast Cancer Res Treat.* 2011;125(2):315–323. Epub 2010 Nov 27.

Dowsett M, Cuzick J, Ingle J, Coates A, Forbes J, Bliss J, Buyse M, Baum M, Buzdar A, Colleoni M, Coombes C, Snowdon C, Gnant M, Jakesz R, Kaufmann M, Boccardo F, Godwin J, Davies C, Peto R. Meta-analysis of breast cancer outcomes in adjuvant trials of aromatase inhibitors versus tamoxifen. *J Clin Oncol.* 2010;28(3): 509–518. Epub 2009 Nov 30.

Duggan C, Irwin ML, Xiao L, Henderson KD, Smith AW, Baumgartner RN, Baumgartner KB, Bernstein L, Ballard-Barbash R, McTiernan A. Associations of insulin resistance and adiponectin with mortality in women with breast cancer. *J Clin Oncol.* 2011;29(1):32–39. Epub 2010 Nov 29.

Early Breast Cancer Trialists' Collaborative Group (EBCTCG). Effects of chemotherapy and hormonal therapy for early breast cancer on recurrence and 15-year survival: an overview of the randomised trials. *Lancet.* 2005;365(9472):1687–1717.

Early Breast Cancer Trialists' Collaborative Group (EBCTCG), Darby S, McGale P, Correa C, Taylor C, Arriagada R, Clarke M, Cutter D, Davies C, Ewertz M, Godwin J, Gray R, Pierce L, Whelan T, Wang Y, Peto R. Effect of radiotherapy after breast-conserving surgery on 10-year recurrence and 15-year breast cancer death: meta-analysis of individual patient data for 10,801 women in 17 randomised trials. *Lancet.* 2011;378(9804):1707–1716. Epub 2011 Oct 19.

Early Breast Cancer Trialists' Collaborative Group (EBCTCG), Peto R, Davies C, Godwin J, Gray R, Pan HC, Clarke M, Cutter D, Darby S, McGale P, Taylor C, Wang YC, Bergh J, Di Leo A, Albain K, Swain S, Piccart M, Pritchard K. Comparisons between different olychemotherapy regimens for early breast cancer: meta-analyses of long-term outcome among 100,000 women in 123 randomised trials. *Lancet.* 2012;379(9814):432–444. Epub 2011 Dec 5.

Flatt SW, Thomson CA, Gold EB, Natarajan L, Rock CL, Al-Delaimy WK, Patterson RE, Saquib N, Caan BJ, Pierce JP. Low to moderate alcohol intake is not associated with increased mortality after breast cancer. *Cancer Epidemiol Biomarkers Prev.* 2010;19(3):681–688. Epub 2010 Feb 16.

Goel S, Sharma R, Hamilton A, Beith J. LHRH agonists for adjuvant therapy of early breast cancer in premenopausal women. *Cochrane Database Syst Rev.* 2009;(4):CD004562.

Guha N, Kwan ML, Quesenberry CP Jr, Weltzien EK, Castillo AL, Caan BJ. Soy isoflavones and risk of cancer recurrence in a cohort of breast cancer survivors: the Life After Cancer Epidemiology Study. *Breast Cancer Res Treat.* 2009;118(2):395–405. Epub 2009 Feb 17.

Hackshaw A, Roughton M, Forsyth S, Monson K, Reczko K, Sainsbury R, Baum M. Long-term benefits of 5 years of tamoxifen: 10-year follow-up of a large randomized trial in women at least 50 years of age with early breast cancer. *J Clin Oncol.* 2011;29(13):1657–1663. Epub 2011 Mar 21.

Holmberg L, Anderson H; HABITS steering and data monitoring committees. HABITS (hormonal replacement therapy after breast cancer—is it safe?), a randomised comparison: trial stopped. *Lancet.* 2004;363(9407):453–455.

Holmes MD, Chen WY, Feskanich D, Kroenke CH, Colditz GA. Physical activity and survival after breast cancer diagnosis. *JAMA.* 2005;293(20):2479–2486.

Ibrahim EM, Abouelkhair KM. Clinical outcome of panitumumab for metastatic colorectal cancer with wild-type KRAS status: a meta-analysis of randomized clinical trials. *Med Oncol.* 2011;28 Suppl 1:S310–S317. doi: 10.1007/s12032-010-9760-4. Epub 2011 Jan 9.

Kroenke CH, Chen WY, Rosner B, Holmes MD. Weight, weight gain, and survival after breast cancer diagnosis. *J Clin Oncol.* 2005;23(7):1370–1378. Epub 2005 Jan 31.

Kroenke CH, Fung TT, Hu FB, Holmes MD. Dietary patterns and survival after breast cancer diagnosis. *J Clin Oncol.* 2005;23(36):9295–9303.

Kushi LH, Doyle C, McCullough M, Rock CL, Demark-Wahnefried W, Bandera EV, Gapstur S, Patel AV, Andrews K, Gansler T; American Cancer Society 2010 Nutrition and Physical Activity Guidelines Advisory Committee. American Cancer Society guidelines on nutrition and physical activity for cancer prevention: reducing the risk of cancer with healthy food choices and physical activity. *CA Cancer J Clin.* 2012;62(1):30–67. doi: 10.3322/caac.20140.

Kwan ML, Kushi LH, Weltzien E, Tam EK, Castillo A, Sweeney C, Caan BJ. Alcohol consumption and breast cancer recurrence and survival among women with early-stage breast cancer: the life after cancer epidemiology study. *J Clin Oncol.* 2010;28(29):4410–4416. Epub 2010 Aug 30.

Li CI, Daling JR, Porter PL, Tang MT, Malone KE. Relationship between potentially modifiable lifestyle factors and risk of second primary contralateral breast cancer among women diagnosed with estrogen receptor-positive invasive breast cancer. *J Clin Oncol.* 2009;27(32):5312–5531. Epub 2009 Sep 8.

Litton JK, Gonzalez-Angulo AM, Warneke CL, Buzdar AU, Kau SW, Bondy M, Mahabir S, Hortobagyi GN, Brewster AM. Relationship between obesity and pathologic response to neoadjuvant chemotherapy among women with operable breast cancer. *J Clin Oncol.* 2008 Sep 1;26(25):4072–4077. doi: 10.1200/JCO.2007. 14.4527.

Mieog JS, van der Hage JA, van de Velde CJ. Neoadjuvant chemotherapy for operable breast cancer. *Br J Surg.* 2007;94(10):1189–2000.

Nichols HB, Trentham-Dietz A, Egan KM, Titus-Ernstoff L, Holmes MD, Bersch AJ, Holick CN, Hampton JM, Stampfer MJ, Willett WC, Newcomb PA. Body mass index before and after breast cancer diagnosis: associations with all-cause, breast cancer, and cardiovascular disease mortality. *Cancer Epidemiol Biomarkers Prev.* 2009;18(5):1403–1409. Epub 2009 Apr 14.

Pierce JP, Natarajan L, Caan BJ, Parker BA, Greenberg ER, Flatt SW, Rock CL, Kealey S, Al-Delaimy WK, Bardwell WA, Carlson RW, Emond JA, Faerber S, Gold EB, Hajek RA, Hollenbach K, Jones LA, Karanja N, Madlensky L, Marshall J, Newman VA, Ritenbaugh C, Thomson CA, Wasserman L, Stefanick ML. Influence of a diet very high in vegetables, fruit, and fiber and low in fat on prognosis following treatment for breast cancer: the Women's Healthy Eating and Living (WHEL) randomized trial. *JAMA.* 2007;298(3):289–298.

Pierce JP, Stefanick ML, Flatt SW, Natarajan L, Sternfeld B, Madlensky L, Al-Delaimy WK, Thomson CA, Kealey S, Hajek R, Parker BA, Newman VA, Caan B, Rock CL. Greater survival after breast cancer in physically active women with high vegetable-fruit intake regardless of obesity. *J Clin Oncol.* 2007;25(17):2345–2351.

Protani M, Coory M, Martin JH. Effect of obesity on survival of women with breast cancer: systematic review and meta-analysis. *Breast Cancer Res Treat.* 2010;123(3): 627–635. Epub 2010 Jun 23.

Regan MM, Neven P, Giobbie-Hurder A, Goldhirsch A, Ejlertsen B, Mauriac L, Forbes JF, Smith I, Láng I, Wardley A, Rabaglio M, Price KN, Gelber RD, Coates AS, Thürlimann B; BIG 1-98 Collaborative Group; International Breast Cancer Study Group (IBCSG). Assessment of letrozole and tamoxifen alone and in sequence for postmenopausal women with steroid hormone receptor-positive breast cancer: the BIG 1-98 randomised clinical trial at 8•1 years median follow-up. *Lancet Oncol.* 2011;12(12):1101–1108. Epub 2011 Oct 20.

van de Velde CJ, Rea D, Seynaeve C, Putter H, Hasenburg A, Vannetzel JM, Paridaena R, Markopoulos C, Hozumi Y, Hille ET, Kieback DG, Asmar L, Smeets J, Nortier JW, Hadji P, Bartlett JM, Jones SE. Adjuvant tamoxifen and exemestane in early breast cancer (TEAM): a randomised phase 3 trial. *Lancet.* 2011;377(9762):321–331.

Voskuil DW, van Nes JG, Junggeburt JM, van de Velde CJ, van Leeuwen FE, de Haes JC. Maintenance of physical activity and body weight in relation to subsequent quality of life in postmenopausal breast cancer patients. *Ann Oncol.* 2010;21(10):2094–2101. Epub 2010 Mar 31.

Yin W, Jiang Y, Shen Z, Shao Z, Lu J. Trastuzumab in the adjuvant treatment of HER2-positive early breast cancer patients: a meta-analysis of published randomized controlled trials. *PLoS One.* 2011;6(6):e21030. Epub 2011 Jun 9.

Appendix A

Smith RA, Saslow D, Sawyer KA, Burke W, Costanza ME, Evans WP 3rd, Foster RS Jr, Hendrick E, Eyre HJ, Sener S; American Cancer Society High-Risk Work Group;

American Cancer Society Screening Older Women Work Group; American Cancer Society Mammography Work Group; American Cancer Society Physical Examination Work Group; American Cancer Society New Technologies Work Group; American Cancer Society Breast Cancer Advisory Group. American Cancer Society guidelines for breast cancer screening: update 2003. *CA Cancer J Clin*. 2003;53(3):141–169.

Appendix B

US Department of Health and Human Services. The Women's Health and Cancer Rights Act (WHCRA) of 1998—helpful tips as of June 27, 2008. US Department of Health and Human Services, Centers for Medicare & Medicaid Services Website. http://www.cms.hhs.gov/HealthInsReformforConsume/Downloads/WHCRA_Helpful_Tips.pdf. Accessed May 25, 2011.

US Department of Labor. Fact sheet: Women's Health and Cancer Rights Act. US Department of Labor, Employee Benefits Security Administration Website. http://www.dol.gov/ebsa/newsroom/fswhcra.html. Accessed May 25, 2011.

US Department of Labor. Your rights after a mastectomy: Women's Health & Cancer Rights Act of 1998. US Department of Labor, Employee Benefits Security Administration Website. http://www.dol.gov/ebsa/Publications/whcra.html. Accessed on May 25, 2011.

Appendix C

No references.

Appendix D

Kushi LH, Doyle C, McCullough M, Rock CL, Demark-Wahnefried W, Bandera EV, Gapstur S, Patel AV, Andrews K, Gansler T; American Cancer Society 2010 Nutrition and Physical Activity Guidelines Advisory Committee. American Cancer Society guidelines on nutrition and physical activity for cancer prevention: reducing the risk of cancer with healthy food choices and physical activity. *CA Cancer J Clin*. 2012;62(1):30–67. doi: 10.3322/caac.20140.

GLOSSARY

accelerated breast irradiation: *see* external beam radiation therapy (EBRT).

acellular dermal matrix: a material derived from human or animal skin that has been treated to remove any cells and certain proteins that can cause an immune reaction. The product works as a type of skin substitute that encourages the formation of new tissue and can serve as a temporary wound covering. Acellular dermal matrix products can be used in a variety of medical applications, including breast reconstruction.

adenocarcinoma: cancer of the glandular tissue, such as in the ducts or lobules of the breast. *See* duct, lobules.

adenoid cystic carcinoma of the breast: a rare type of cancer that accounts for less than 0.2 percent of all breast cancers. Under the microscope, this cancer looks similar to a type of cancer of the salivary glands. This type of cancer is often found at an early stage, is considered to be somewhat less aggressive than infiltrating ductal carcinoma, and has a good prognosis. Also called adenocystic carcinoma.

adenosquamous carcinoma: a rare type of invasive breast cancer. Adenosquamous carcinoma contains two types of atypical cells: squamous cells (flat, thin cells that line certain organs) and gland-like cells. It is a variant of metaplastic carcinoma that is often slow growing and has a better prognosis than infiltrating ductal carcinoma.

adjuvant therapy: treatment used in addition to the main treatment. It usually refers to hormone therapy, chemotherapy, or radiation therapy added after surgery to increase the chances of curing the disease or prevent it from recurring.

adrenal glands: triangle-shaped glands that sit on top of the kidneys. They make hormones, such as cortisol, aldosterone, epinephrine, and norepinephrine, that control metabolism, fluid balance, and blood pressure and are essential for life. In addition, the adrenal glands produce small amounts of "male" hormones (androgens).

alternative therapy: an unproven medication or therapy that is recommended instead of standard (proven) therapy. Some alternative therapies have dangerous or even life-threatening side effects. With others, the main danger is that the patient may lose the opportunity to benefit from standard therapy. The American Cancer Society recommends that patients considering the use of any alternative or complementary therapies discuss them with their medical team. *Compare with* complementary therapy.

American Joint Committee on Cancer (AJCC) staging system: a system for describing the extent of a cancer's spread by using the number 0 and the Roman numerals I through IV. Also called the TNM system. *See also* staging.

anemia: a low red blood cell count.

anesthesia: the loss of feeling or sensation as a result of drugs or gases. General anesthesia causes loss of consciousness (puts you to sleep). Local or regional anesthesia numbs only a certain area of the body.

aneuploid: *see* ploidy.

angiogenesis: the formation of new blood vessels. Some cancer treatments work by blocking angiogenesis, thus preventing blood from reaching the tumor.

angiosarcoma: a type of cancer that begins in the cells that line blood vessels or lymph vessels. Cancer that begins in blood vessels is called hemangiosarcoma. Cancer that begins in lymph vessels is called lymphangiosarcoma.

antibody: a protein produced by the body's immune system cells and released into the blood. Antibodies defend the body against foreign agents, such as bacteria. These agents contain certain substances called antigens. Each antibody works against a specific antigen.

antigen: a substance that causes the body's immune system to respond. This response often involves making antibodies. For example, the immune system's response to antigens that are a part of bacteria and viruses helps people resist infections. Cancer cells have certain antigens that can be found in laboratory tests. These antigens are important in cancer diagnosis and in watching response to treatment. Other antigens play a role in the body's resistance to cancer.

areola: the area of dark-colored skin on the breast that surrounds the nipple.

aromatase inhibitor: a drug that prevents the formation of estradiol, a female hormone, by interfering with an aromatase enzyme. Aromatase inhibitors are used as a type of hormone therapy for postmenopausal women who have hormone–dependent breast cancer.

atypical: not usual; abnormal. Often refers to the appearance of cancerous or precancerous cells.

atypical ductal hyperplasia: a benign condition in which there are small areas (smaller than 2 mm) of mildly atypical cells with an abnormal growth pattern that distend the ducts. This has some (but not all) of the features of ductal carcinoma in situ. Having atypical ductal hyperplasia increases the risk of breast cancer. Also called ADH and atypical ductal breast hyperplasia.

atypical lobular hyperplasia: a benign condition in which there are small areas of slightly atypical cells in clusters in the lobules of the breast. Atypical lobular hyperplasia has some (but not all) of the features of lobular carcinoma in situ. Having atypical lobular hyperplasia increases the risk of breast cancer. Also called ALH and atypical lobular breast hyperplasia, it is grouped with lobular carcinoma in situ as lobular neoplasia.

autologous reconstruction: breast reconstruction using a woman's own tissue—skin, fat, blood vessels, and sometimes muscle—to form the breast shape. The tissue, called a flap, can come from the belly, back, inner thigh, or buttock to create the reconstructed breast. Autologous reconstruction can occur at the same time as mastectomy or after mastectomy and other treatments. Also called autogenous reconstruction. *See also individual flap procedure names.*

axillary lymph node: a lymph node in the armpit.

axillary lymph node dissection: removal of the lymph nodes in the armpit (axillary nodes). They are examined under a microscope to determine whether they contain cancer. *See also* lymph nodes.

benign: not cancerous. *Compare with* malignant.

biopsy: the removal of a sample of tissue to see whether cancer cells are present. There are several kinds of biopsies. *See also* surgical biopsy, needle biopsy, stereotactic needle biopsy, incisional biopsy.

bisphosphonates: drugs that turn off osteoclasts, the cells that break down bone. They are sometimes given to cancer patients whose disease has spread to the bones to slow the breakdown of bone, lower the rate of bone fractures, and alleviate bone pain. They can also be given to prevent and treat osteoporosis. *See also* bone-directed therapy.

blood tumor marker: a substance that can be found in the blood when cancer is present. There are many different types of tumor markers.

blood vessel: a tube through which the blood circulates in the body. Blood vessels include a network of arteries, arterioles, capillaries, venules, and veins.

bone-directed therapy: a combination of anticancer therapy and medications such as bisphosphonates or a RANKL inhibitor like denosumab that help maintain bone integrity and prevent skeletal complications caused by bone metastasis. *See also* bisphosphonates.

bone marrow: the soft tissue in the hollow center of some bones of the body that produces new blood cells. Bone marrow is often affected by chemotherapy. *See also* platelets, red blood cells, white blood cells.

bone scan: an imaging method that gives important information about the bones, including the location of cancer that may have spread to the bones. It can be done as an outpatient procedure and is painless, except for the needle stick when a low-dose radioactive substance is injected into a vein. Special pictures are taken to see where the radioactivity collects, pointing to an abnormality.

brachytherapy: internal radiation treatment given by placing radioactive material directly into the tumor or close to it. Also called interstitial radiation therapy or seed implantation. *Compare with* external beam radiation therapy.

BRCA1: a gene that when damaged (mutated) places a woman at much greater risk of developing breast, ovarian, and other cancers, compared with women who do not have the mutation.

BRCA2: a gene that when damaged (mutated) puts the carrier at a much higher risk for developing breast, ovarian, and other cancers than the general population.

breast: a glandular organ located on the chest. The breast is made up of connective tissue, fat, and breast tissue that contains the glands that can make milk. Also called mammary gland.

breast-conserving surgery: surgery to remove breast cancer and a small amount of normal tissue around the cancer (margin), without removing any other part of the breast. The lymph nodes under the arm may be removed. Radiation therapy is often administered after the surgery. This method is also called lumpectomy, partial mastectomy, segmental excision, limited breast surgery, or tylectomy. *See also* lymph nodes. *Compare with* mastectomy.

breast form: an artificial body part worn either inside the bra or attached to the body to simulate the appearance and feel of a natural breast.

breast implant: a sac used to increase breast size or restore the shape of the breast after mastectomy. The sac is filled with silicone gel (a synthetic material) or sterile saltwater (saline).

breast reconstruction: surgery done to rebuild the breast after mastectomy. A breast implant or the patient's own tissue is used. If desired, the nipple and areola may also be recreated. Reconstruction can be done at the time of mastectomy (immediate reconstruction) or any time later (delayed reconstruction). *Compare with* breast form.

breast self-examination (BSE): a method of checking one's breasts for lumps or suspicious changes. BSE is an option for women in their twenties and older. The goal with BSE is to know what your breast tissue feels and looks like and to be able to report any breast changes to a doctor or nurse right away.

calcifications: tiny calcium deposits within the breast, either alone or in clusters, usually found by mammography. They are a sign of changes within the breast that may need to be followed by more mammograms or by a biopsy. Calcifications may be caused by benign breast conditions or by breast cancer. The ones most closely linked to breast cancer are called **microcalcifications**, while the larger **macrocalcifications** are more often linked to benign changes.

cancer: cancer is not just one disease but a group of diseases. All forms of cancer cause cells in the body to change and grow out of control. Most types of cancer cells form a lump or mass called a tumor. The tumor can invade and destroy healthy tissue. Cells from the tumor can break away and travel to other parts of the body where they can continue to grow—a process called metastasis. When cancer spreads, it is still named after the part of the body where it started. For example, if breast cancer spreads to the lungs, it is still called breast cancer, not lung cancer.

Some cancers, such as blood cancers, do not form a tumor. A tumor is not always cancer; a tumor that is not cancer is called benign. Benign tumors do not grow and spread the way cancer does. Benign tumors are usually not a threat to life. Another word for cancerous is malignant.

capsular contracture: scar tissue that forms around the implant and squeezes it. There are four grades of contracture (Grades I–IV) that range from normal and soft to hard, painful, and distorted.

carcinoma: any cancerous tumor that begins in the lining layer of organs. At least 80 percent of all cancers are carcinomas.

cell: the basic unit of which all living things are made. Cells replace themselves by splitting and forming new cells (mitosis). The processes that control the formation of new cells and the death of old cells are disrupted in cancer.

chemoprevention: prevention or reversal of disease by using drugs, chemicals, vitamins, or minerals. Whereas this idea is not ready for widespread use, it is a very promising area of study.

chemotherapy: treatment with drugs to destroy cancer cells. Chemotherapy is often used, either alone or with surgery or radiation therapy, to treat cancer that has spread or recurred, or when there is a strong chance that it could recur.

chromogenic in situ hybridization (CISH): a laboratory test that uses labeled small deoxyribonucleic acid (DNA) probes to identify certain genes (or gene sequences). Unlike fluorescence in situ hybridization (FISH), a fluorescent microscope is not needed. CISH is an alternative to FISH in testing for gene alterations such as HER2/neu status in cells (such as breast cancer cells), though it is not yet used as commonly as FISH. *See also* fluorescence in situ hybridization.

clinical breast examination: an examination of the breasts done by a health care professional such as a doctor or nurse. Clinical breast exams (CBE) are recommended every three years for women in their twenties and thirties, and every year for women aged forty and older.

clinical stage: an estimate of the extent of cancer based on physical examination, biopsy results, and imaging tests. *See also* pathologic stage, staging.

clinical trials: research studies in people. They may be used to test new drugs or to compare current, standard treatments with others that may be better. Before a new treatment is used on people, it is studied in the laboratory. If laboratory studies suggest the treatment will work, the next step is to test its value for patients. These human studies are called clinical trials. The main questions the researchers want to answer are these:

- Does this treatment work?
- Does it work better than what we're currently using?
- What side effects does it cause?
- Do the benefits outweigh the risks?
- Which patients are most likely to find this treatment helpful?

comedocarcinoma: a form of breast cancer in which plugs of necrotic malignant cells may be expressed from the ducts. *See* necrosis.

comedonecrosis: In ductal carcinoma in situ (DCIS), an area of dead cells (necrosis) occupying most of the central area of a duct. It is called "comedo" because it often contains a whitish material. In cases of DCIS, comedonecrosis can be an indication that the DCIS is high-grade, meaning that the person would be at higher risk for recurrence and invasive cancer. *See also* necrosis.

complementary therapy: treatment used in addition to standard therapy. Some complementary therapies may help relieve certain symptoms of cancer, relieve side effects of standard cancer therapy, or improve a patient's sense of well-being. The American Cancer Society recommends that patients considering the use of any alternative or complementary therapies discuss them with their medical team, since many of these treatments are unproven and some can be harmful. *Compare with* alternative therapy.

computed tomography: an imaging test in which many x-rays are taken of a part of the body from different angles. These images are combined by a computer to produce cross-sectional pictures of internal organs. Except for the injection of a contrast dye (needed in some but not all cases), this is a painless procedure that can be done in an outpatient clinic. It is often referred to as "CT" or "CAT" scanning.

cone views with magnification: a special mammogram image used to "zoom in " on a certain area of the breast so that the doctor can visualize the area more clearly.

core needle biopsy: *see* needle biopsy.

Cowden syndrome: an inherited condition characterized by lesions that form on various organs, especially in the breast, thyroid, colon, skin, oral mucosa, and intestines. Cowden syndrome is associated with a higher risk of malignancies developing in the organs involved. Also called Cowden disease.

CT scan or CAT scan: *see* computed tomography.

deep inferior epigastric artery perforator (DIEP) flap: a type of breast reconstruction procedure that uses fat and skin from the abdomen to form the breast mound. A DIEP flap is similar toa TRAM flap but does not take muscle from the abdomen.

deoxyribonucleic acid: *see* DNA.

diethylstilbestrol (DES): a man-made form of estrogen. Taking this drug during pregnancy may put women at a slightly higher risk for breast cancer.

digital mammogram: a method of storing an x-ray of the breast as a computer image rather than on the usual x-ray film. Digital mammography can be combined with computer-aided detection (CAD), a process in which the radiologist uses a computer program to help interpret the mammogram. Also known as full-field digital mammogram (FFDM). *See also* x-ray, mammogram.

dimpling: a pucker or indentation of the skin. On the breast, it may be a sign of cancer.

diploid: *see* ploidy.

DNA: deoxyribonucleic acid. DNA is the genetic "blueprint" found in the nucleus of each cell. It holds genetic information on cell growth, division, and function.

dose-dense chemotherapy: a treatment plan in which drugs are given with less time between the doses than is traditional. Often this means chemotherapy cycles being given every two weeks instead of every three. *See also* chemotherapy.

duct: a hollow passage for gland secretions. In the breast, milk passes from the lobule (which makes the milk) through the ducts to the nipple.

ductal carcinoma: the most common type of breast cancer. It begins in the cells that line the milk ducts in the breast.

ductal carcinoma in situ (DCIS): cancer that starts in cells in the ducts (milk passages) and does not break through the duct walls into the nearby tissue. This is a precancerous (or noninvasive) form of breast cancer that is highly curable. It is treated with surgery, sometimes combined with radiation therapy and/or hormone therapy. Also called intraductal carcinoma.

ductal lavage: a method used to collect cells from milk ducts in the breast. A hair-size catheter (tube) is inserted into the nipple, and a small amount of salt water is released into the duct. The water picks up breast cells and is removed. The cells are checked under a microscope.

ductogram: a test in which a fine plastic tube is inserted into the nipple and contrast dye injected to outline the shape of the duct. X-rays are then taken to see if there is a mass. Also called a galactogram.

epithelial cells: cells that line the internal and external surfaces of the body.

estrogen: a female sex hormone produced mainly by the ovaries, and in smaller amounts by fat tissue in the body. In women, levels of estrogen and other hormones work together to regulate the development of secondary sex characteristics, including breasts; regulate the monthly cycle of menstruation; and prepare the body for fertilization and reproduction. In breast cancer, estrogen may promote the growth of cancer cells. *See also* estrogen replacement therapy, hormone therapy.

estrogen receptors: *see* hormone receptor.

estrogen replacement therapy (ERT): the use of estrogen from sources other than the body. Estrogen may be administered after a woman's body no longer makes its own supply. This type of hormone therapy is often used to relieve symptoms of menopause in women who no longer have a uterus. It has also been shown to help protect against bone thinning (osteoporosis). Estrogen nourishes some types of breast cancer, but so far giving it alone (without progesterone) does not seem to increase the risk of breast cancer very much, if at all. It does increase the risk of vascular diseases, such as stroke.

excisional biopsy: *see* surgical biopsy.

external beam radiation therapy (EBRT): radiation that is focused from a source outside the body on the area affected by the cancer. It is much like getting a diagnostic x-ray, but for a longer time and at a higher dose. Radiation to the breast can be delivered from outside the body in different ways.

fatigue: a common symptom during cancer treatment, a bone-weary exhaustion that doesn't get better with rest. For some, this condition can last for some time after treatment.

FDA: *see* US Food and Drug Administration.

fibroadenoma: a breast tumor made of fibrous and glandular tissue that is not cancer. On a clinical breast examination or breast self-examination, it usually feels like a firm, round, smooth lump. Fibroadenomas usually occur in young women.

fibrocystic changes: an older term for the combination of fibrosis and cysts that is found in many healthy women and is not related to cancer. Symptoms are breast swelling or pain. The breasts often feel lumpy or nodular. Because these signs sometimes resemble breast cancer, more tests may be needed to show that there is no cancer. Also called fibrocystic disease.

fibrosis: formation of excessive fibrous tissue, the same material that ligaments and scar tissues are made of. Areas of fibrosis feel rubbery, firm, or hard to the touch. Fibrosis in breast tissue is common. It does not increase the risk of breast cancer and does not need any special treatment.

fine needle aspiration (FNA): *see* needle biopsy.

first-degree relative: a parent, sibling, or child. *Compare with* second-degree relative.

five (5)-year survival rate: the percentage of people with a specific cancer who survive five years or longer with the disease. Five-year survival rates have some drawbacks. Although the rates may be based on the most recent information available, they have to be based on patients treated at least five years earlier. Treatment advances since then may mean that patients treated now would be expected to have better outcomes. Also, they are based on large groups of people, but cannot predict what will happen in any one individual case.

fluorescence in situ hybridization: a laboratory technique used to look at genes or chromosomes in cells and tissues. Pieces of DNA that contain a fluorescent dye are made in the laboratory and added to cells or tissues on a glass slide. When these pieces of DNA bind to parts of specific genes (on chromosomes) on the slide, they light up when viewed under a microscope with a special light. Also called FISH. *See also* gene, genetic testing, genetic counselor, chromogenic in situ hybridization.

founder mutation: a specific gene mutation that is found with high frequency in a group that is or was geographically or culturally isolated, which reflects that one or more of the ancestors in that group was a carrier of the mutant gene. Because the group was isolated, the mutation spread from the founder to his or her many descendants. Knowing that a founder mutation exists can allow for easier (and often less expensive) genetic testing for people within that group, because the test can just look for that one mutation, instead of having to sequence the entire gene. Also, because many people have the exact same mutation, it is easier to determine the risks associated with it by looking at their history. *See also* mutation, DNA, gene, genetic risk factor, gene expression profile.

free flap: surgery in which the tissue for reconstruction is moved entirely from another area of the body and the blood and nerve supplies are surgically reattached with special microscopes.

full-field digital mammogram (FFDM): *see* digital mammogram.

gadolinium: a metal element that is used in magnetic resonance imaging (MRI) and other imaging methods. It is a contrast agent that helps reveal abnormal tissue in the body during an imaging procedure.

galactogram: *see* ductogram.

gene: a segment of DNA that contains the code for hereditary characteristics such as hair color, eye color, and height, as well as susceptibility to certain diseases. *See also* DNA.

gene expression profile: the measurement and determination of the pattern of expression of many genes at once by certain cells or under certain conditions. All cells contain the same genes—what makes cells different is which genes are expressed or active. A gene expression profile may be used to see what type of cancer is contained in a tumor. It can also be used to see whether cells are actively dividing or dying, which can help determine whether a certain treatment is working. *See also* gene, genetic testing, genetic counselor, genetic risk factor.

genetic counseling: the process of counseling people who may have a gene that makes them more susceptible to cancer. The purpose of the counseling is to help them decide whether they wish to be tested, to explore what the genetic test results might mean, and to support them before and after the test.

genetic counselor: a specially trained health care professional who helps people as they consider genetic testing, as they adjust to the test results, and as they consider whatever screening and preventive measures are best for them.

genetic risk factor: a change in a gene that you were born with that alters your risk of getting cancer. This gene changes in the DNA of every cell in the body and is often inherited from a parent. A risk factor is anything that changes a person's chance of a disease developing such as cancer. Risk factors can be lifestyle-related or environmental, or genetic (inherited). Having a risk factor, or several risk factors, does not mean that a person will get the disease. *See also* risk factor.

genetic testing: tests performed to determine whether a person has certain gene changes known to increase cancer risk. Such testing is not recommended for everyone, but specifically for individuals with specific types of family history. Genetic counseling should be part of the process. *See also* genetic risk factor, gene expression profile.

glandular tissue: tissue that makes or secretes a substance.

gluteal free flap or gluteal artery perforator (GAP) flap: a newer type of breast reconstruction procedure that uses tissue and muscle from the buttock to create the breast shape.

grade: a measure of how abnormal cancer cells look under the microscope and how fast they are dividing. There are several grading systems for breast cancer, and each grading system divides cancer into those with the greatest abnormality, the least abnormality, and those in between. Grading is done by a pathologist who examines the tissue from the biopsy.

Grading is important because higher-grade cancers tend to grow and spread more quickly and have a worse prognosis (outlook). Along with the cancer's stage, the grade is used to help determine the best treatment options. Histologic tumor grade (sometimes called the Bloom-Richardson grade, Nottingham grade, Scarff-Bloom-Richardson grade, or Elston-Ellis grade) is based on the arrangement of the cells in relation to each other: whether they form tubules, how closely they resemble normal breast cells (nuclear grade), and how many of the cancer cells are in the process of dividing (mitotic count). This system of grading is used for invasive cancers but not for in situ cancers. DCIS is also graded, but the grade is based only on how abnormal the cancer cells appear (nuclear grade). *See also* stage, staging.

helical CT: *see* spiral CT.

hematoma: a collection of blood outside a blood vessel caused by a leak or injury. A hematoma that occurs in the breast after injury or after surgery may feel like a lump.

HER2 gene: a gene that produces a type of receptor that helps cells grow. This receptor is present in very small amounts on the outer surface of normal breast cells and some other cells in the body. About 25 percent to 30 percent of breast cancers have too many of these receptors. These cancers tend to be more aggressive, but the outlook for these cancers improves if certain drugs that target HER2 are used, such as trastuzumab (Herceptin). *See also* oncogene.

hormone: a chemical substance released into the body by the endocrine glands, such as the thyroid, adrenal glands, or ovaries. Hormones travel through the bloodstream and set in motion various bodily functions. For example, prolactin, which is produced in the pituitary gland, begins and continues milk production in the breast after childbirth. *See also* estrogen, progesterone.

hormone receptor: a protein on or in a cell to which a specific hormone binds. The hormone causes many changes to take place in the cell.

hormone replacement therapy (HRT): a term used for therapy in which estrogen and progesterone are given to women after menopause to replace the hormones no longer produced by the body. Also called PHT (postmenopausal hormone therapy) or MHT (menopausal hormone therapy).

hormone therapy (HT): treatment with hormones, with drugs that interfere with hormone production or hormone action, or the surgical removal of hormone-producing glands to kill cancer cells or slow their growth. Selective estrogen receptor modifiers and aromatase inhibitors are examples of hormone therapy drugs used to treat breast cancer.

hospice: a special kind of care for people in the final phase of illness, their families, and caregivers. The care may take place in the patient's home or in a home-like facility.

hot spots: areas of diseased bone that show up on bone scans. The hot spots can be bone metastasis, but they may also be arthritis, infection, or other bone diseases.

hysterectomy: an operation to remove the uterus. Hysterectomy can be performed through a large incision in the abdomen (abdominal hysterectomy); through the vagina (vaginal hysterectomy); or by making a few very small incisions in the lower abdomen (laparoscopic hysterectomy). Removal of the ovaries (oophorectomy) and the fallopian tubes (salpingectomy) may be done at the same time.

imaging tests: methods used to produce pictures of internal body structures. Some imaging methods used to help diagnose or stage cancer are x-rays, CT scans, magnetic resonance imaging (MRI), and ultrasound.

immunohistochemistry (IHC): a laboratory test that uses special antibodies (manmade versions of immune system proteins) that attach only to specific molecules on the cell surface. These antibodies cause color changes that can be seen under a microscope. This test may be helpful in testing biopsy samples in distinguishing different types of cancer from one another and from other diseases. It is also used in basic research to understand how cells grow and differentiate. *See also* monoclonal antibody.

incisional biopsy: a surgical procedure in which part of an abnormal area of tissue is removed so that it can be examined by a pathologist. The pathologist may study the tissue under a microscope or perform other tests. When an entire lump or suspicious area is removed, the procedure is called an excisional biopsy. When a sample of tissue or fluid is removed with a needle, the procedure is called a needle biopsy, core biopsy, or fine needle biopsy (aspiration).

infiltrating ductal carcinoma (IDC): cancer that starts in the ducts (milk passages) of the breast and then breaks through the duct wall and spreads into the fatty tissue of the breast. When it reaches this point, it can spread elsewhere in the breast, as well as to other parts of the body through the bloodstream and lymphatic system. Invasive ductal carcinoma is the most common type of breast cancer, accounting for about 80 percent of breast malignancies. Also called invasive ductal carcinoma. *See also* lymphatic system.

infiltrating lobular carcinoma (ILC): a cancer that starts in the lobules (milk-producing glands) of the breast and then breaks through the lobule walls to spread into nearby fatty tissue. From this site, it may then spread elsewhere in the breast. About 10 percent of invasive breast cancers are invasive lobular carcinomas. It is often difficult to detect by physical examination or even by mammography. Also called invasive lobular carcinoma.

inflammatory breast cancer: a type of invasive breast cancer with spread to lymph vessels in the skin covering the breast. The skin of the affected breast is red, feels warm, and may thicken to look and feel like an orange peel. About 1 percent of invasive breast cancers are inflammatory breast cancers. Also called inflammatory carcinoma. *See also* invasive breast cancer, lymphatic system.

informed consent: a legal document that explains a course of treatment, the risks, benefits, and possible alternatives; the process by which patients agree to treatment.

infraclavicular lymph nodes: lymph nodes located beneath the clavicle (collarbone). *See also* lymph nodes, supraclavicular lymph nodes.

inherited (familial) cancer: cancer that originates from mutated genes that have been passed from parents to their offspring (children).

in situ: literally, in place. When referring to cancer, it means that the cancer cells have not grown out of the layer of cells in which they started. This is often called precancer or noninvasive cancer.

internal mammary lymph nodes: *see* mammary lymph nodes.

intracavitary radiation therapy: a type of internal radiation therapy in which radioactive material sealed in needles, seeds, wires, or catheters is placed directly into a body cavity such as the cavity left after a tumor is removed. *See also* radiation therapy, brachytherapy. *Compare with* external beam radiation therapy.

intraductal carcinoma: *see* ductal carcinoma in situ.

intraductal papillomas: small, finger-like, noncancerous growths in the breast ducts that may cause a clear or bloody nipple discharge. These are most often found in women forty-five to fifty years of age. A woman with a history of many papillomas is at slightly higher risk for breast cancer.

intraoperative radiation therapy: radiation treatment given during surgery before the operation is finished. Also called IORT.

intravenous (IV) line: a method of supplying fluids and medications by using a needle or a thin tube (called a catheter), which is inserted into a vein.

invasive breast cancer: cancer that grows out of the layer of cells of the breast tissue in which it began and invades nearby tissues. It then can spread to lymph nodes and other organs. *Compare with* noninvasive breast cancer.

irradiation: the use of high-energy radiation from x-rays, gamma rays, neutrons, protons, and other sources to kill cancer cells and shrink tumors. Radiation may come from a machine outside the body (external beam radiation therapy), or it may come from radioactive material placed in the body near cancer cells (internal radiation therapy). Systemic irradiation uses a radioactive substance, such as a radiolabeled monoclonal antibody, that travels in the blood to tissues throughout the body. Also called radiation therapy and radiotherapy.

Ki-67 test: a test that measures the levels of an antigen (Ki-67) in cells that indicates how many are dividing. This test is done on a sample of tumor tissue, to help predict prognosis.

latissimus dorsi (LAT) flap: a breast reconstruction procedure that tunnels muscle, fat, and skin from the upper back to the chest to create a breast mound.

Li-Fraumeni syndrome: a rare, inherited predisposition to multiple cancers (including breast cancer), caused by an alteration in the *TP53* tumor suppressor gene.

lobular carcinoma: cancer that begins in the lobules (milk-producing glands) of the breast.

lobular carcinoma in situ (LCIS): a condition that increases the risk of breast cancer. It is not a true cancer or precancer, although in the past it was sometimes classified as a type of noninvasive cancer. It develops within the milk-producing glands (lobules) of the breast and does not break through the wall of the lobules. Having LCIS puts a woman at a higher risk for an invasive breast cancer developing later in either breast. For this reason, it's important for women with LCIS to have an annual mammogram and clinical breast exam. Also called lobular neoplasia. *See also* clinical breast examination, infiltrating lobular carcinoma, mammogram.

lobular neoplasia: *see* lobular carcinoma in situ.

lobules: milk-producing glands of the breast.

local therapy: treatment of cancer at its site, so that the rest of the body is not affected. Surgery and radiation therapy are examples of local therapy. *Compare with* systemic therapy.

lumpectomy: surgery to remove the breast tumor and a small amount of the normal tissue around it. *See also* breast-conserving surgery.

luteinizing hormone-releasing hormone: a hormone made by the hypothalamus that controls the release of other hormones (follicle-stimulating hormone [FSH] and luteinizing hormone [LH]) by the pituitary gland. FSH and LH regulate the production of sex hormones in the testicles (in men) and the ovaries (in women). Also called LHRH or gonadotropin-releasing hormone (GnRH).

lymph: clear fluid that flows through the lymph vessels and contains cells known as lymphocytes. These cells are important in fighting infections and may also have a role in fighting cancer. *See also* lymphatic system, lymph nodes, lymph vessel, lymphadenectomy.

lymphadenectomy: surgical removal of one or more lymph nodes. After removal, the lymph nodes are examined under a microscope to determine whether the cancer has spread. Also called lymph node dissection. *See also* lymph, lymphatic system, lymph nodes.

lymphatic system: a network of tissues and organs (including lymph nodes, spleen, thymus, and bone marrow) that produce and store lymphocytes (cells that fight infection) and the channels that carry the lymph fluid. The lymphatic system is an important part of the body's immune system, as its function is to fight infection. Invasive cancers sometimes penetrate the lymphatic vessels (channels) and spread (metastasize) to lymph nodes. *See also* lymph, lymph nodes, lymph vessel, lymphadenectomy.

lymphedema: swelling due to a collection of excess fluid, most often in the arms or legs. This may happen after the lymph nodes and vessels are removed or are injured by radiation, and it can happen many years after treatment. It may also happen when a tumor disrupts normal fluid drainage. Lymphedema can persist and interfere with activities of daily living. *See also* lymph, lymphatic system, lymph nodes.

lymph nodes: small bean-shaped collections of immune system tissue such as lymphocytes, found along lymph vessels. They remove cell waste, germs, and other harmful substances from lymph. They help fight infections and also have a role in fighting cancer, although cancers sometimes spread through lymph nodes. Also called lymph glands. *See also* lymph, lymph vessel, lymphatic system, lymphadenectomy.

lymphoma: cancer that begins in cells of the immune system called lymphocytes (or in cells destined to become lymphocytes). Lymphoma can cause a tumor in the breast, but it is not actually breast cancer, and so it is treated differently.

lymph vessel: a thin vessel (or tube) that carries lymph and white blood cells. *See also* lymph, lymph nodes, lymphatic system.

macrocalcifications: *see* calcifications.

macrometastasis: a relatively large area of cancer spread (larger than 2.0 mm). *See also* metastasis. *Compare with* micrometastasis.

magnetic resonance imaging (MRI): a method of taking pictures of the inside of the body by using a powerful magnet to send radio waves through the body (instead of using x-rays). The images appear on a computer screen, as well as on film. Like x-rays, the procedure is physically painless, but some people may feel confined inside the MRI machine.

malignant: cancerous. *Compare with* benign.

mammary lymph nodes: lymph nodes that are near the sternum or breastbone, inside the chest. *See* lymph nodes.

mammogram, mammography: an x-ray of the breast; a way to find breast cancers that cannot be felt. Mammograms are done with a special type of x-ray machine that is used only for this purpose. A mammogram can show a developing breast tumor before it is large enough to be felt by a woman or even by a highly skilled health care professional. A **screening mammogram** is used to help find breast cancer early in women without any signs or symptoms. A **diagnostic mammogram** helps the doctor learn more about breast masses that have been found by clinical breast examination or learn more about what's causing other breast symptoms.

margin: the edge of the cancerous tissue or lump removed during surgery. A negative surgical margin is a sign that no cancer was left behind. A positive surgical margin means that cancer cells are found at the outer edge of the removed sample and is usually a sign that some cancer is still in the body.

mastectomy: surgery to remove all or part of the breast and sometimes other tissue. There are different types of mastectomy:

Extended radical mastectomy removes the breast, skin, nipple, areola, chest muscles (pectoral major and minor), and all axillary and internal mammary lymph nodes on the same side.

Halsted radical mastectomy removes the breast, skin, nipple, areola, both pectoral muscles, and all axillary lymph nodes on the same side.

Modified radical mastectomy removes the breast, skin, nipple, areola, and most of the axillary lymph nodes on the same side, leaving the chest muscles intact.

Nipple-sparing mastectomy removes the breast tissue but leaves behind the nipple and/or areola and as much breast skin as possible.

Partial mastectomy removes less than the whole breast, taking only the part of the breast in which the cancer occurs and a margin of healthy breast tissue surrounding the tumor. This is sometimes called a lumpectomy or breast-conserving surgery.

Prophylactic mastectomy is a mastectomy done before any evidence of cancer can be found, to prevent cancer. This procedure is sometimes recommended for women at very high risk for breast cancer. Also called risk-reducing mastectomy.

Quadrantectomy is a partial mastectomy in which the quarter of the breast that contains a tumor is removed.

Segmental mastectomy is a partial mastectomy.

Simple mastectomy or total mastectomy removes only the breast and overlying skin, including the nipple and areola, but no lymph nodes.

Skin-sparing mastectomy removes the breast tissue, leaving as much of the breast skin as possible to improve the appearance of the reconstructed breast.

mastitis: an infection in the breast that results in swelling, pain, warmth, and redness. Mastitis most commonly occurs in women who are breastfeeding.

medullary breast carcinoma: a type of infiltrating breast cancer that has a rather well-defined boundary between tumor tissue and normal tissue. It also has other special features, including a growth pattern called "syncytial" without glandular formation and the presence of immune system cells in the tumor. Medullary carcinoma accounts for about 3 to 5 percent of breast cancers. The prognosis for this kind of breast cancer is generally better than that of more common types of invasive breast cancer.

menopausal hormone therapy: *see* hormone replacement therapy.

menopause: the time in a woman's life when monthly cycles of menstruation stop and hormone production by the ovaries stops. Menopause usually occurs naturally when a woman is in her late forties or early fifties (the average age is fifty-one years), but it can also be caused by surgical removal of both ovaries, radiation to the ovaries, and by some chemotherapies that destroy ovarian function. Women who are past menopause are called menopausal or postmenopausal. Women who are still menstruating are called premenopausal. Those who have begun to have signs of menopause, but have not completely stopped menstruating are said to be perimenopausal.

metaplastic carcinoma: a very rare type of invasive ductal cancer. These tumors include cells that are normally not found in the breast, such as cells that look like skin cells (squamous cells) or cells that make bone or muscle. These tumors tend to have a worse outlook than regular infiltrating ductal carcinoma of the breast. Metaplastic carcinoma is also known as carcinoma with metaplasia.

metastasis: cancer cells that have spread to one or more sites elsewhere in the body, often by way of the lymphatic system or bloodstream. Regional metastasis is cancer that has spread to the lymph nodes, tissues, or organs close to the primary site. Distant metastasis is cancer that has spread to organs or tissues that are farther away (such as when breast cancer spreads to the bones or liver). *See also* primary site, lymph nodes, lymphatic system.

metastasize: the spread of cancer from one part of the body to another.

metastatic cancer: a way to describe cancer that has spread from the primary site (where it started) to other structures or organs, nearby or far away (distant). *See also* primary site, metastasis.

microcalcifications: *see* calcifications.

microinvasion: in breast cancer, the spread (or invasion) of cancer cells into adjacent tissue in areas smaller than 1.0 mm. Most often used to describe tiny areas of invasive cancer in areas of ductal carcinoma in situ.

micrometastasis: areas of cancer spread that measure between 0.2 millimeters and 2.0 millimeters. *See also* metastasis. *Compare with* macrometastasis.

micropapillary carcinoma: a rare type of breast cancer in which the cells are arranged in small, finger-like projections in a clear space when viewed under the microscope. Unlike papillary carcinoma, the finger-like projections are not arranged around a fibrovascular core. Micropapillary carcinoma has a very high rate of lymph node metastasis and has a poorer prognosis than typical infiltrating ductal carcinoma.

mixed carcinoma: tumors that contain a variety of carcinoma cell types, such as invasive ductal cancer combined with invasive lobular cancer. In this situation, the tumor is treated as if it were an invasive ductal cancer.

modified radical mastectomy: *see* mastectomy.

monoclonal antibody: a type of antibody manufactured in the laboratory. Monoclonal antibodies are designed to lock onto specific antigens (substances that can be recognized by the immune system). Monoclonal antibodies that have been attached to chemotherapy drugs or radioactive substances are being studied for their potential to seek out antigens unique to cancer cells and go directly to the cancer, thus killing the cancer cells and not harming healthy tissue. Monoclonal antibodies are often used to help detect and classify cancer cells under a microscope. Other studies are being done to determine whether radioactive atoms attached to monoclonal antibodies can be used in imaging tests to detect and locate small groups of cancer cells. *See* antibody, antigen, immunohistochemistry.

MRI: *see* magnetic resonance imaging.

mucinous carcinoma: a rare type of invasive breast cancer formed by mucus-producing cancer cells. This type of breast cancer is more common in older women, with an average age at diagnosis in the seventies or eighties. The prognosis for mucinous carcinoma is usually better than for the more common types of invasive breast cancer. Also known as colloid carcinoma.

multimodality therapy: a therapeutic approach that combines more than one method of treatment, such as surgery and chemotherapy. Also called combination therapy and multimodality treatment.

mutation: an abnormal change in the DNA of a cell. Mutations may be caused by mistakes during cell division, or they may be caused by exposure to DNA-damaging agents in the environment. Mutations can be harmful, beneficial, or have no effect. If they occur in cells that make eggs or sperm, they can be passed on to offspring (inherited); if mutations occur in other types of cells, they are not inherited. Certain mutations may lead to cancer or other diseases. *See also* DNA.

necrosis: the death of living tissues. Necrotic refers to tissue that has died.

needle biopsy: removal of fluid, cells, or tissue with a needle for examination under a microscope. There are two types: **fine needle aspiration (FNA)** and **core biopsy**. FNA uses a thin needle to draw up (aspirate) fluid or small tissue fragments from a cyst or tumor. A core needle biopsy uses a thicker needle to remove a cylindrical sample of tissue from a tumor.

neoadjuvant therapy: treatment given before the main treatment. *Compare with* adjuvant therapy.

neuropathy: nerve abnormality or damage that causes numbness, tingling, pain, muscle weakness, or even swelling. It may be caused by injury, infection, disease (cancer, diabetes, kidney failure, or poor nutrition, for example), or by drugs. Peripheral neuropathy is a type of neuropathy that starts in nerves farthest away from the brain, such as the hands and feet.

nipple: the tip of the breast; the pigmented projection in the middle of the areola. The nipple contains the opening of milk ducts from the breast.

nipple aspiration: the collection of fluid containing cells from the lining of the milk ducts. The fluid is collected by using gentle suction from a device similar to the breast pumps used by nursing women.

nipple discharge: any fluid coming from the nipple. It may be clear, milky, bloody, tan, gray, or green. In a nipple discharge examination, fluid is collected and examined under the microscope to determine whether any cancer cells are present. *See also* ductal lavage, ductogram.

nipple retraction: a turning inward of the nipple.

noninvasive breast cancer: a precancer of the breast, with cancer cells only present in the layer of cells in which they started and not growing into other tissues of the breast. Because it is noninvasive, the cancer cannot spread outside the breast to lymph nodes or other organs or tissues. Also known as in situ carcinoma or ductal carcinoma in situ. *Compare with* invasive breast cancer, metastatic cancer.

nonsteroidal anti-inflammatory drug: a drug that decreases fever, swelling, pain, and redness. Also called NSAID.

NSAID: *see* nonsteroidal anti-inflammatory drug.

nuclear grade: *see* grade.

oncogene: a mutated or changed form of a normal gene that, in its new form, promotes cell growth and multiplication. The original form of the gene, called a proto-oncogene, is normally present in the cell, but it then may undergo changes that activate it, causing cells to grow too quickly and form tumors.

oncoplastic surgery: the combination of surgery for cancer treatment and plastic surgery intended to remodel, repair, or restore body parts, especially by the transfer of tissue. *See also* autologous reconstruction.

oophorectomy: surgery to remove one or both ovaries.

opioid: a substance related to morphine used to treat moderate to severe pain. Opioids are similar to opiates, but are not made from opium. Opioids bind to opioid receptors in the central nervous system. Sometimes called narcotics.

osteonecrosis: the destruction and death of bone tissue.

osteoporosis: a condition that is marked by a decrease in bone mass and density, causing bones to become fragile and break more easily. A milder form of weak bones is known as osteopenia.

p53: the protein made by TP53. *See also* TP53.

Paget disease of the nipple (formerly called Paget's disease): a rare form of breast cancer that begins in the milk ducts and spreads to the skin of the nipple and areola, which may cause oozing or look crusted, scaly, or red. Paget disease is almost always associated with either ductal carcinoma in situ (DCIS) or infiltrating ductal carcinoma. The outlook is usually better if these nipple changes are the only sign of breast disease, no lump can be felt, and infiltrating ductal carcinoma is not present. *See* duct, nipple.

palliative treatment: treatment that relieves symptoms, such as pain, but is not expected to cure the disease. Its main purpose is to improve the patient's quality of life. Sometimes, chemotherapy and radiation therapy are used as palliative treatments.

papillary carcinoma: a rare type of breast cancer in which the cells are arranged in small, finger-like projections around a fibrovascular core when viewed under the microscope. These cancers are most often considered to be a subtype of ductal carcinoma in situ (DCIS) and are treated as such. In rare cases, they are invasive, in which case they are treated like invasive ductal carcinoma, although the outlook is likely to be better. These cancers tend to be diagnosed in older women, and they make up no more than 1 to 2 percent of all breast cancers.

partial (segmental) mastectomy: *see* mastectomy.

pathologic stage: an estimate of the extent of cancer by direct study of the samples removed during surgery. *See also* clinical stage, staging.

pectoral muscles: muscles attached to the front of the chest wall and upper arms. The larger one is called pectoralis major, and the smaller one is called pectoralis minor. Because these muscles are next to the breast, breast cancer may spread to them, although this rarely happens.

pedicle flap: tissue that is surgically removed, but the blood vessels remain attached and are tunneled from the original site to the area where the tissue is to be attached.

percutaneous: passing through the skin, as an injection or a topical medicine.

peripheral neuropathy: damage to the nerves that can cause numbness, tingling, sensitivity to heat or cold, or even pain, most often in the hands and feet. It can also lead to muscle weakness and balance problems. Although it usually begins in the hands or feet, it can affect other areas of the body, as well. When it affects the throat and esophagus, it can lead to trouble swallowing. Peripheral neuropathy is a side effect of some anticancer drugs and will tend to get worse if the drugs are continued. It can also be caused by certain medical conditions, such as diabetes. Also called neuropathy.

PET scan: *see* positron emission tomography.

phyllodes tumor: a type of breast tumor that forms from the cells of the breast stroma (supporting and connective tissue). It often grows quickly and can become large and bulky. Most phyllodes tumors are benign, but they can be malignant and can spread to other parts of the body. Phyllodes tumors of the breast are rare. They are typically treated with surgery. Also called phylloides tumor and cystosarcoma phyllodes.

phytoestrogen: an estrogen-like substance found in some plants and plant products. Some people believe that phytoestrogens may have anticancer effects. *See also* estrogen.

placebo: an inert, inactive substance, such as sugar, distilled water, or saline solution, that may be used in studies (clinical trials) to compare the effects of a given treatment with no treatment.

The placebo effect is a phenomenon in which a placebo can sometimes improve a person's condition simply because the person has the expectation that the treatment will be helpful.

platelet: a part of the blood that plugs up holes in blood vessels after an injury and helps the blood clot. Chemotherapy can cause a drop in the platelet count, resulting in a condition called thrombocytopenia, which carries a risk of excessive bleeding.

pleural effusion: an abnormal collection of fluid between the thin layers of tissue (pleura) coating the lung and lining the wall of the chest cavity.

ploidy: the number of sets of chromosomes within a cell. Ploidy is a marker that helps predict how quickly a cancer is likely to spread. Cancers with the same number of chromosomes as normal cells are called **diploid**, and those with either more or less than that amount are **aneuploid**. Patients with diploid cancers have longer disease-free intervals and a better prognosis, but about two of three breast cancers are aneuploid. This test is done by using lasers and computers, a process called flow cytometry.

positron emission tomography (PET): a PET scan creates an image of the body (or of biochemical events) after the injection of a very low dose of a radioactive form of a substance such as glucose (sugar). Cells that use more sugar take in more glucose and concentrate the radioactivity, which can be detected with a special camera. In general, high-grade tumors use more sugar than low-grade tumors. PET scans are especially useful for finding areas of cancer spread and are often combined with CT scans for that purpose. PET scans may also be used to see how well the tumor is responding to treatment.

postmastectomy pain syndrome (PMPS): a painful condition affecting women who have had breast surgery. It is called PMPS because it was first seen in women who had had a mastectomy, but it can occur after breast-conserving surgery, as well. The pain is thought to be linked to damage done to the nerves in the armpit and chest during surgery, but the causes are not known. Symptoms can include a burning, achy feeling around the breasts and chest, limitations in movement of the shoulder and arm, tenderness around the area, and pain and tingling in the scar tissue.

postmenopausal hormone therapy (PHT): *see* hormone replacement therapy.

primary site: the place where cancer begins. Primary cancer is usually named after the organ in which it starts. For example, cancer that starts in the breast is always breast cancer even if it spreads (metastasizes) to other organs, such as the lungs, bones, or liver.

progesterone: a female sex hormone released by the ovaries during every menstrual cycle to prepare the uterus for pregnancy and the breasts for milk production. *See also* hormone, estrogen.

progesterone receptors: *see* hormone receptor.

prognosis: a prediction of the course of disease; the outlook for the chances of survival.

progression-free survival (PFS): the length of time, both during and after cancer treatment, that a person lives with the disease and it does not get worse. In clinical trials, measuring progression-free survival is one way to measure the effectiveness of a new treatment. *See also* clinical trials.

proliferative lesions with atypia: excessive growth of cells in the ducts or lobules of the breast tissue in which the cells deviate from normal cells when examined under the microscope. These lesions are benign but are linked to a moderate increase in breast cancer risk. *Compare with* proliferative lesions without atypia.

proliferative lesions without atypia: excessive growth of cells in the ducts or lobules of the breast tissue in which the cells do not deviate from normal cells when examined under the microscope. These lesions are benign but are linked to a slight increase in breast cancer risk. *Compare with* proliferative lesions with atypia.

prosthesis: an artificial part used to replace or improve the function of a body part. A breast form is an example of a prosthesis.

quadrantectomy: *see* mastectomy.

quality of life: overall enjoyment of life, which includes a person's sense of well-being and ability to do the things that are important to him or her.

rad: a basic unit of measurement of the amount of radiation transmitted during radiation therapy.

radiation: energy released in the form of particles or electromagnetic waves. Common sources of radiation include radon gas, cosmic rays from outer space, medical x-rays, and energy given off by a radioisotope.

radiation therapy: treatment with high-energy rays (such as x-rays) or particles (like protons) to kill or shrink cancer cells. The radiation may come from outside of the body (external beam radiation) or from radioactive materials placed directly in the tumor (brachytherapy or internal radiation). Radiation therapy may be used as the main treatment for a cancer, to reduce the size of a cancer before surgery, or to destroy any remaining cancer cells after surgery. In advanced cancer cases, it may also be used as palliative treatment. *See also* external beam radiation therapy, brachytherapy, palliative treatment.

radical mastectomy: *see* mastectomy.

randomized or randomization: a process used in clinical trials that uses chance to assign participants to different groups that compare treatments. Randomization means that each person has an equal chance of being in either the treatment or comparison groups. This helps reduce the chance of bias that might happen if, for example, the healthiest people all were assigned to a particular treatment group. *See also* control group, clinical trials.

receptor activator of nuclear factor kappa-B ligand (RANKL or RANK-ligand): a molecule important in bone metabolism, which activates cells involved in breaking down bone. Overproduction of RANKL can occur in cancer, but it is also associated with a variety of degenerative bone diseases, such as rheumatoid arthritis and psoriatic arthritis. RANKL also has a function in the immune system, where it is thought to be involved in cell maturation. The drug denosumab targets this molecule.

reconstruction: *see* breast reconstruction.

recurrence: the return of cancer after treatment. **Local recurrence** means that the cancer has come back in or near the same place as the original cancer. **Regional recurrence** means that the cancer has come back after treatment in the lymph nodes near the primary site. **Distant recurrence**, also known as metastatic recurrence, is when cancer metastasizes after treatment to distant organs or tissues (such as the lungs, liver, bone marrow, or brain). *See also* primary site, metastasis, metastasize.

red blood cells: blood cells that contain hemoglobin, the substance that carries oxygen to all of the cells of the body. *See also* anemia.

risk factor: anything that affects a person's chance of getting a disease such as cancer. Different cancers have different risk factors. For example, unprotected exposure to strong sunlight is a risk factor for skin cancer; smoking is a risk factor for lung, mouth, larynx, and other cancers. Some risk factors, such as smoking, can be controlled. Others, like a person's age, cannot be changed.

sarcoma: a cancer starting in connective tissues, such as cartilage, fat, muscle, or bone. Several types of sarcoma (such as angiosarcoma, liposarcoma, and malignant phyllodes tumor) can develop in the breast, although this is rare.

scan: a test used to produce images of internal body organs, often using x-rays or radioactive isotopes.

scintimammography: a breast imaging test that is used to detect cancer cells in the breasts of some women who have had abnormal mammograms or who have dense breast tissue. It is not used for screening or as a substitute for a mammogram. With scintimammography, a woman receives an injection of a small amount of a radioactive substance called technetium 99, which is taken up by cancer cells, and a gamma camera is used to take pictures of the breasts.

screening: the search for disease, such as cancer, in people without symptoms. For example, screening measures recommended by the American Cancer Society for breast cancer include clinical breast examinations and mammograms. Screening may also refer to coordinated programs in large populations.

second-degree relative: an aunt, uncle, grandparent, grandchild, niece, nephew, or half-sibling. *Compare with* first-degree relative.

selective serotonin reuptake inhibitors (SSRIs): a category of drugs that are primarily used to treat depression. SSRIs work by affecting chemical messengers, called neurotransmitters, used to communicate between brain cells. SSRIs block the reabsorption of the neurotransmitter serotonin in the brain. This leaves more serotonin in the area between nerve cells (called the synapse) which affects mood. SSRIs are called selective because they seem to primarily affect serotonin, not other neurotransmitters.

sentinel lymph node biopsy: a diagnostic procedure involving the removal of the first lymph node (or nodes) to which cancer cells are likely to spread from the primary tumor. In some cases, there can be more than one sentinel lymph node. For this procedure, a radioactive substance and/or dye is injected into the tumor, near the tumor, or in the area around the nipple. These will collect in one or more lymph nodes, which are then removed at surgery and examined for the presence of cancer cells. *See also* lymph node.

seroma: a tumor-like collection in the tissues of the clear liquid part of the blood that remains after blood cells and clotting proteins have been removed.

skin-sparing mastectomy: *see* mastectomy.

S-phase fraction: a laboratory test that shows the percentage of cells that are replicating or reproducing their DNA. DNA replication is usually a sign that a cell is getting ready to split into two new cells. A low S-phase fraction is a sign that a tumor is slow-growing; a high S-phase fraction shows that the cells are dividing rapidly and the tumor is growing quickly. *See* DNA.

spiral CT: the most common type of CT scanner. Also called helical CT. *See also* computed tomography.

stage: the extent of a cancer in the body. *See* staging.

staging: the process of finding out whether cancer has spread and, if so, how far. The system used for breast cancer is the AJCC/TNM system. The TNM system gives three key pieces of information:
- T refers to the size of the tumor
- N describes how far the cancer has spread to nearby lymph nodes
- M shows whether the cancer has spread (metastasized) to other organs of the body

Letters or numbers after the T, N, and M give more details about each of these factors. To make this information more clear, the TNM descriptions can be grouped together into a simpler set of stages, labeled with the number 0 (zero) or the Roman numerals I to IV. In general, the lower the number, the less the cancer has spread. A higher number means a more serious cancer. The two types of staging are clinical staging and pathologic staging. *See also* clinical stage, pathologic stage.

stereotactic needle biopsy: a method of needle biopsy that is useful in some cases where there are calcifications or a mass that can be seen on mammogram but cannot be felt. A computer maps the location of the mass to guide the placement of the needle. When this type of biopsy is done with a larger needle, it may be called a stereotactic core needle biopsy. *See also* needle biopsy.

stereotactic wire localization: a procedure used to guide a surgical breast biopsy when the lump is hard to find or when there is an area that looks suspicious on a mammogram. A thin hollow needle is placed into the breast, and computer images are taken to guide the needle to the area in question. A fine thin wire is inserted through the center of the needle. A small hook at the end of the wire keeps it in place. The hollow needle is then removed, and the surgeon uses the path of the wire as a guide to find the abnormal area to be removed. *See also* biopsy, mammogram, x-ray.

stroma: fatty and connective tissue.

subcutaneous mastectomy: *see* mastectomy.

supraclavicular lymph nodes: lymph nodes just above the collarbone (clavicle). *See* lymph nodes.

surgical biopsy: a method of biopsy in which all or part of a lump is removed by a surgeon for examination. *See also* biopsy, stereotactic wire localization.

surgical margin: *see* margin.

systemic therapy: treatment that reaches and affects cells throughout the entire body, for example, chemotherapy.

tamoxifen: a drug used to prevent breast cancer in high-risk women; decrease the risk of getting invasive breast cancer in women with ductal cancer in situ (DCIS); help keep cancer from coming back after surgery, radiation therapy, and chemotherapy; and to treat advanced breast cancer. It is also used to treat other types of cancer and may be used for other conditions.

targeted therapy: treatment that attacks the part of cancer cells that makes them different from normal cells, as opposed to treatment that harms all cells. Targeted therapy tends to have different and sometimes fewer side effects than some standard treatments such as chemotherapy.

tissue: a collection of cells, united to perform a particular function in the body.

tissue expander: a balloon implanted under the skin and used to keep living tissues under tension. This causes new cells to form and stretches the tissue. The surgeon puts the expander beneath the skin where the breast should be and, over a period of weeks or months, injects a saline solution to slowly expand the overlaying skin to make space for a breast implant.

tissue flap reconstruction: tissue for reconstruction that is surgically removed from another area of the body. It can be a pedicle (left attached to its base and then tunneled under the skin) or free flap (cut free from its base and transplanted to the chest).

total mastectomy: *see* mastectomy.

TP53: an important tumor suppressor gene that is not working properly in many cancers. The protein that this gene makes (called p53) normally causes damaged cells to die. Mutations, or changes, in this gene can be inherited or they can occur during a person's life. The changes, or mutations, that are inherited can lead to a condition called Li-Fraumeni syndrome, which is linked to an increased risk for many types of cancer. *See* mutation, tumor suppressor genes.

transverse rectus abdominis muscle (TRAM) flap: a breast reconstruction procedure that uses tissue and muscle from the lower abdominal wall to reconstruct a breast mound. It can be a pedicle (left attached to its base and then tunneled under the skin) or free flap (cut free from its base and transplanted to the chest).

transverse upper gracilis (TUG) flap: a breast reconstruction technique that uses tissue from the inner upper thigh near the natural groin crease, as well as the gracilis muscle in the thigh, to create breast tissue. TUG flap reconstruction is usually done if a woman does not have adequate skin and tissue in the abdomen or buttock region, or has had previous abdominal surgeries that may have interfered with blood vessels that the DIEP flap requires. The ideal candidate for the TUG flap is a woman with small breasts who does not require a significant amount of volume for the reconstruction.

triple-negative breast cancer: a type of breast cancer, usually an invasive ductal carcinoma, in which the cells lack estrogen and progesterone receptors and do not have an excess of HER2 protein on their surfaces. Hormone therapy and drugs that target HER2 are not effective for treating this type of cancer. *See also* hormone receptor, hormone therapy, *HER2* gene.

tubular carcinoma: a less common type of invasive ductal carcinoma. They are called tubular because the cells are arranged in tiny tubes when seen under the microscope. Tubular carcinomas were diagnosed rarely before mammography, but they account for about 8 percent of all breast cancers found in populations screened with mammography. Now, they most often are diagnosed on mammography as small tumors (about 1.0 cm or smaller). They tend to grow and spread slowly and have a better prognosis than typical infiltrating ductal carcinomas.

tumor: an abnormal lump or mass of tissue. Tumors can be benign (noncancerous) or malignant (cancerous).

tumor marker: a substance found in tissue, blood, or other body fluids that may be a sign of cancer or certain benign (noncancerous) conditions. Most tumor markers are made by both normal cells and cancer cells, but they are made in larger amounts by cancer cells. A tumor marker may help to diagnose cancer, plan treatment, or find out how well treatment is working or if cancer has come back. Examples of tumor markers include CA 15-3 and CA 27-29.

tumor suppressor genes: genes that slow down cell division or cause cells to die at the appropriate time. Alterations of these genes can lead to too much cell growth and development of cancer.

ultrasound: an imaging method in which high-frequency sound waves are used to outline a part of the body. The sound wave echoes are picked up and displayed on a screen. Also called ultrasonography.

US Food and Drug Administration (FDA): an agency of the United States Department of Health and Human Services. The FDA is responsible for regulating drugs, tobacco products, biological medical products, blood products, medical devices, and radiation-emitting devices, along with other products.

white blood cells: cells that work as part of the immune system to help defend the body against infections. This is one of many types of blood cells made in the bone marrow. Certain cancer treatments (especially chemotherapy) can reduce the number of these cells (a condition called neutropenia) and make a person more likely to get infections. *See also* bone marrow.

x-ray: one form of radiation that can be used at low levels to produce an image of the body on film or at high levels to destroy cancer cells.

INDEX

Numbers in *italics* indicate images.

aneuploid cells, 51
angiolymphatic invasion, 79
angiosarcoma, 14, 168, 419
anthracyclines, 204
anti-anxiety drugs, 264, 267
antibody-drug conjugate, 190
anticonvulsants, 209, 264
antidepressants, 290, 402
    hot flashes and, 274
    pain and, 263, 264, 266, 267
antiemetics, 258, 260
anti-estrogens, 184–185
antioxidants, 241
antiperspirants, 33
anxiety, 266–267, 393–394
    art therapy and, 233–234
    hypnosis and, 234
    massage and, 235
    meditation and, 236
    music therapy and, 236
    prayer and, 237
    relaxation and, 237
    yoga and, 239
apocrine metaplasia, 24, 437
appetite
    changes in, 179, 249–250
    loss of, 166
Aredia, 192, 193, 203
areola reconstruction, 304, 305, 316
areola-sparing mastectomy, 134
Arimidex, 185
arm, weakness in, 166
Aromasin, 185
aromatase, 185
aromatase inhibitors (blockers), 184, 185–186, 192, 199, 201, 211, 417, 418
aromatherapy, 233
arrhythmia, 176
art therapy, 233–234
Ashkenazis, breast cancer among, 20
aspirin, 263
ataxia-telangiectasia, 21
ATEC (Automated Tissue Excision and Collection), 47
Ativan, 264
ATM gene, 21
atypical ductal hyperplasia, 25, 425, 439–440
atypical hyperplasia, 435
atypical lobular hyperplasia, 25, 425, 439–440
autogenous reconstruction techniques, 308
autologous reconstruction techniques, 308
Avastin, 191
Avicenna, 233
Avinza, 263

axillary lymph node dissection, 139–140, 141, 142, 143, 144, 146, 197, 198, 200, 422
axillary lymph nodes, 7, 8, 139
axillary web syndrome, 142
Axxent, 164, 165

B
bankruptcy, 354
Bannayan-Riley-Ruvalcaba syndrome, 21, 425
BardPort, 173
behavioral therapy, 274, 297
belladonna, 274
Bellergal, 274
benign breast conditions, 8, 24–25, 435–440
benign phyllodes tumors, 15, 24, 436
bevacizumab, 191
bilateral mastectomy, 197
bilateral salpingo-oophorectomy, 22
bills, paying, 353
biofeedback, 234, 258
bioidentical hormones, 28
biopsy, 37, 38
    breast, 43–52
    needle, 43–47
    pathology report from, 59–62, 78–83, 147
    samples from, testing, 48–52
    surgical, 47–48
    types of, 43–48
birth control, need for, 275
birth control pills, as risk factor, 27
Bisphenol-A, 31
bisphosphonates, 129, 186, 192–193, 203, 206, 207
black cohosh, 274
bleeding
    after biopsy, 48
    chemotherapy devices and, 175
    vaginal, 184
blood, donating, before surgery, 143
blood calcium
    high levels of, 207
    low levels of, 193
blood cell counts, low, 178, 189, 191, 192
blood chemical tests, 55
blood clots, 28, 177, 184–185, 187, 191
blood lipids, increase of, 192
blood pressure
    hypnosis and, 234
    tai chi and, 239
blood sugars, increase of, 192
blood tests, 55–56
Bloom-Richardson grade, 49
board certification, 108
body image, acceptance of, 293–294, 295, 400–401

five-year survival rate, 76–77
flap procedure, 304, 305, 308–315, 318
fluid leak, catheters and, 176
fluorescence in situ hybridization, 50, 51, 83
fluorouracil, 170, 171
fluoxetine, 274
fluoxymesterone, 187
FMLA. *See* Family and Medical Leave Act
FNA. *See* fine needle aspiration
Folex, 170
follow-up care, 120, 372–374, 413–414
food stamps, 327
foot pain, 268
founder mutations, 20–21
fraternal organizations, 340
fraudulent treatments, 229, 230
free flap, 310
friends, talking to, about the diagnosis, 91–92
frozen shoulder, 142
full-field digital mammogram, 36
fulvestrant, 185
futility analysis, 221

G

gabapentin, 264
gadolinium, 55
Gail model, 426
galactogram, 43
GAP flap. *See* gluteal free (gluteal artery) perforator flap
gemcitabine, 171
gender, as risk factor, 19
gene expression profiling, 51–52
gene-pattern tests, 203
genes, 18
 mutations in, 20–22
 patterns of, 51–52
genetic counselor, 102
genetics, as risk factor, 20–22
genetic testing, 22, 102
genital herpes, 182
genital wart infections, 182
germline deleterious mutations, 21
Gerson diet, 238
gifts, tax-free, 347
ginger tea, 227
gluteal free (gluteal artery) perforator flap, 308, 315
goserelin, 187
grade 1 (well-differentiated) cancer, 49
grade 1 cells, 62
grade 2 (moderately differentiated) cancer, 49
grade 2 cells, 62
grade 3 (poorly differentiated) cancer, 49
grade 3 cells, 62

Groshong, 175
Groshong Midline, 175
gross description, 60
group insurance, 429
growth factor, 171
guaranteed-issue insurance plan, 340
guided imagery, 235, 258
guided relaxation, 240

H

HABITS study, 418
hair loss, 178, 254–256
Halaven, 170
Hallelujah diet, 238
hamartoma, 24, 438
hand-foot syndrome, 179, 190, 268
Hatha yoga, 240
headaches, 190, 191
health care power of attorney, 351
health care proxy, 351
health care service plans, 340
Health Consequences of Involuntary Exposure to Tobacco Smoke, The (US Surgeon General), 31
health insurance, 332–333. *See also* Women's Health and Cancer Rights Act
Health Insurance Portability and Accountability Act of 1996, 338–339
health maintenance organizations, 334, 336, 340
hearing loss, 183
heart, damage to, 168, 180, 190
heat, avoiding, 283
help, asking for, 290–291
hemangiomas, 24, 438
hematomas, 132, 136, 308
herbal medicines, 229
herbs, 240, 241, 274
Herceptin, 190, 198, 416–417. *See also* trastuzumab
HER-positive cancer, 205
HER2/neu gene, 50
HER2/neu-negative breast cancer, 192, 199
HER2/neu-positive breast cancer, 50–51, 188–189, 190, 199, 200, 202, 203, 204–205, 416–417
HER2/neu protein, 12, 50, 188
Hickman, 175
high blood pressure, 191
 breast reconstruction and, 302–304
 meditation and, 236
high-fat diet, 31
high-grade cancer, 199
high-grade cells, 62
Hill-Burton Program, 337, 339
HIPAA. *See* Health Insurance Portability and Accountability Act of 1996

ABOUT THE EDITORS

Ruth O'Regan, MD, is professor of Hematology and Medical Oncology at the Winship Cancer Institute of Emory University and chief of Hematology and Medical Oncology, Georgia Cancer Center for Excellence at Grady Memorial Hospital. Dr. O'Regan also holds the Louisa and Rand Glenn Family Chair in Breast Cancer Research; is the director of the Translational Breast Cancer Research program at Winship; and is the director of the Hematology and Oncology Fellowship program, Emory University School of Medicine.

A native of Dublin, Ireland, Dr. O'Regan earned her medical degree at University College in Dublin, conducted a residency in internal medicine and a fellowship in oncology at the Mater Hospital in Dublin, and did her US residency and fellowship at Northwestern University. While at Northwestern, she studied the mechanisms of selective estrogen receptor modulator, or SERM, resistance.

Since joining the faculty at the Emory Winship Cancer Institute, Dr. O'Regan has continued her research in SERM resistance. Additionally, her laboratory focuses on the evaluation of novel targeted approaches for triple-negative breast cancer, which has led to the development of novel trials for patients with this subtype of breast cancer.

With the help of Avon Foundation, Dr. O'Regan has developed a multidisciplinary breast cancer clinic at the Georgia Cancer Center of Excellence. She is also the director of the Jean Sindab Endowment Research Team, which focuses on developing scientific research into breast cancer in African American women.

Dr. O'Regan is a widely published author in peer-reviewed scientific journals and speaks nationally and internationally on topics related to breast cancer, including the use of hormone and targeted therapies.

Sheryl G. A. Gabram-Mendola, MD, FACS, is the surgeon-in-chief for Grady Health System, principal investigator on the AVON Foundation grant, and director of the AVON Comprehensive Breast Center at Grady (AFCBC). Dr. Gabram completed medical school at Georgetown University, surgical residency at the Washington Hospital Center, and a fellowship at the University of Connecticut, Hartford Hospital.

Dr. Gabram's current research focuses on decreasing disparities for breast cancer patients. She serves as the medical liaison for the AVON community education outreach initiative and navigation program and is responsible for clinical access to high-quality care for patients seen in the AFCBC. She collaborates with the Rollins School of Public Health at Emory University on the delivery of breast cancer treatments to Medicaid patients. To date, she has authored or coauthored more than eighty-five peer-reviewed journal publications.

Dr. Gabram is the recipient of numerous awards and honors. She has been named by the patient resource guide *Castle Connolly* as one of America's Top Doctors for nine consecutive years and American's Top Cancer Doctors for seven consecutive years. She has received the Arthur G. Michel, MD, Award for Excellence in Breast Care from the Y-ME National Breast Cancer Organization and was selected as one of Atlanta Magazine's Top Doctors in 2007 and 2009. In the November 2008 *Women's Health* magazine, she was named one of five top oncologists for women in the South.

Terri Ades, DNP, FNP-BC, AOCN, is director of Cancer Information for the American Cancer Society in Atlanta. In this position, she oversees the development and maintenance of the Society's cancer information that is available through the Society's website, toll-free call center, patient education/consumer awareness materials, and translations. Dr. Ades is an expert in health literacy and is certified as an advanced practice oncology nurse and family nurse practitioner. She is an adjunct faculty member of Emory University Nell Hodgson Woodruff School of Nursing and the Winship Cancer Institute of Emory Healthcare, where she continues in clinical practice.

Rick Alteri, MD, has been a medical editor at the American Cancer Society in Atlanta for twelve years. During this time, he has helped develop and maintain the Society's extensive cancer information database, the source of the information available through the Society's website and toll-free call center. He has also helped develop several of the Society's consumer-focused books and other publications. Prior to joining the Society, Dr. Alteri helped coordinate patient care in clinical trials for breast and other cancers at a large private oncology practice in the Atlanta area.

Joan L. Kramer, MD, is a medical editor at the American Cancer Society in Atlanta and helps to develop and maintain the Society's extensive cancer information database. Dr. Kramer is board certified in medical oncology and hematology and continues in clinical practice in the Breast Cancer Outpatient Clinic at Grady Memorial Hospital.

Kimberly A. Stump-Sutliff, MSN, RN, AOCNS, is an associate medical editor at the American Cancer Society in Atlanta. She received her bachelor of science in nursing degree from Thomas Jefferson University and her master's degree from Georgia State University. She is certified as an Advanced Oncology Clinical Nurse Specialist. Her nursing background includes hematology/oncology inpatient and bone marrow transplant care, home infusion care and home management of peripheral stem cell transplant patients, and transplant and infusion therapy in the outpatient setting.

OTHER BOOKS PUBLISHED BY
THE AMERICAN CANCER SOCIETY

Available everywhere books are sold and online at **cancer.org/bookstore**

Information

American Cancer Society Complete Guide to Complementary and Alternative Cancer Therapies, Second Edition
American Cancer Society Complete Guide to Nutrition for Cancer Survivors, Second Edition
Breast Cancer Clear & Simple
QuickFACTS™ Breast Cancer

Day-to-Day Help

American Cancer Society Complete Guide to Family Caregiving, Second Edition
Cancer Caregiving A to Z: An At-Home Guide for Patients and Families
Cancer in Our Family: Helping Children Cope with a Parent's Illness
What to Eat During Cancer Treatment: 100 Great-Tasting, Family-Friendly Recipes to Help You Cope

Emotional Support

Chemo and Me: My Hair Loss Experience
I Can Survive
Picture Your Life After Cancer
Rad Art: A Journey Through Radiation Treatment
The Survivorship Net: A Parable for the Family, Friends, and Caregivers of People with Cancer
What Helped Get Me Through: Cancer Survivors Share Wisdom and Hope

For Children

Because… Someone I Love Has Cancer
Let My Colors Out
Mom and the Polka-Dot Boo-Boo
Nana, What's Cancer?
Our Mom Has Cancer
Our Mom Is Getting Better
What's Up with Bridget's Mom? Medikidz Explain Breast Cancer
    (available in English and Spanish)

Healthy Eating

The American Cancer Society's Healthy Eating Cookbook: A Celebration of Food, Friends, and Healthy Living, Third Edition
Celebrate! Healthy Entertaining for Any Occasion
The Great American Eat-Right Cookbook
Maya's Secrets: Delightful Latin Dishes for a Healthier You

Visit **cancer.org/bookstore** for a full listing
of books published by the American Cancer Society.